Handbook of Clinical and Practical Pediatric Nutrition

Kadakkal Radhakrishnan
Editor

Handbook of Clinical and Practical Pediatric Nutrition

Springer

Editor
Kadakkal Radhakrishnan
Division of Pediatric Gastroenterology, Hepatology & Nutrition
Cleveland Clinic Children's Hospital
Cleveland, OH, USA

Section Editors
Senthilkumar Sankararaman
Pediatric Nutrition Support
Division of Pediatric Gastroenterology, Hepatology, and Nutrition
Cleveland Clinic Children's Hospital
Cleveland, OH, USA

Christina DeTallo
Pediatric Nutrition Support
Division of Pediatric Gastroenterology, Hepatology, and Nutrition
Cleveland Clinic Children's Hospital
Cleveland, OH, USA

ISBN 978-3-031-97758-9 ISBN 978-3-031-97759-6 (eBook)
https://doi.org/10.1007/978-3-031-97759-6

This Springer imprint is published by the registered company Springer Nature Switzerland AG
The registered company address is: Gewerbestrasse 11, 6330 Cham, Switzerland

Preface

This is a unique handbook on pediatric nutrition with a specific goal to provide the pediatric practitioner an up-to-date, easy, and quick read on various nutrition-related topics in children. The idea for this book stemmed from the desire of various pediatric providers, physicians, dietitians, and trainees, to have a one-stop read on various topics, which covers all relevant aspects of pediatric nutritional needs including macro- and micronutrients.

There is clearly a perceived gap among pediatric clinicians, with regard to clinical assessment of nutritional status, biochemical testing in the evaluation of malnutrition, as well as insights into macro- and micronutrient needs in children. Though there are few books available for pediatric providers, there seems to be a dearth of easy-to-read, quick bedside references. This book was conceptualized to address these gaps.

Nutritional management is key in ensuring optimal growth and development in children. It is even more indispensable in managing children with chronic medical disorders, as optimization of nutritional status in this population results in improved outcomes and can be therapeutic as well in select circumstances. For example, managing a child with chronic liver disease requires a good understanding of the pathophysiology leading to adverse nutritional status. Further, in this situation, nutritional assessment can be challenging due to fluid retention and requires an in-depth knowledge of available nutrition assessment tools and meticulous management of both macro- and micronutrient deficiencies.

This book has been divided into six parts or sections. Part I addresses basic concepts and is meant to provide insight into nutritional assessment, pertinent calculations and formulas in dietetics, breastfeeding concepts, modes of enteral therapy, and parenteral nutrition. Part II (the section on macronutrients) is meant to provide the reader with a wholesome approach to basic concepts, digestion, absorption, and disorders related to the digestion and absorption of fat, carbohydrates, and proteins. Parts 3 to 6 cover trace elements, water-soluble vitamins, fat-soluble vitamins, and nutrition in disease-specific states, respectively.

We have solicited contributions from advanced practice providers, registered dietitians, and physicians working in the field of pediatric gastroenterology, hepatology, and nutrition, from across the United States. The book is edited for easy reading and to ensure that the reader gets a well-rounded concept on the above-mentioned topics. Although the chapters have been written and edited well to keep the concepts up-to-date, we respectfully request the reader to do their own research for further intricate details on any topic. We have made a concerted effort to look at avenues for future research possibilities on many areas, to help further research opportunities.

The editors would like to express their sincere gratitude to all the contributors for their hard work, as well as editors (Sharath Rangarajan), and other editorial staff from Springer for their kind help and support.

Cleveland, OH, USA Kadakkal Radhakrishnan
Cleveland, OH, USA Christina DeTallo
Cleveland, OH, USA Senthilkumar Sankararaman

Contents

Part I Normal Nutrition and Nutrition Support

1 **Nutrition Intake Across Ages** 3
Audrey Matuska and Merideth Miller

2 **Nutrition Assessment** 17
Hanna Leikin and Danielle Melton

3 **Breastfeeding and the Use of Human Milk** 37
Anfal Marafie, Jennifer Hyland, Audrey Matuska, and Heidi Szugye

4 **Formulas Including Special Formulas** 49
Margherita Shook

5 **Enteral Nutrition Support** 57
Sara Bewley, Christine Bowen, Elizabeth Robinson, and Senthilkumar Sankararaman

6 **Parenteral Nutrition** 69
Andrea Adler and Christina DeTallo

Part II Macronuttrients

7 **Fat** 85
Kritika Sukumar, Kyleigh Rodriguez, and Kadakkal Radhakrishnan

8 **Proteins and Amino Acids** 97
Meenal Karuvannur, Kristina Pytlak, and Kadakkal Radhakrishnan

9 **Carbohydrates** 111
Mira Younis, Kristina Pytlak, and Kadakkal Radhakrishnan

Part III Micronutrients

10 **Iron** 129
Haig Manougian and Ravi Talati

11 **Calcium** 153
Andrea Mucci

12 **Phosphorus** 165
Anuradha Viswanathan

13 **Magnesium** 177
Andrew R. Lavik

14 **Copper** 195
Anthony Anani

15 **Zinc** 211
Aditi Mittal

16 **Manganese** 219
Michael James Schmalz

17 **Selenium** 227
Praveen Kumar Conjeevaram Selvakumar

18 **Iodine, Cobalt, Molybdenum, and Chromium** 235
Rasha Abi Radi Abou Jaoudeh and Kadakkal Radhakrishnan

Part IV Water Soluble Vitamins

19 **Vitamin B1: Thiamine** 249
Noy Lapidot Alon and Kadakkal Radhakrishnan

20 **Vitamin B2: Riboflavin** 265
Jennifer Donais and Kadakkal Radhakrishnan

21 **Vitamin B3: Niacin** 271
Tsering Yangchen Dirkhipa and Reema Gulati

22 **Vitamin B5: Pantothenic Acid** 277
Mohammad Nasser Kabbany

23 **Vitamin B_6: Pyridoxine** 281
Natalie Bhesania

24 **Biotin** 289
Christine Seif Pasquarella

25 **Vitamin B12** 295
Amala Alenchery and Kadakkal Radhakrishnan

26 **Folic Acid** 305
Nila Mistry Ambani

27 **Vitamin C** 311
Suruchi Ramanujan and Kadakkal Radhakrishnan

28 **Carnitine in Pediatric Nutrition** 317
Elizabeth Hilow

29 **Coenzyme Q10 in Pediatric Nutrition** 327
Nishaben Patel

30 **Alpha Lipoic Acid** 335
Elizabeth Robinson and Kadakkal Radhakrishnan

Part V Fat Soluble Vitamins

31 **Vitamin A** 343
Charles B. Chen

32 **Vitamin D** 351
Rishi Gupta

33 **Vitamin E** 359
Sanu Raja Yadav

34 Vitamin K 367
Supraja Swamy, Senthilkumar Sankararaman, and Kadakkal Radhakrishnan

Part VI Medical Nutrition Therapy

35 Congenital Heart Disease: Nutritional Considerations 377
Rukmini Komarlu and Christina DeTallo

36 Diabetes in Children: Nutritional Considerations . . . 397
Sumana Narasimhan and Jennifer Hyland

37 Pediatric Obesity 417
Roy Kim and Evelyn Benden

38 Nutrition and Inflammatory Bowel Disease 427
Diana Schnee, Maria Haught, Jacob A. Kurowski, and Sandra C. Kim

39 Failure to Thrive and Feeding Problems 441
Jessica Barry, Evelyn Benden, and Christine Bowen

40 Nutritional Considerations in Pediatric Liver Disease 451
Vera Hupertz and Andrea Adler

41 Short Bowel Syndrome and Intestinal Failure 461
Ali Salar Khalili, Nicole Lidyard, and Andrea Adler

42 Food Allergies and Eosinophilic GI Disorders: Nutritional Management 485
Sophia Patel, Brian Schroer, Maria Haught, and Diana Schnee

43 Nutrition in Pancreatic Disorders 497
Senthilkumar Sankararaman, Terri Schindler, and Aravind Thavamani

44 Nutritional Considerations in Celiac Disease 515
Elizabeth Collyer and Rachel Goodwin

45 Protein-Losing Enteropathy in Children 545
Chetan Mandelia and Donna Clement

46 Nutrition Requirements in Neurological Disorders . . 555
Amanda Abou-Fadel and Catherine Wills

47 Neonatal Nutrition and Prematurity 569
Taylor Rice, Audrey Ruthenberg, and Subhash Puthuraya

48 Pediatric Pulmonary Disorders and Nutritional Concerns 589
Parevi Majmudar, Sara Bewley, Kristina Pytlak, and Diana Schnee

49 Nutritional Considerations in Kidney Disease 601
Raed Bou Matar and Merideth Miller

50 Nutrition in Malignancy and Stem Cell Transplant . 615
Rachel N. Zeno, Seth Rotz, Sara Bewley, and Alexis Payton

51 Eating Disorders in the Child and Adolescent 625
Ellen S. Rome, Veronica E. Issac, Jennifer Hyland, and Hanna Leikin

52 Nutrition in Disorders of Gut-Brain Interaction and Motility 643
Sujithra Velayuthan, Ben Freiberg, Diana Schnee, and Maria Haught

Index 665

Contributors

Amanda Abou-Fadel, MD Pediatric Gastroenterology, Hepatology and Nutrition, Akron Children's Hospital, Akron, OH, USA

Andrea Adler Pediatric Nutrition Support, Division of Pediatric Gastroenterology, Hepatology, and Nutrition, Cleveland Clinic Children's Hospital, Cleveland, OH, USA

Amala Alenchery Division of Pediatric Gastroenterology, Hepatology and Nutrition, Cleveland Clinic Children's Hospital, Cleveland, OH, USA

Noy Lapidot Alon Division of Pediatric Gastroenterology, Hepatology, and Nutrition, Cleveland Clinic Children's Hospital, Cleveland, OH, USA

Department of Gastroenterology Nutrition and Liver Diseases, Schneider Children's Medical Center of Israel, Petach Tikva, Israel

Sackler Faculty of Medicine, Tel Aviv University, Tel Aviv, Israel

Nila Mistry Ambani Division of Pediatric Gastroenterology, Hepatology, and Nutrition, Cleveland Clinic Children's Hospital, Cleveland, OH, USA

Anthony Anani Department of Pediatric Gastroenterology, Cook Children's Medical Center Prosper, Prosper, TX, USA

Jessica Barry Division of Pediatric Gastroenterology, Hepatology, & Nutrition, Cleveland Clinic Children's Hospital, Cleveland, OH, USA

Evelyn Benden Pediatric Gastroenterology, Hepatology, and Nutrition, Pediatric Nutrition Support, Children's Institute, Cleveland, OH, USA

Pediatric Nutrition Support, Division of Pediatric Gastroenterology, Hepatology, & Nutrition, Cleveland Clinic Children's Hospital, Cleveland, OH, USA

Cleveland Clinic, Cleveland, OH, USA

Sara Bewley Pediatric Nutrition Support, Division of Pediatric Gastroenterology, Hepatology, and Nutrition, Cleveland Clinic Children's Hospital, Cleveland, OH, USA

Division of Pediatric Hematology, Oncology, and BMT, Cleveland Clinic Children's Hospital, OH, USA

Natalie Bhesania Division of Gastroenterology, Hepatology, and Nutrition, Children's Hospital Los Angeles, Los Angeles, CA, USA

Christine Bowen Pediatric Nutrition Support, Division of Pediatric Gastroenterology, Hepatology, & Nutrition, Cleveland Clinic Children's Hospital, Cleveland, OH, USA

Charles B. Chen Division of Gastroenterology, Department of Pediatrics, University of Missouri School of Medicine, Columbia, MO, USA

Donna Clement Division of Pediatric Gastroenterology, Department of Pediatrics, Brody School of Medicine, East Carolina University, Greenville, NC, USA

Elizabeth Collyer Celiac Disease Specialty Clinic at Phoenix Children's Hospital, Phoenix, AZ, USA

Christina DeTallo Pediatric Nutrition Support, Division of Pediatric Gastroenterology, Hepatology, and Nutrition, Cleveland Clinic Children's Hospital, Cleveland, OH, USA

Tsering Yangchen Dirkhipa Department of Pediatrics, MetroHealth Medical Center, Case Western Reserve University, Cleveland, OH, USA

Jennifer Donais Department of Pediatrics, Cleveland Clinic Children's Hospital, Cleveland, OH, USA

Ben Freiberg Division of Pediatric Gastroenterology, Hepatology, and Nutrition, Cleveland Clinic Children's Hospital, Cleveland, OH, USA

Rachel Goodwin Celiac Disease Specialty Clinic at Phoenix Children's Hospital, Phoenix, AZ, USA

Reema Gulati Pediatric Gastroenterology, Department of Pediatrics, MetroHealth Medical Center, Case School of Medicine, Case Western Reserve University, Cleveland, OH, USA

Rishi Gupta Division of Pediatric Gastroenterology, Hepatology and Nutrition, Golisano Children's Hospital at University of Rochester Medical Center, Rochester, NY, USA

Maria Haught Pediatric Nutrition Support, Division of Pediatric Gastroenterology, Hepatology, and Nutrition, Cleveland Clinic Children's Hospital, Cleveland, OH, USA

Elizabeth Hilow Department of Pediatric Gastroenterology, Phoenix Children's Hospital, Phoenix, AZ, USA

Vera Hupertz Division of Pediatric Gastroenterology, Hepatology, and Nutrition, Cleveland Clinic Children's Hospital, Cleveland, OH, USA

Jennifer Hyland Pediatric Nutrition Support, Division of Pediatric Gastroenterology, Hepatology, and Nutrition, Cleveland Clinic, Children's Hospital, Cleveland, OH, USA

Veronica E. Issac Center for Adolescent Medicine, Cleveland Clinic Children's Hospital, Cleveland, OH, USA

Cleveland Clinic Lerner College of Medicine, Cleveland, OH, USA

Rasha Abi Radi Abou Jaoudeh Department of Pediatrics, Cleveland Clinic Children's Hospital, Cleveland, OH, USA

Mohammad Nasser Kabbany Department of Pediatric Gastroenterology, Hepatology and Nutrition, University of Chicago, Chicago, IL, USA

Meenal Karuvannur Division of Pediatric Gastroenterology, Hepatology and Nutrition, Cleveland Clinic Children's Hospital, Cleveland, OH, USA

Ali Salar Khalili Case Western Reserve University School of Medicine, Pediatric Gastroenterology, University Hospitals Cleveland Medical Center, Rainbow Babies and Children's Hospital, Cleveland, OH, USA

Roy Kim Section for Pediatric Endocrinology, Cleveland Clinic Children's Hospital, Cleveland, OH, USA

Sandra C. Kim Division of Pediatric Gastroenterology, Hepatology and Nutrition, Cleveland Clinic Children's Hospital, Cleveland, OH, USA

Rukmini Komarlu Division of Pediatric Cardiology and Cardiovascular Medicine, Department of Heart, Vascular and Thoracic Cleveland Clinic, Children's Institute, Cleveland, OH, USA

Jacob A. Kurowski Pediatric Inflammatory Bowel Diseases, Division of Pediatric Gastroenterology, Hepatology & Nutrition, Cleveland Clinic Children's Hospital, Cleveland Clinic, Cleveland, OH, USA

Andrew R. Lavik Section of Pediatric Endocrinology, Cleveland Clinic Children's Hospital, Cleveland, OH, USA

Hanna Leikin Pediatric Nutrition Support, Pediatric Gastroenterology, Hepatology and Nutrition, Cleveland Clinic, Children's Institute, Cleveland, OH, USA

Nicole Lidyard University Hospitals Cleveland Medical Center, Rainbow Babies & Children's Hospital, Department of Pediatric Gastroenterology, Hepatology and Nutrition, Case Western Reserve University, Public Health Nutrition/Dietetics, Cleveland, OH, USA

Parevi Majmudar Center for Pediatric Pulmonology, Cleveland Clinic Children's Hospital, Cleveland, OH, USA

Chetan Mandelia Division of Pediatric Gastroenterology, Department of Pediatrics, Brody School of Medicine, East Carolina University, Greenville, NC, USA

Haig Manougian Division of Pediatric Hematology/Oncology and Bone Marrow Transplantation, Cleveland Clinic Children's Hospital, Cleveland, OH, USA

Anfal Marafie Pediatric Residency Program, Department of Pediatrics, Cleveland Clinic Children's Hospital, Cleveland, OH, USA

Raed Bou Matar Center for Pediatric Nephrology, Cleveland Clinic Children's Hospital, Cleveland, OH, USA

Audrey Matuska Pediatric Nutrition Support, Division of Pediatric Gastroenterology, Hepatology, and Nutrition, Cleveland Clinic Children's Hospital, Cleveland, OH, USA

Danielle Melton Center for Functional Medicine, Cleveland Clinic, Cleveland, OH, USA

Merideth Miller Pediatric Nutrition Support, Division of Pediatric Gastroenterology, Hepatology, and Nutrition, Cleveland Clinic Children's Hospital, Cleveland, OH, USA

Center for Pediatric Nephrology, Cleveland Clinic Children's, Cleveland, OH, USA

Aditi Mittal Presbyterian Healthcare Services, Department of Pediatric Gastroenterology, Albuquerque, NM, USA

Andrea Mucci Section of Pediatric Endocrinology, Cleveland Clinic Children's Hospital, Cleveland, OH, USA

Sumana Narasimhan Cleveland Clinic Lerner College of Medicine, Case Western Reserve University, Cleveland, OH, USA

Section of Pediatric Endocrinology, Cleveland Clinic Children's Hospital, Cleveland, OH, USA

Christine Seif Pasquarella Pediatric Gastroenterology, Hepatology and Nutrition, Akron Children's Hospital, Akron, OH, USA

Nishaben Patel Department of Pediatric Gastroenterology, Hepatology and Nutrition, University of Rochester Medical Center, Golisano Children's Hospital, Rochester, NY, USA

Sophia Patel Division of Pediatric Gastroenterology, Cleveland Clinic Children's Hospital, Cleveland, OH, USA

Alexis Payton Division of Pediatric Hematology, Oncology, and BMT, Cleveland Clinic Children's Hospital, Cleveland, OH, USA

Subhash Puthuraya Neonatology, Cleveland Clinic Lerner College of Medicine of Case Western Reserve University, Cleveland, OH, USA

Kristina Pytlak Pediatric Nutrition Support, Division of Pediatric Gastroenterology, Hepatology and Nutrition, Cleveland Clinic Children's Hospital, Cleveland, OH, USA

Kadakkal Radhakrishnan Division of Pediatric Gastroenterology, Hepatology & Nutrition, Cleveland Clinic Children's Hospital, Cleveland, OH, USA

Suruchi Ramanujan Department of Medicine, University of California San Diego, San Diego, CA, USA

Taylor Rice Pediatric Nutrition Support, Division of Pediatric Gastroenterology, Hepatology, and Nutrition, Cleveland Clinic Children's Hospital, Cleveland, OH, USA

Elizabeth Robinson Division of Pediatric Gastroenterology, Hepatology and Nutrition, Cleveland Clinic Children's Hospital, Cleveland, OH, USA

Kyleigh Rodriguez Pediatric Nutrition Support, Division of Pediatric Gastroenterology, Hepatology and Nutrition, Cleveland Clinic Children's Hospital, Cleveland, OH, USA

Ellen S. Rome Center for Adolescent Medicine, Cleveland Clinic Children's Hospital, Cleveland, OH, USA

Cleveland Clinic Lerner College of Medicine, Cleveland, OH, USA

Seth Rotz Division of Pediatric Hematology, Oncology, and BMT Cleveland Clinic Children's Hospital, Cleveland, OH, USA

Audrey Ruthenberg Pediatric Nutrition Support, Division of Pediatric Gastroenterology, Hepatology, and Nutrition, Cleveland Clinic, Cleveland, OH, USA

Cleveland Clinic Children's Healthy, Cleveland, OH, USA

Senthilkumar Sankararaman Division of Pediatric Gastroenterology, Hepatology, and Nutrition, Cleveland Clinic Children's Hospital, Cleveland, OH, USA

Terri Schindler Division of Pediatric Pulmonology, University Hospitals Rainbow Babies and Children's Hospital, Cleveland, OH, USA

Michael James Schmalz GI Associates, LLC, Pediatric Gastroenterology, Milwaukee, WI, USA

Diana Schnee Pediatric Nutrition Support, Division of Pediatric Gastroenterology, Hepatology, and Nutrition, Cleveland Clinic Children's Hospital, Cleveland, OH, USA

Brian Schroer Center of Pediatric Allergy and Immunology, Cleveland Clinic Children's Hospital, Cleveland, OH, USA

Praveen Kumar Conjeevaram Selvakumar Bon Secours Pediatric Gastroenterology Associates, Richmond, VA, USA

Margherita Shook Pediatric Nutrition Support, Division of Pediatric Gastroenterology, Hepatology, and Nutrition, Cleveland Clinic Children's Hospital, Cleveland, OH, USA

Kritika Sukumar Division of Pediatric Gastroenterology, Hepatology and Nutrition, Cleveland Clinic Children's Hospital, Cleveland, OH, USA

Supraja Swamy Department of Pediatric Gastroenterology, Wake Forest University, Winston Salem, NC, USA

Heidi Szugye Pediatric Nutrition Support, Division of Pediatric Gastroenterology, Hepatology, and Nutrition, Cleveland Clinic, Children's Hospital, Cleveland, OH, USA

Breastfeeding Medicine Section, Cleveland Clinic Children's Hospital, Cleveland, OH, USA

Ravi Talati Division of Pediatric Hematology/Oncology and Bone Marrow Transplantation, Cleveland Clinic Children's Hospital, Cleveland, OH, USA

Aravind Thavamani Division of Pediatric Gastroenterology, Hepatology, and Nutrition, University Hospitals Rainbow Babies and Children's Hospital, Cleveland, OH, USA

Sujithra Velayuthan Division of Pediatric Gastroenterology, Hepatology and Nutrition, Cleveland Clinic Children's Hospital, Cleveland, OH, USA

Anuradha Viswanathan Section of Pediatric Endocrinology, Cleveland Clinic Children's Hospital, Cleveland Clinic Learner College of Medicine, Case Western Reserve University, Cleveland, OH, USA

Catherine Wills, MS, RDN, LD, CNSC Pediatric Gastroenterology, Hepatology and Nutrition, Akron Children's Hospital, Akron, OH, USA

Sanu Raja Yadav Division of Pediatric Gastroenterology, Department of Pediatrics, University of Missouri School of Medicine, Columbia, MO, USA

Mira Younis Division of Pediatric Gastroenterology, Hepatology & Nutrition, Cleveland Clinic Children's Hospital, Cleveland, OH, USA

Rachel N. Zeno Division of Pediatric Hematology, Oncology, and BMT, Cleveland Clinic Children's Hospital, OH, USA

Part I

Normal Nutrition and Nutrition Support

Nutrition Intake Across Ages

1

Audrey Matuska and Merideth Miller

Infants

Energy Needs for Infants

- The Dietary Reference Intake (DRI) is recommended for healthy infants in determining estimated energy and protein needs. Please see Chap. 2 for more specific predictive equation recommendations.
- The World Health Organization (WHO) growth chart should be utilized for 0–24 months when assessing growth for weight, length, head circumference, and weight for length [1] (Table 1.1).

A. Matuska · M. Miller (✉)
Pediatric Nutrition Support, Division of Pediatric Gastroenterology, Hepatology, and Nutrition, Cleveland Clinic Children's Hospital, Cleveland, OH, USA
e-mail: MATUSKA@ccf.org; MILLERM5@ccf.org

K. Radhakrishnan (ed.), *Handbook of Clinical and Practical Pediatric Nutrition*, https://doi.org/10.1007/978-3-031-97759-6_1

Table 1.1 Average growth rates based on age [1]

Age (months)	Weight gain goals (g/day)	Length goals (cm/month)	Head circumference goals (cm/month)
0–3 months	28–33	3.5–3.8	1.8–2
3–6 months	16–17.5	2.0–2.1	0.9–1.0
6–9 months	10–11	1.5	0.5–0.6
9–12 months	8	1.3	0.4

Progression of Feeding/Solids (Table 1.2)

- Infants should be primarily breast or formula fed for the first 4–6 months of life.
- It is recommended that complementary foods be introduced no earlier than 4–6 months, ideally after 6 months of age.
- Breast feeding may be continued as desired according to the American Academy of Pediatrics (AAP) and the WHO. Prior to initiation of solid foods, infants should exhibit signs of readiness (see Table 1.2).
- It is recommended, infants be introduced to a variety of foods from all food groups (grains, fruits, vegetables, proteins, and dairy).
- Note, cow's milk should not be introduced until >12 months of age.
- It is recommended to introduce complementary foods that are rich in iron and zinc sources first as infants >6 months of age are at risk for deficiency [2]. Please refer to Chaps. 10 and 15, respectively, for iron- and zinc-rich food sources.
- Complementary foods should be introduced one single ingredient at a time to monitor for possible reactions/food allergens.
- Introduction of high allergen foods should be initiated early in the first year of life as this may reduce the risk for developing allergies. High allergen foods include cow's milk, soy, egg, peanuts, nuts/seeds, wheat, fish/shellfish (shrimp, crab, lobster, clams, mussels, oysters, scallops).
- Juice is not indicated in infants <12 months of age as breast milk/formula is the primary source for hydration [3].

Table 1.2 Development of feeding and recommended intakes [4–6]

Age (months)	Feeding skills	Types of food	Recommended intakes
0–3	Coordinates suck, swallow, breath Brings hands to mouth Limited head control	Breast milk or formula	8–12 feeds per day every 2–3 h
4–6	Good head control Opens and closes mouth for spoon Moves food to the back of tongue to swallow Begins to grasp objects Tracks food with eyes Begins sitting with less support	Breast milk or formula Iron + zinc rich Fortified infant cereals Pureed meats	6–8 times per day every 3–4 h
6–8	Sits upright without support Pincer grasp objects Swallow foods with closed mouth	Breast milk or formula Mashed foods with progressively larger lumps, soft chew, and finger foods (vegetables, fruits, meats) Fortified infant cereals	5–8 times per day every 3–4 h
9–12	Move food side to side with tongue Chewing in rotary pattern Feeds self with spoon Refined pincer grasp Picks up cup and drinks	Breast milk or formula Hader/lumpier solids, soft meats, small pieces	2–5 times per day

[a]Note infants should not be introduced to solid foods until showing signs of readiness

Important Nutrients of Concern

Vitamin D

- While breast milk provides primarily all nutrient needs, Vitamin D is not well transferred from mother to infant in breast milk.
- Primarily breast-fed infants should supplement with 400 IU Vitamin D daily to meet the RDA [7].
- Please refer to Chap. 32 for further details on vitamin D.

Iron

- Most healthy infants do not require iron supplements before 4–6 months of age. However, after 6 months of age, breast fed infants are at higher risk or iron deficiency. Iron-rich food sources are recommended >6 months.
- Supplementation may be necessary if infants do not eat iron-rich food sources [8, 9].
- Please see Chap. 10 on iron for more information.

Toddlers (Aged 1–4 Years)

- During the toddler years, the growth rate slows and thus energy needs decrease concurrently.
- Vitamins and minerals continue to be a high priority for growth and development but may be difficult to attain with increasing autonomy.
- Toddlers generally transition to whole milk at 1 year of age from formula or breast milk.
- If they do not consume whole milk at this time, their caloric and protein intake may be significantly decreased, allowing for down trending on growth charts.
- Children in this age group tend to have multiple locations where they eat: home, daycare, preschool, etc. Intake may vary based on where and who they are eating with; ensure to include all venues the child may be offered foods [10].

Growth Charts

Children 0–24 months of age are plotted on the WHO 0–24 months growth charts.

Weight, length, head circumference, and weight/length.

Children 2–4 years of age are plotted on the Centers for Disease Control (CDC) 2–20 years growth charts.

Weight, height, and BMI/age (Tables 1.3 and 1.4).

Table 1.3 Average growth rates based on age (girls) [1]

Anthropometric (average gain per year)	12–≤24 months	2–3 years	4 years
Weight	2.4 kg (5.3 lbs)	1.8 kg (4 lbs)	2 kg (4.5 lbs)
Height/length	12.3 cm (4.8 in)	8.9 cm (3.5 in)	6.3 in (2.5 in)
Head circumference	2.3 cm (0.9 in)	NA	NA

Table 1.4 Average growth rates based on age (boys) [1]

Anthropometric (average gain per year)	12–≤24 months	2–3 years	4 years
Weight	2.3 kg (5.1 lbs)	1.6 kg (3.5 lbs)	2 kg (4.5 lbs)
Height/length	12 cm (4.7 in)	8.5 cm (3.3 in)	6.3 in (2.5 in)
Head circumference	2.2 cm (0.9 in)	NA	NA

Table 1.5 Development of feeding skills [16]

Age	Age appropriate feeding skills
12–18 months	Begins rotary chew (accomplished by 36 months)
15 months	Helps hold cup with both hands; use a lid or assist with a regular cup Discards the bottle Self feeds with a spoon with frequent spills (offer thicker foods)
18 months	Uses a regular cup well (lifts, drinks, replaces) Turning the spoon over before it reaches mouth Mostly feeds self (increased food refusals) Hands empty dish to caregiver when requested
21 months	Eats part of meal with a fork
30 months	Pours well from glass to glass
36 months	Sucks through a straw well

Table 1.6 Average macronutrient needs for toddlers [10, 17]

Age	12–≤24 months	2–3 years	4 years
Calories	800–1400 calories/day	800–1400 calories/day	1300–1600 calories/day
Protein	13 g/day	13 g/day	13–19 g/day
Fat needs	30–40% of total calories	30–40% of total calories Saturated fat <10% of total calories	30–40% of total calories Saturated fat <10% of total calories

[a]See chapter on estimating needs for specific equations based on age

Table 1.7 Nutrients of concern

Nutrient	DRI	Rationale/recommendations	Foods high in iron
Iron [12]	1–3y: 7 mg	Due to inadequate iron intake, toddlers are at significant risk for iron deficiency anemia Excessive milk intake (≥32 oz./day) due to calcium's decreasing absorption of iron Screening for anemia at 12 months of age	Fortified breads and cereals, beans, nuts, red meat, and dried fruit
Zinc [13]	1–3 y: 3 mg	Due to dislike or lower intake of zinc-rich foods Offer easy to chew or ground meats	Red meat, legumes, peanut butter, oats, and tofu
Vitamin D [10]	1–3 y: 400 IU	Poor transition to milk/milk substitute Wearing sunscreen Indoor activities/limited sun exposure	Fortified milk, milk products, and milk substitutes; fatty fish
Calcium [10]	1–3 y: 500 mg	Poor transition to milk/milk substitute Encourage yogurt, enriched juice	Dairy products, milk substitutes, tofu, broccoli, kale, and spinach
Vitamin A [10]	1–3 y: 300 mcg RAE	Decreased intake of fruits and vegetables	Dairy products, fish, carrots, and sweet potatoes

[a]See chapter on specific nutrients for more details

Tips for Feeding Toddlers [11]

- Provide a quiet, pleasant, distraction free, safe space to eat.
- Help toddlers wash hands before eating.
- Let them help shop and prepare meals and snacks.
- Allow messes—let toddlers explore their food.
- Provide meals and snacks at consistent times.
  – Allow 2 h between meals/snacks to avoid grazing.
- Have child sit at a table or in a highchair to avoid walking around or playing.
- Use child-sized plates and cups.
- Model healthy habits—children are more likely to try a food if the parents are eating it.
- Remember that a toddler's appetite changes from day to day—occasional skipping of meals is within the norm.
- Provide favorite foods as well as new or disliked foods.
- Reintroduce disliked foods after several days or weeks.
- Try foods separate instead of mixed together—for example, a deconstructed sandwich.
- Provide soft foods, finger foods, and/or pieces that are easily picked up of handled on a utensil.

Young Children (5–12 years)

Energy Needs

- Energy needs for young children vary both based on age and sex/gender as well as activity level.
- Average energy needs for children 5–7 years ranges between 1200 and 1800 calories per day and children 8–11 years ranges between 1400 and 2200 calories per day according to the Dietary Guidelines for Americans [9].
- For best calculations of energy needs, utilization of the DRI equation is recommended, found in Chap. 2.
- Average protein needs of children from 5 to 11 years is 0.95 g/kg/day according to the DRI [15].

Growth Goals

- The CDC growth charts should be used to assess individual growth for weight, height, and BMI/age.
- Disease-specific growth charts may be necessary depending on specific growth trends.
- On average, optimal growth is between the 5th and < 85th percentile on the CDC growth chart [16].

Nutrients of Concern

- Dietary intake may vary greatly across this population with continued growth that requires consistent energy intakes and varied diet.
- However, depending on daily intakes, food habits, and food preference, young children may require a multivitamin if not meeting nutrient needs.
- Common nutrients of concern include Vitamin D, iron, and calcium (please refer to Chap. 11 for more details).
- Please note that common nutrition concerns for young children may also warrant additional specific nutrient needs such as undernutrition/malnutrition, obesity, eating disorders, and iron-deficiency anemia [16].
- Iron-deficiency anemia may be treated orally or intravenously depending on severity. Recommend oral dosing for iron-deficiency anemia is dependent on age and sex, please refer to Chap. 10 for specific dosing guidelines [12].

Adolescents (Aged 13–18 Years)

- Rapid growth and development of lean body mass occur during the adolescent years.
- Puberty changes body shape and mass leading to the possibility of body image concerns.

- Eating disorders are a concern at this stage in development (see chapter on eating disorders for more information).
- Adolescents are more autonomous in the foods, they eat at school, around friends, and at home.
- Social media plays a large role in what adolescents think about nutrition with influencers and content creators sharing their nutrition choices and views [10].
- The prevalence of overweight and obesity has more than quadrupled in adolescence over the past 30 years. It is important to address this diagnosis with care due to body image concerns in this age group. Education should be focused on healthy eating choices and habits [14]. See chapter on obesity for more information.
- Encourage activity that is engaging and enjoyable.
- It is recommended that adolescents get 60 min of exercise per day including both cardiovascular and strength training [10].

Growth Chart

Children 12–18 years of age are plotted on the CDC 2–20 years growth charts.

Weight, height, and BMI/age (Tables 1.8 and 1.9).

Average Macronutrient Needs for Adolescents

- Calorie needs are calculated based on gender, age, weight, height, and activity level using standard equations (see chapter on estimated energy needs for equations).
- Protein needs are based on weight and age. The amount of protein required will vary based on age, presence of acute or chronic illnesses, and activity level (Tables 1.10 and 1.11).

Table 1.8 Average growth rates per year based on age (girls) [14]

Anthropometric	12–13 years	13–14 years	14–15 years	15–17 years	17–18 years
Weight	4.2–4.4 kg (9.2–9.7 lbs)	3.5 kg (7.7 lbs)	2.7 kg (5.9 lbs)	1.3–1.8 kg (2.9–4 lbs)	1 kg (2.2 lbs)
Height	6 cm (2.4 in)	3.2 cm (1.26 in)	1.5 cm (0.6 in)	0.4–0.7 cm (0.16–0.3 in)	0.2 cm (0.08 in)

[a]Based on 50th percentile on the girls CDC 2–20 years growth chart

Table 1.9 Average growth rates per year based on age (boys) [14]

Anthropometric	12–14 years	14–15 years	15–16 years	17–18 years	17–18 years
Weight	5.1–5.5 kg (11–12 lbs)	5.2 kg (11.4 lbs)	4.7 kg (8.8 lbs)	3.6 kg (7.9 lbs)	2.6 kg (5.7 lbs)
Height	7–7.8 cm (2.75–3.1 in)	6.1 cm (2.4 in)	3.6 cm (1.4 in)	0.9 cm (0.35 in)	0.2 cm (0.08 in)

[a]Based on 50th percentile on the boys CDC 2–20 years growth chart

Table 1.10 DRI for protein in adolescents (boys and girls) [10, 17]

Age	13–14 years	14–18 years
Protein	0.85 g pro/kg/day	0.95 g pro/kg/day

Table 1.11 Nutrients of concern [10]

Nutrient	DRI	Rationale/ recommendations	Foods high in iron
Iron	12–13 years: 8 mg 14–18 years: Male: 11 mg Female: 15 mg	Due to demands from growth in males and menstruating in females Change in eating habits	Fortified breads and cereals, beans, nuts, red meat, and dried fruit
Vitamin D	12–18 years: 600 IU	Poor milk/milk substitute intake Wearing sunscreen Greater amounts of melanin in skin Indoor activities/limited sun exposure	Fortified milk, milk products, and milk substitutes; fatty fish
Calcium	1–3 years: 500 mg	Poor milk/milk substitute intake Rapid bone growth Encourage yogurt, enriched juice	Dairy products, milk substitutes, tofu, broccoli, kale, and spinach

[a]See other chapters on specific nutrients for more details

References

1. Ebrahim GJ. WHO child growth standards. Growth velocity based on weight, length and head circumference. * Methods and development. J Trop Pediatr. 2009;56(2):136.
2. American Academy of Pediatrics. Infant Food and Feeding [Internet] wwwaaporg. 2023. Available from: https://www.aap.org/en/patient-care/healthy-active-living-for-families/infant-food-and-feeding/.
3. Infant and Toddler Nutrition [Internet]. Centers for disease control and prevention; 2022 [cited 2024 Jul 8]. Available from: https://www.cdc.gov/nutrition/infantandtoddlernutrition/index.html.

4. Reverri EJ, Arensberg MB, Murray RD, Kerr KW, Wulf KL. Young child nutrition: knowledge and surveillance gaps across the Spectrum of feeding. Nutrients. 2022;14(15):3093. https://doi.org/10.3390/nu14153093. PMID: 35956275; PMCID: PMC9370290.
5. Goday PS, Walia CLS. Chapter 5 Infant nutrition. In: Pediatric nutrition for dietitians. 1st ed. Boca Raton: CDR Press; 2022. p. 65–78.
6. American Academy of Pediatrics. Starting solid foods [internet]. HealthyChildrenorg. 2019. Available from: https://www.healthychildren.org/English/ages-stages/baby/feeding-nutrition/Pages/Starting-Solid-Foods.aspx
7. Meek JY, Noble L. Section on breastfeeding; policy statement: breastfeeding and the use of human Milk. Pediatrics. 2022;150(1):e2022057988. https://doi.org/10.1542/peds.2022-057988.
8. Office of dietary supplements – iron [Internet]. U.S. Department of Health and Human Services; [cited 2024 Jul 8]. Available from: https://ods.od.nih.gov/factsheets/iron-healthprofessional/#h6.
9. USDA Dietary guidelines for Americans 2020–2025 [Internet]. Dietary guidelines for Americans. USDA; 2020 Dec. Available from: https://www.dietaryguidelines.gov/sites/default/files/2021-03/Dietary_Guidelines_for_Americans-2020-2025.pdf.
10. Pediatric nutrition care manual. Edited by Aida Miles, AND, 29 May 2024. Accessed 1 Aug 2024.
11. American Academy of Pediatrics. Feeding & Nutrition Tips: your 2-year-old. HealthyChildrenorg. 2019. www.healthychildren.org/English/ages-stages/toddler/nutrition/Pages/Feeding-and-Nutrition-Your-Two-Year-Old.aspx.
12. National Institutes of Health. "Iron." NIH, 5 Apr 2022. http://ods.od.nih.gov/factsheets/Iron-HealthProfessional/.
13. National Institutes of Health. "Zinc." NIH, 28 Sep 2022, Zinc – Health Professional Fact Sheet (nih.gov)
14. World Health Organization "Obesity and overweight." World Health Organization, 1 Mar 2024, www.who.int/news-room/fact-sheets/detail/obesity-and-overweight.
15. Goday PS, Walia C. Pediatric nutrition for dietitians. Milton, Taylor & Francis Group; 2022. p. 2–3, 10.
16. American Dietetic Association. Pediatric Nutrition Care Manual®. School-aged Children. https://www.nutritioncaremanual.org/. Accessed 15 Aug 2024.
17. Institute of Medicine. Dietary reference intakes for energy, carbohydrate, fiber, fat, fatty acids, cholesterol, protein, and amino acids (macronutrients). National Academies Press. 2005:659. Full text.

Nutrition Assessment

2

Hanna Leikin and Danielle Melton

Definitions

BMR Daily rate of energy metabolism an individual needs to sustain to preserve the integrity of vital functions without the influence of external environmental conditions, under thermal neutrality, void of physical movement, and the effects of food or drugs. It is typically expressed as heat production or oxygen consumption per unit of body size, and standard estimations are measured with a spirometer to assess O_2 consumption and CO_2 production [7].

DRI Set of reference values used to calculate nutrient requirements for healthy children who are metabolically normal. Dietary reference intakes (DRI) for protein is used for children with normal growth, body composition, and activity. Protein requirements were calculated based on the amount of protein needed for nitrogen equilibrium [1] (Table 2.1).

H. Leikin (✉)
Pediatric Nutrition Support, Division of Pediatric Gastroenterology, Hepatology, and Nutrition, Cleveland Clinic, Children's Institute, Cleveland, OH, USA
e-mail: LEIKINH@ccf.org

D. Melton
Center for Functional Medicine, Cleveland Clinic, Cleveland, OH, USA
e-mail: BEAUDOD@ccf.org

K. Radhakrishnan (ed.), *Handbook of Clinical and Practical Pediatric Nutrition*, https://doi.org/10.1007/978-3-031-97759-6_2

Table 2.1 DRI [1]

Calorie (kg)	
Infant and young children	
0–3 months	((89 × wt [kg]—100) + 175)/wt [kg]
4–6 months	((89 × wt [kg]—100) + 56)/wt [kg]
7–12 months	((89 × wt [kg]—100) + 22)/wt [kg]
13–36 months	((89 × wt [kg] –100) + 20)/wt [kg]
Ages 3–8 years—Boys	
(88.5 – (61.9 × age [y]) + PA × (26.7 × wt [kg] + 903 × ht. [m]) + 20)/wt [kg]	
Ages 3–8 years – Girls	
(135.3 – (30.8 × age [y]) + PA × (10 × wt [kg] + 934 × ht. [m]) + 20)/wt [kg]	
Ages 9–18 years—Boys	
(88.5—(61.9 × age [y]) + PA × (26.7 × wt [kg] + 903 × ht. [m]) + 25)/wt [kg]	
Ages 9–18 years—Girls	
(135.3 – (30.8 × age [y]) + PA × (10 × wt [kg] + 934 × ht. [m]) + 25)/wt [kg]	

Peterson's Failure to Thrive (FTT) Used for infants and children who present underweight and need to achieve catch-up growth. Upon initial assessment, limit estimated calories to 125 kcal/kg due to risk of refeeding syndrome [25] (Table 2.2).

Schofield equation is a method used to calculate BMR and is typically used for healthy children, who are acutely ill in the hospital setting. Limitations to this equation are lack of consideration of body composition, physical activity, or population specificity. Studies have shown that this equation also may over- or underes-

Table 2.2 Peterson's FTT [25]

Calorie (kg)	(calories for weight age[a] [kcal/kg] x IBW [kg])/ actual weight [kg]
Protein (kg)	(protein for weight age[a] [g/kg] x IBW [kg])/ actual weight [kg]

[a]Weight age is a value that compares a child's weight to the expected weight of a healthy child (at the 50th percentile based on appropriate growth charts—see Chap. 1 for more information on growth charts) of the same age and sex

Table 2.3 Schofield [3]

Calorie (kg)	
Males	
0–3 years	((0.167 × wt [kg]) + (15.174 × ht. [cm])—617.6)/wt [kg]
3–10 years	((19.59 × wt [kg]) + (1.303 × ht. [cm]) + 414.9)/wt [kg]
10–18 years	((16.25 × wt [kg]) + (1.372 × ht. [cm]) + 515.5)/wt [kg]
>18 years	((15.057 × wt [kg]) + (1.0004 × ht. [cm]) + 705.8)/wt [kg]
Females	
0–3 years	((16.252 × wt [kg]) + (10.232 × ht. [cm]) – 413.5)/wt [kg]
3–10 years	((16.969 × wt [kg]) + (1.618 × ht. [cm]) + 371.2)/wt [kg]
10–18 years	((8.365 × wt [kg]) + (4.65 × ht. [cm]) + 200)/wt [kg]
>18 years	((13.623 × wt [kg]) + (2.83 × ht. [cm]) + 98.2))/wt [kg]

timate needs in certain patient populations [22]. It is important that the equations be practically applied in the appropriate clinical setting with serial monitoring of patient to ensure that the recommendations are appropriate (Table 2.3).

TEE Includes BMR, energy expended during physical activity and diet-induced thermogenesis [4].

TEF The increase in metabolism after a meal—accounts for ~10% of total energy expenditure (TEE). Thermic effect of food (TEF) may be influenced by age, physical activity, meal volume, composition frequency, and timing [8].

WHO Resting energy expenditure (REE) equation is defined by the WHO as the energy expended by a person at rest. These calculations are commonly used for acutely ill children in the hospital setting. Approximately 80% of variability in REE is related to variances in lean body mass [4]. Studies have found that this predictive equation may over- or underestimate needs [22]. Additional limitations include misrepresentative of all ethnicities and does not consider body composition, height, or activity level (Table 2.4).

Nutrient calculations should be used as an initial estimate to determine energy and protein requirements. Clinical judgment is advised to adjust patients estimated nutrient needs based on growth and presence of malnutrition, which is discussed later in this chapter. Sex, age, and body composition are variables that differentiate energy needs. Coexisting pathological conditions reduce or increase calorie requirements [4].

Table 2.4 WHO (REE) [2]

Calorie (kg)		
Age	Male	Female
0–3 years	((60.9 × wt [kg]) – 54)/wt [kg]	((61 × wt [kg]) – 51)/wt [kg]
3–10 years	((22.7 × wt [kg]) + 495)/wt [kg]	((22.5 × wt [kg]) + 499)/wt [kg]
10–18 years	((17.5 × wt [kg]) + 651)/wt [kg]	((12.2 × wt [kg]) + 746)/wt [kg]

Activity factors	Stress factors	
Paralyzed: 1.0	Surgery: 1.2–1.5	Burn: 1.5–2.5
Confined to bed: 1.1	Infection: 1.2–1.6	Starvation: 0.7
Ambulatory: 1.2–1.3	Trauma: 1.1–1.8	Growth failure: 1.5–2.0

Phases associated with post-traumatic metabolic changes:

1. Ebb phase:
   (a) Initial shorter phase (~12–24 h)
   (b) Decrease in metabolic rate that is influenced by decreased oxygen consumption and reduced body temperature [5]
2. Flow phase:
   (a) As the blood volume is restored post hemorrhage, the flow phase or catabolic phase begins
   (b) Increase in total energy expenditure
   (c) Muscle and fat catabolism are present, which lead to a negative nitrogen balance and gluconeogenesis [6]

Energy Calculations

Physical activity coefficient

	Sedentary	Low active	Active	Very active
Ages 3–18 years—Boys	1.0	1.13	1.26	1.42
Ages 3–18 years—Girls	1.0	1.16	1.31	1.56

Indirect Calorimetry (IC) [9]

- Gold standard for measuring individual energy needs, as predictive equations may over- or underestimate needs.
- Chemical energy is released from nutrients via the oxidation of food substrates. Carbon-based nutrients are converted into CO_2, H_2O, and heat in the presence of O_2.
- IC measures the amount of oxygen consumed (VO_2) and carbon dioxide released (VCO_2) by the body to assess energy expenditure.

- A metabolic cart collects the VO_2 and VCO_2 values, which are then plugged into the following equation:

$$Energy\,expenditure\left(kcal / day\right) = [\left(VO_2 \times 3.941\right) + \left(VCO_2 \times 1.11\right) \times 1440$$

Limitations Multiple factors may impact the effectiveness of IC. It is important to keep the following in mind when evaluating IC calculations:

- Mechanical ventilation settings or air leakages may affect the presence of additional gases impeding IC results. Thoracic drains may also lead to air leakage.
- Clinical instability has the potential to change metabolic requirements, including agitation, fever, sedatives, and inotropic support.
- Organ support systems, including continuous renal replacement therapy (CRRT) and extracorporeal membrane oxygen (ECMO), can impact gas exchange [24] (Table 2.5).

Table 2.5 DRI protein [1]

Protein (kg)	
Age	Dosage (g/kg)
0— < 6 months	1.52
6–12 months	1.2
1–<4 years	1.05
4–<14 years	0.95
14–18 years	0.85

Protein Calculations

Protein requirements for critically Ill and injured children has been defined by the American Society for Parenteral and Enteral Nutrition (ASPEN) [26]. Metabolic stress increases catabolism and breakdown of lean body mass. To meet the increased stress demands and spare lean body mass, a greater amount of protein is needed until the underlying stress has been overcome [26, 27] (Tables 2.6 and 2.7).

Table 2.6 Protein requirements for critically ill and injured children [26, 27]

Protein (gkg)	
0–2 years	2–3
2–13 years	1.5–2
13–18 years	1.5

Table 2.7 Fluid calculations (Holliday–Segar method) [19]

Body weight (kg)	Maintenance fluid needs/day
0–10	100 mL/kg
11–20	1000 mL + 50 mL/kg for each kg >10 kg
>20	1500 mL + 20 mL/kg for each kg >20 kg

Note: Fluid needs are altered in patients with decreased mobility, hypermetabolism, and increased GI losses. Use discretion and adjust accordingly

Malnutrition

- In 2015, the American Society of Parenteral and Enteral Nutrition and the Academy of Nutrition and Dietetics defined pediatric malnutrition indicators for assessment [10] (see Table 2.8).
- For a complete nutrition assessment, evaluation of growth charts (see Chap. 1 for more information on growth charts), nutrient intake, and physical assessment is required.
- A nutrition-focused physical exam uses inspection and palpation as primary techniques. The practitioner will assess for bone protrusion, hallowed cheeks, and hallowing of muscle to identify subcutaneous fat loss and muscle wasting. Regions for assessment include orbital, buccal, temple, upper arm (area under triceps muscle), clavicle bone, acromion bone, scapular bone and spine, thoracic and lumbar, anterior thigh, patellar, posterior calf, and buttocks [18].
- Mid-upper arm circumference (MUAC) measures muscle and subcutaneous fat in the upper arm region. This measurement is a reliable tool to strengthen a malnutrition diagnosis and has been recognized as a more sensitive prognostic marker for mortality than weight-for-height in malnourished pediatric patients [21].
- Triceps skin fold (TSF) can be used to monitor changes in body fat composition.
- MUAC and TSF measurements can be used to calculate arm fat area and arm muscle area. Percentile ranges for these calculations are available for comparison [23] (Tables 2.8, 2.9, and 2.10).

Waterlow criteria for malnutrition is based on percentage of ideal body weight [12]. This method of use is outdated, as *z* score assessment is more descriptive.

Table 2.8 Pediatric malnutrition criteria

Malnutrition in context of: Acute illness/injury Chronic illness/injury Acute on chronic illness/injury Non-illness-related factors (behavioral/socioeconomic/environmental)	Mild malnutrition	Moderate malnutrition	Severe malnutrition
Anthropometrics: Z scores for BMI for age, weight for length, length/height for age*	−1 to −1.9 *z* score or a decline of 1 *z* score	−2 to −2.9 *z* score or decline of 2 *z* scores	<−3 *z* score or decline of 3 *z* score −3 *z* score length/height for age*
Weight gain velocity: <2 years of age	Less than 75% of the norm for expected weight gain	Less than 50% of the norm for expected weight gain	Less than 25% of the norm for expected weight gain
Weight loss: 2–20 years	5% weight loss	7.5% weight loss	10% weight loss
Inadequate nutrient intake: RD obtains diet history and estimated needs	51–75% estimated energy/protein need	26–50% estimated energy/protein need	≤25% estimated energy/protein need
Physical assessment: Mid-upper arm circumference	−1 to −1.9 *z* score	−2 to −2.9 *z* score	−3 *z* score or below
Physical assessment: Loss/absence of subcutaneous fat stores and muscle mass	Mild depletion	Moderate depletion	Severe depletion

Adapted from Becker et al. [10]

Table 2.9 Etiology-related definitions of pediatric malnutrition

Illness-related malnutrition	Non-illness-related malnutrition
Etiology: Illness-related malnutrition caused by malabsorption, increased nutrient losses, hypermetabolism, or altered nutrient utilization in the setting of disease or trauma. Diseases that are at risk for malnutrition are those with a cystic fibrosis, anorexia nervosa (see Chap. 51 for more information on eating disorders and refeeding syndrome), gastrointestinal conditions (chronic diarrhea, inflammatory bowel disease), food allergies, prematurity, long-term nutrition support, congenital heart disease, intestinal failure, liver disease, chylothorax, burns, cancer and renal disease [13]	Etiology: Non-illness-related malnutrition is caused by reduced nutrient intake in the setting of behavioral factors (i.e., anorexia), socioeconomic factors (i.e., food insecurity), or environmental factors (i.e., neglect)
Adverse clinical outcomes such as immune dysfunction, delayed wound healing, prolonged hospitalizations, or developmental delays can occur in the setting of malnutrition [11]	

Adapted from Mehta et al. [13]. Available from: https://www.ncbi.nlm.nih.gov/pubmed/23528324

- >90% normal
- 80–90% mild wasting
- 70–79% moderate wasting
- <70% severe wasting

Table 2.10 Macro- and micronutrient deficiencies based on physical examination

Exam area	Physical sign	Potential nutrient deficiency
Hair	Alopecia	Protein, zinc, biotin, essential fatty acid, selenium deficiency
	Easily pluckable	Protein deficiency
	Lanugo	Energy deficiency
Eyes	Pale conjunctiva	Anemia (iron, folate, and/or vitamin B_{12}), copper deficiency
	Night blindness; dull dry membrane with foamy spots (Bitot's spots)	Vitamin A deficiency
	Dry itchy, cracked, red corners	Riboflavin, niacin deficiency
Mouth	Dry, cracked, red lips	Riboflavin, niacin, vitamin B_6 deficiency
	Bleeding gums	Vitamin C deficiency
	Dry mouth	Zinc deficiency
	Inflamed mucosa	Vitamin B complex, iron, vitamin C deficiency
	Glossitis	Niacin, folate, riboflavin, iron, vitamin B_{12}, vitamin B_6 deficiency
	Beefy red tongue	Niacin, folate, riboflavin, iron, vitamin B_{12} deficiency
Nails	Koilonychia (spoon-shaped nails)	Iron deficiency
	Lackluster, dull	Protein deficiency
	Mottled, pale nails; poor blanching	Vitamin A, vitamin C deficiency

(continued)

Table 2.10 (continued)

Exam area	Physical sign	Potential nutrient deficiency
Skin	Pallor	Iron, folate, vitamin B_{12} deficiency
	Dry scaly skin	Vitamin A, essential fatty acid deficiency
	Dermatitis	Essential fatty acid, zinc, niacin, riboflavin, or tryptophan deficiency
	Nonhealing wound	Zinc, vitamin C, or protein deficiency
Face	Moon face	Protein-calorie deficiency
	Bilateral temporal wasting	Protein-calorie deficiency
Neck	Enlarged thyroid (goiter)	Iodine deficiency

Table adapted from ASPEN | Practitioner's Guide to Nutrition-Focused Physical Exam of Infants, Children, and Adolescents [Internet]. Nutritioncare.org. 2019 [cited 2024 Sep 25]. Available from: https://www.nutritioncare.org/NFPEPediatrics/ and Green Corkins K. Nutrition-focused physical examination in pediatric patients. Nutrition in Clinical Practice: Official Publication of the American Society for Parenteral and Enteral Nutrition [Internet]. 2015 Apr 1;30 (2):203–9. Available from: https://pubmed.ncbi.nlm.nih.gov/25739708/

Biochemical Data and Malnutrition

Note that laboratory tests alone do not give a complete assessment of nutrition status. While serum albumin and prealbumin have historically been assessed to determine the presence of malnutrition, these markers are influenced by inflammation; therefore, current practices should include the evaluation of C-reactive protein and Erythrocyte sedimentation rate, and so on in conjunction with biochemical indicators of malnutrition [15] (Tables 2.11 and 2.12).

Table 2.11 Laboratory tests and malnutrition

Hypoalbuminemia (<2.5 g/dL) [14, 15]	Poor indicator of malnutrition in acute setting as a negative acute-phase protein with short half-life	Can by caused by: ↓ energy or amino acids supply Impaired liver synthesis ↑ loss ↑ tissue catabolism Distributional issues Sepsis, infection, trauma, major surgery Complications: ↓ oncotic pressure resulting in ↑ ECF ↓ immune function Possible impact on drug utilization
Potential micronutrient deficiencies [18, 20] (see sections on micronutrients and vitamins for more information)	Fat soluble vitamins: Vitamin A 25-OH vitamin D* Vitamin E Vitamin K Water soluble vitamins Vitamin C Vitamin B1, B2, B3, B6, B7, B12 MMA Folic acid Trace minerals Copper Zinc* Manganese Chromium Selenium Essential fatty acids [20] Linoleic acid (LA, omega- 6) Alpha-linolenic acid (ALA, Omega-3) Triene/Tetraene (T/T) ratio, calculated as Mead acid to arachidonic acid, and is ↑ in EFAD Carnitine profile Free and total carnitine Iron studies* Iron TIBC Ferritin *recommend obtaining initially, followed by other labs as warranted	
Refeeding surveillance [15] (see Chap. 51 for more information)	CMP (potassium, magnesium, phosphorus) Baseline levels and daily monitoring is recommended with the advancement of nutrition, until goal intake is achieved, and labs are stable May require oral or IV repletion	

Table 2.12 Types of malnutrition

<table>
<tr><th>Kwashiorkor [16]</th><th>Marasmus [16]</th></tr>
<tr><td>“Protein malnutrition”—Inadequate protein intake.
Often occurs after acute infection.
Gastrointestinal infections lead to damaged intestinal mucosa, reducing absorption.
Complicated by septicemia and bacteremia.
Characteristics:
Edema
Depigmentation of skin
Enlarged and/or fatty liver, aflatoxin detected
Liver dysfunction leads to impaired plasma protein synthesis and export (total protein, albumin, transferrin)
↓ glutathione and methionine
↑ free circulating iron and Na+/K+ pump sites
Pathogenic gut microbiota disturbances
Inflammatory response
Treatment with antibiotics beneficial for survival</td><td>“Severe undernutrition”—Prolonged inadequate carbohydrate and fat intake.
More chronic illness, deprivation syndrome, most prevalent type of severe acute malnutrition.
Characteristics:
Loss of subcutaneous fat
Dry skin, wrinkled, and loose
Reduced gut Bacteroidetes</td></tr>
<tr><td colspan="2">Both Kwashiorkor and Marasmus have a high mortality rate in children.
Metabolic changes:
↑ plasma concentrations of free fatty acids (higher in kwashiorkor)
Cholesterol, plasma fasting triglyceride, and phospholipid changes (lower in kwashiorkor)
Fasting glucose in low-normal range, low fasting serum insulin level, impaired glucose tolerance [16]
Total body water (TBW) is increased as a percentage of body weight
Manifests as edema in kwashiorkor
Possible greater loss of body solids in marasmus thought to preserve extracellular fluid volume (ECF), resulting in higher TBW than kwashiorkor without obvious edema
ECF changes may also be related to energy intake and phase of malnutrition recovery rather than anthropometric changes alone
TBW increased in early rapid weight gain may be the result of potassium repletion, glycogen synthesis, and alterations in cellular membrane Na + and K+ transport [17]</td></tr>
<tr><td colspan="2">Protein-calorie malnutrition—a combination of Kwashiorkor and Marasmus [16]</td></tr>
</table>

Case Scenarios

Scenario 1 2-year-old female with severe iron-deficiency anemia with increased work on breathing, moderate heart failure, and moderate malnutrition. Currently receiving ¼ liter oxygen and bolus nasogastric tube feeds at 120 mL 5 times per day.

Anthropometrics:
Weight: 11.5 kg
Height: 92 cm
BMI: 13.6 kg/m^2, z score = −2.44
Weight-for-age: 24 months
Ideal body weight: 13.9 kg

Estimated Needs:
Enteral energy goal 99 cal/kg/day (Peterson's FTT)
Protein goal 1.5–2 g pro/kg/day (ASPEN)

Predictive equations and rational for use: this patient would require calories based on Peterson's FTT equation, as they would benefit from increased caloric intake to achieve catch up growth. Protein needs based on ASPEN critical care, as this is a critically ill child.

Scenario 2 15-year-old male with Crohn's disease, admitted with melena, weight loss, and poor appetite. Prior to admission, family reports decreased PO intake, consuming two meals per day.

Anthropometrics:
Weight: 45 kg (weight trends: 50 kg 3 months prior).
Height: 162 cm.
BMI: 17.1 kg/m^2, z score = −1.26.

Estimated Needs:
Enteral energy goals 45–49 cal/kg/day (DRI x 1.1–1.2 due to flare/weight loss).
Protein goal 1.3 g pro/kg/day (DRI x 1.5 due to flare).

Predictive equations and rational for use: energy needs increase during a flare especially in the setting of weight loss/malnutrition. Based on patient's worsening nutrition status (weight loss, decline in oral intake) and flare, he would benefit from 110–120% of the DRI for optimal caloric intake during an inflammatory state. In addition, during a flare, protein needs may increase to 150% of the DRI due to inflammation.

Scenario 3 11-year-old Class III obese female presenting with acute respiratory distress, chest pain, and vomiting, now concerning for possible myocarditis and heart failure. She is intubated and sedated on neuromuscular blockade and inotropic support. Course complicated by wounds and acute kidney injury, requiring CRRT and has been placed on ECMO. Patient unable to be fed enterally, thus parenteral nutrition support initiated.

Anthropometrics:
Weight: 99.8 kg
Height: 153 cm
BMI: 42.6 kg/m^2, >99%ile, z score = 4.4
Dose weight: 70 kg—weight used for estimated needs based on obesity status

Estimated Needs:
Parenteral energy goals 18 cal/kg/day (Enteral energy goals −10% due to lack of thermic effect of food)
Enteral energy goals 20 cal/kg/day (Schofield using dose weight × 1.3 for wound factor)
Protein goal 1.5–2 g pro/kg/day (ASPEN)

Predictive equations and rational for use: IC or metabolic cart is the gold standard in estimating this medically complex patient's needs if available. As patient is acutely ill in the hospital setting, the Schofield energy equation would also be appropriate in estimating her needs with a stress factor for trauma of 110–180% above her needs. Protein needs based on ASPEN critical care, as this patient is critically ill.

Scenario 4 9-year-old female with Cerebral Palsy Gross Motor Function Classification System 5, gastrostomy tube dependent, admitted with respiratory syncytial virus and need for high-flow nasal cannula. No presence of malnutrition identified.

Anthropometrics:
Weight: 26 kg
Height: 125 cm
BMI: 16.6 kg/m^2, z score = 0.17

Estimated Needs:
Enteral energy goals 42 cal/kg/day (WHO)
Protein goal 0.95 g pro/kg/day (DRI)

Predictive equations and rational for use: for patients with limited mobility, the WHO equation best estimates patient's energy requirements, as it calculates energy expended by a person at rest. The DRI for protein is appropriate for this patient, as no malnutrition is present.

References

1. Medicine I of. Dietary Reference Intakes for Energy, Carbohydrate, Fiber, Fat, Fatty Acids, Cholesterol, Protein, and Amino Acids [Internet]. nap.nationalacademies.org. 2002. Available from: https://nap.nationalacademies.org/catalog/10490/dietary-reference-intakes-for-energy-carbohydrate-fiber-fat-fatty-acids-cholesterol-protein-and-amino-acids
2. Energy and protein requirements. Report of a joint FAO/WHO/UNU expert consultation. World Health Organization Technical Report Series [Internet] 1985;724:1–206. Available from: https://pubmed.ncbi.nlm.nih.gov/3937340/.
3. Schofield WN. Predicting basal metabolic rate, new standards and review of previous work. Hum Nutr Clin Nutr [Internet]. 1985;39(Suppl 1):5–41. Available from: https://pubmed.ncbi.nlm.nih.gov/4044297/
4. Allowances NRC (US) S on the TE of the RD. Energy [Internet] wwwncbinlmnihgov National Academies Press (US); 1989. Available from: https://www.ncbi.nlm.nih.gov/books/NBK234938/.
5. Cuthbertson DP, Angeles Valero Zanuy MA, León Sanz ML. Post-shock metabolic response. 1942. Nutricion Hospitalaria [Internet].

2001;16(5):176–82; discussion 175–176. Available from: https://pubmed.ncbi.nlm.nih.gov/11708288/.
6. Sobotka L, Soeters PB. e-SPEN. Euro e-J Clin Nutr Metabol. 2009;4:e1–3.
7. Henry C. Basal metabolic rate studies in humans: measurement and development of new equations. Public Health Nutr. 2005;8(7a):1133–52.
8. Calcagno M, Kahleova H, Alwarith J, Burgess NN, Flores RA, Busta ML, et al. The thermic effect of food: a review. J Am Coll Nutr. 2019;38(6):547–51.
9. Haugen HA, Chan LN, Li F. Indirect calorimetry: a practical guide for clinicians. Nutr Clin Pract. 2007;22(4):377–88.
10. Becker P, Carney LN, Corkins MR, Monczka J, Smith E, Smith SE, et al. Consensus statement of the academy of nutrition and dietetics/American Society for Parenteral and Enteral Nutrition. Nutr Clin Pract. 2014;30(1):147–61.
11. Bouma S. Diagnosing pediatric malnutrition: paradigm shifts of etiology-related definitions and appraisals of the indicators. ASPEN. 2017;32(1):52–67.
12. Waterlow JC. Classification and definition of protein-calorie malnutrition. BMJ. 1972;3(5826):566–9.
13. Mehta NM, Corkins MR, Lyman B, et al. Defining pediatric malnutrition: a paradigm shift toward etiology-related definitions. JPEN J Parenter Enteral Nutr. 2013;37(4):460–81.
14. Gatta A, Verardo A, Bolognesi M. Hypoalbuminemia. Intern Emerg Med. 2012;7(S3):193–9.
15. da Silva JSV, Seres DS, Sabino K, Adams SC, Berdahl GJ, Citty SW, et al. ASPEN consensus recommendations for refeeding syndrome. Nutr Clin Pract [Internet]. 2020;35(2):178–95. Available from: https://aspenjournals.onlinelibrary.wiley.com/doi/10.1002/ncp.10474
16. Difference between kwashiorkor and marasmus: comparative meta-analysis of pathogenic characteristics and implications for treatment. Microbial Pathogen [Internet] 2021 ;150:104702. Available from: https://www.sciencedirect.com/science/article/pii/S0882401020310688.
17. Patrick J, Reeds PJ, Jackson AA, Seakins A, Picou DIM. Total body water in malnutrition: the possible role of energy intake. Br J Nutr. 1978;39(3):417–24.
18. Green Corkins K, Teague EE. Pediatric nutrition assessment. Nutr Clin Pract. 2016;32(1):40–51.
19. Meyers RS. Pediatric fluid and electrolyte therapy. J Pediat Pharmacol Therap: JPPT: Off J PPAG [Internet]. 2009;14(4):204–11. Available from: https://www.ncbi.nlm.nih.gov/pmc/articles/PMC3460795/
20. Selbuz S, Kırsaçlıoğlu CT, Kuloğlu Z, Yılmaz M, Penezoğlu N, Sayıcı U, et al. Diagnostic workup and micronutrient deficiencies in children with failure to thrive without underlying diseases. Nutr Clin Pract. 2019;34(4):581–8.

21. Rasmussen J, Andersen A, Fisker AB, Ravn H, Sodemann M, Rodrigues A, et al. Mid-upper-arm-circumference and mid-upper-arm circumference z-score: the best predictor of mortality? Eur J Clin Nutr. 2012;66(9):998–1003.
22. Carpenter A, Pencharz P, Mouzaki M. Accurate estimation of energy requirements of young patients. J Pediat Gastroenterol Nutr [Internet]. 2015;60(1):4–10. Available from: https://www.naspghan.org/files/documents/pdfs/cme/jpgn/Accurate_Estimation_of_Energy_Requirements_of.5.pdf.
23. Frisancho AR. Triceps skin fold and upper arm muscle size norms for assessment of nutritional status. Am J Clin Nutr. 1974;27:1052–8.
24. Delsoglio M, Achamrah N, Berger MM, Pichard C. Indirect calorimetry in clinical practice. J Clin Med. 2019;8(9):1387.
25. Peterson KE, Washington J, Rathbun JM. Team management of failure to thrive. Journal of the American Dietetic Association [Internet]. 1984;84(7):810–5. Available from: https://pubmed.ncbi.nlm.nih.gov/6736509/
26. Mehta NM, Compher CASPEN. Clinical guidelines: nutrition support of the critically ill child. J Parenter Enter Nutr. 2009;33(3):260–76.
27. Jaksic T. Effective and efficient nutritional support for the injured child. Surg Clin N Am. 2002;82(2):379–91.

Breastfeeding and the Use of Human Milk

3

Anfal Marafie, Jennifer Hyland,
Audrey Matuska, and Heidi Szugye

Note About Inclusive Language

The authors chose to use the words breastfeeding when referring to a child directly getting human milk from a lactating parent's chest and human milk feeding when referring to the consumption of human milk via other modalities such as a bottle. However, the authors recognize and emphasize the importance of using terminology preferred by the patient (i.e., some parents may prefer the term chest over breast).

A. Marafie
Pediatric Residency Program, Department of Pediatrics, Cleveland Clinic Children's Hospital, Cleveland, OH, USA

J. Hyland · A. Matuska
Pediatric Nutrition Support, Division of Pediatric Gastroenterology, Hepatology, and Nutrition, Cleveland Clinic, Children's Hospital, Cleveland, OH, USA
e-mail: HYLANDJ2@ccf.org; MATUSKA@ccf.org

H. Szugye (✉)
Pediatric Nutrition Support, Division of Pediatric Gastroenterology, Hepatology, and Nutrition, Cleveland Clinic, Children's Hospital, Cleveland, OH, USA

Breastfeeding Medicine Section, Cleveland Clinic Children's Hospital, Cleveland, OH, USA
e-mail: SZUGYEH@ccf.org

K. Radhakrishnan (ed.), *Handbook of Clinical and Practical Pediatric Nutrition*, https://doi.org/10.1007/978-3-031-97759-6_3

Recommendations for Duration of Human Milk Feeding and Benefits

- The Center for Disease Control (CDC), World Health Organization (WHO), and American Academy of Pediatrics (AAP) recommend exclusive breastfeeding for the first 6 months of life and support human milk feeding until 2 years of age and beyond due to its benefits to the child and lactating parent [1–3]:
  - *Benefits to child*: Lower risk of asthma, childhood obesity, type 2 diabetes, Sudden Infant Death Syndrome (SIDS), otitis media, eczema, severe diarrhea/vomiting, respiratory infections, inflammatory bowel disease, and childhood leukemia [3]
  - *Benefits to lactating parent*: Decreased risk of breast, thyroid, and ovarian cancer, type 2 diabetes, and hypertension [3]

Stages of Human Milk Production [4, 5]

	Colostrum	Transitional milk	Mature milk
General Timing postpartum (can vary based on maternal factors)	1–5 days	5 days to 2 weeks	>2 weeks
Contents	Often referred to as "liquid gold" High in immunologic components (antibodies, antioxidants, immunoglobulins) and protein Lower in fat and carbs High sodium content	Often described as "milk coming in" signaling lactogenesis II Slow increase in lactose, fat, and total calories Shift to lower sodium content	Established milk supply Highest water content (90%) and most calorically dense Highest in lactose and fat
Appearance	Thick, clear, gold colored	Lighter yellow, thicker than mature milk	Generally white, thinner although can vary in color

Human Milk Composition

- The average energy composition of human milk is 20 kcal/oz. when calculating energy intake of human milk-fed infants although it can vary based on child's age and from human to human [5].
- Milk differs in content throughout breastfeeding and is referred to as foremilk and hindmilk [6].
  - *Foremilk*: "First milk" obtained by infant when human milk feeding. Higher in water and protein content compared to hindmilk.
  - *Hindmilk*: "Last milk" obtained by infant when human milk feeding. Contains higher fat content than foremilk.
- While oversupply can cause an imbalance of foremilk and hindmilk the infant ingests and this can lead to gastrointestinal upset such as voluminous stools, gas, and spitting up, it is not a cause for poor infant weight gain. Resolution should be aimed at reducing oversupply.
- Breast milk is made up of water, proteins, fats, carbohydrates, vitamins, and minerals (Table 3.1).

Table 3.1 Human milk components [4, 7]

Water	~87–88%
Lipids	~50%; primarily triglycerides making up 99% of fat composition (triacylglycerol, phospholipids, sterols, docosahexaenoic acid "DHA," arachidonic acid)
Carbohydrates	~40%; primarily lactose but also milk oligosaccharides "HMOs"
Proteins	~10%; 60:40 whey:Casein (casein, whey, immunoglobulins, mucins, sialic acid-containing glycoproteins, free amino acids)
Hormones	Thyroid hormones, adipokines (leptin, ghrelin, adiponectin), estrogens, progesterone, calcitonin, somatostatin, adiponectin prolactin, erythropoietin, epidermal growth factor (EGF), prostaglandins, relaxin, bile salts

(continued)

Table 3.1 (continued)

Antimicrobial factors	Lactoferrin, lysozyme, polyamines, nonprotein nitrogen, immunoglobulins (IgG, IgA, IgM), T-cells, lymphocytes, macrophages, VEGF, IGF, cytokines, chemokines
Enzymes	Amylase, lipase, G6PD, lactic acid, malic acid dehydrogenases, lactose synthetase, lysozyme, lactose synthetase, phosphatases, proteases and antiprotease, xanthine oxidase
Minerals	Sodium, potassium, chloride, calcium, magnesium, phosphorus
Trace elements	Iron, zinc, copper, selenium, chromium, manganese, molybdenum, nickel, fluorine, iodine
Vitamins	Human milk contains vitamins A, D, E, K, C, B complex

[a]Micronutrient, vitamin, and mineral content may vary depending on maternal diet and body stores

Important Nutritional Content Considerations

- *Vitamin K*: Vitamin K is not transferred in sufficient quantities from lactating parent to human milk. At birth, infants must be given IM supplementation [8].
- *Vitamin D*: Vitamin D becomes rapidly depleted in infants after birth and all human milk-fed infants require supplementation of 400 IU/day through the first year of life. An alternative strategy to vitamin D supplementation of the infant is to supplement the mother who is human milk feeding with 6400 IU/day of vitamin D. [3]
- *Iron*: Full-term human milk-fed infants do not require iron supplementation. Iron stores in infants begin to deplete at 4–6 months of age. Therefore, it is recommended to include iron-rich or iron-fortified foods when initiating solids. Please see Chap. 10 for specific iron intake recommendations [8].
- *B vitamins*: May be insufficient if the mother's diet is insufficient in these nutrients and can be a cause for failure to thrive in infants (Vitamin B12 deficiency for example) [8].

Recommended Diet By Age [9]

0–1 month	Human milk/formula only 8–12 times/day OR every 1–3 h At day 1 of life, the baby's stomach can hold 1 tsp. at a time, 4–5 tsp. by day 3, 1.5–2.0 oz by 1 week of life, 2.0-3.0 oz by 2–3 weeks of life, and 3.0–4.0 oz by 3–4 weeks of life
1–2 months	Human milk/formula only 8–12 times/day OR every 2–3 h 3–4 oz per feed (volumes and frequency may vary depending on if taken directly via breast vs bottle, human milk vs formula and parental breast storage capacity)
2–4 months	Human milk/formula only 6–12 times/day OR every 2–4 h 3–4 oz per feed
4–6 months	Human milk/formula 6–8 times/day OR every 3–4 h 3–4 oz per feed
6–7 months	Human milk/formula 5–8 times per day (3–4 h) 4 oz per feed Complementary food introduced
7–8 months	Human milk/formula 4–7 times/day 6–8 oz per feed Complementary food
8–12+ months	Human milk/formula 2–5 times per day 7–8 oz per feed Complementary food

Factors Positively Associated with Human Milk Feeding Initiation and Continuation [10]

- Vaginal delivery
- Rooming in
- Skin-to-skin initiation
- Breastfeeding education
- Baby-friendly hospital initiative 10 steps to successful breastfeeding adherence [11]

Safe Storage, Sharing, and Handling of Human Milk [12, 13]

Room temperature	Refrigerator	Freezer
4 h	4 days	6–12 months

- **Freezing:**
  - Freeze in small batches (2–4 ounces)
  - Leave about 1-inch of space at the top as milk will expand when frozen
- **Thawing:**
  - Thaw oldest human milk first
  - Thaw in the refrigerator overnight
  - In warm or lukewarm water
  - Under lukewarm running water
- **Cleaning:**
  - Bottles should be cleaned after every feed
  - All bottle parts should be taken apart
  - All parts should be rinsed under running water, then washed in a basin with soap and water that is used only for infant feeding items
  - Each part should airdry on a clean washcloth (washcloth is preferred to using a dry rack as a dry rack can have areas of mold buildup)
  - The wash basin and brush should be rinsed after each use and allowed to airdry. These items should be washed every 3 days in hot water

Assessment and Treatment of Breastfed or Human Milk-Fed Baby with Poor Weight Gain

When a baby with poor weight gain presents to your clinic, steps to take to protect the human milk feeding experience before initiating formula supplementation include:

1. Poor infant weight gain can be due to inadequate intake of calories, loss of calories, or increased caloric demand that can

include organic and inorganic causes. Please refer to the Chap. 39 on failure to thrive for a full differential to consider. The following recommendations are for full-term infants. For recommendations on treatment of neonates, see Chap. 47.

2. Try to identify if the problem is the lactating parent's milk production, baby's inability to transfer milk, limited offering of human milk (inadequate frequency or volumes), or a combination of the above. To determine this:
   (a) Obtain an accurate and thorough feeding history
   (b) Observe an infant feeding to look for signs of a good latch and transfer
   (c) Conduct a weighted feed to assess transfer of milk
   (d) Measure expressed human milk after infant feeding to assess maternal supply and infant's ability to transfer milk available to them
3. Try to maximize volume through increased frequency of direct feeding on both sides or pumping and/or increased volume offerings via bottles of expressed milk.
4. Work with a lactation consultant or Breastfeeding Medicine early on to assist the lactating parent in increasing milk production and optimize infant transfer of milk.
5. If the infant is unable to gain optimal weight despite maximizing human milk volumes, human milk enrichment should be considered. See below for details on fortification.
6. Lastly, one may recommend additional supplementation with formula if adequate human milk volumes are not available.

Fortification and Human Milk Enrichment

- There are different types of milk fortifiers [9, 14]:
  - *Preterm liquid human milk fortifier*: used in the neonatal intensive care unit to add extra calories for babies born prematurely. Not routinely used for long-term home use
  - *Preterm enriched powdered formula*: used for babies born prematurely who need extra calories
  - *Term infant powdered formula*: used for babies born full term who need extra calories

Table 3.2 Human milk enrichment recipes

20 calorie/ounce human milk	No fortification
22 calorie/ounce human milk	Add 1 teaspoon formula to 150 mL of breast milk (5 ounces)
24 calorie/ounce human milk	Add 1 teaspoon formula to 75 mL of breast milk (2.5 ounces)
27 calorie/ounce human milk	Add 1 teaspoon formula to 45 mL of breast milk (1.5 ounces)
30 calorie/ounce human milk	Add 1 teaspoon formula to 30 mL of breast milk (1 ounce)

[a] Based on 20 kcal/oz United States FDA-approved formula

  - *Hypoallergenic powdered formula*: used for babies with cow's milk protein allergy
  - *Amino acid powdered formula*: used for babies who cannot tolerate intact protein due to malabsorption, severe food allergies or other gastrointestinal problems
- Breast milk can be enriched by adding powdered formula directly to it. The powder dissolves into the breast milk, without adding significant volume. Each teaspoon of formula adds approximately 10.5 calories.*
- When fortifying human milk, it is important to closely follow with the medical team. Incorrect mixing, or inappropriate use, can lead to dehydration and electrolyte imbalances (Table 3.2).

Most Common Reasons for Early Cessation of Human Milk Feeding [15, 16]

- Perceived inadequate milk supply (infant weight gain)
- Latching problems/breast pain/nipple pain
- Concerns about medications and human milk feeding
- Lack of parental leave
- Unsupportive hospital policies
- Include information on disparities, social barriers

Contraindications to Human Milk Feeding [17]

- Maternal factors:
  - T-cell lymphotropic virus type I or type II
  - HIV &:
    Not on Antiretroviral Therapy (ART)
    On ART but viral load remains elevated
  - Suspected or confirmed Ebola virus
  - Illicit drug use (opioids, PCP (phencyclidine) or cocaine)
- Infant factors:
  - Classic galactosemia

Reasons to Temporarily Stop Human Milk Feeding and Not Give Infant Expressed Human Milk [17]

- Active HSV lesions on the breast
- Active brucellosis
- Monkey pox virus infection
- Undergoing certain nuclear medicine imaging (radioactive iodine, technetium 99 m)
- Taking certain medications
- Undergoing chemotherapy/radiation

Reasons to Temporarily Stop Human Milk Feeding But Safe to Feed Infant Expressed Human Milk [17]

- Mothers with untreated, active TB (may be resumed once no longer contagious)
- Mothers with active varicella infection (that developed between 5 days before delivery and 2 days following delivery)

Donor Breastmilk Safety Considerations and Recommendations [18, 19]

- Priority of donor breastmilk should be given to infants <1500 g
- Donor breastmilk must be pasteurized, and donors must be screened
- Obtaining breastmilk from a direct source, internet, or human milk sharing is not recommended due to the risk of bacterial or viral contamination and potential exposure to medications, drugs, or herbs
- Milk banks reduce the risk of exposure to contaminants by pooling milk from many mothers

Resources for Medication Safety in Breastfeeding [20–22]

- LactMed for medications during lactation website
- Infant Risk—hotline and app
- Hale's Medications and Mother's Milk

General Resources for Healthcare Providers [23–27]

- The Little Green Book of Breastfeeding Management for Physicians and Other Healthcare Providers
- AAP: Breastfeeding Practice Tools for Health Professionals
- Academy of Breastfeeding Medicine (ABM) protocols
- WIC breastfeeding support
- IABLE website (https://lacted.org)

References

1. Centers for Disease Control and Prevention. Breastfeeding recommendations and guidance. 2023 Dec. Centers for Disease Control and Prevention [Internet]. [cited 2024 Aug 30]. Available from: https://www.cdc.gov/breastfeeding/php/guidelines-recommendations/index.html.

2. World Health Organization. Infant and young child feeding [Internet]. 2023 Dec. World Health Organization; [cited 2024 Aug 30]. Available from: https://www.who.int/news-room/fact-sheets/detail/infant-and-young-child-feeding.
3. Meek JY, Noble L. Section on Breastfeeding. Policy statement: breastfeeding and the use of human milk. Pediatrics. 2022;150(1) https://doi.org/10.1542/peds.2022-057988.
4. Lawrence RA, Lawrence RB. Biochemistry of human milk. In: Breastfeeding: a guide for the medical professional. 9th ed. St. Louis (MO): Elsevier Inc.; 2022. p. 93–144.
5. Kim SY, Yi DY. Components of human breast milk: from macronutrient to microbiome and microRNA. Clin Exp Pediatr. 2020;63(8):301–9. https://doi.org/10.3345/cep.2020.00059. Epub 2020 Mar 23. PMID: 32252145; PMCID: PMC7402982.
6. Nielsen SD, Beverly RL, Dallas DC. Peptides released from foremilk and hindmilk proteins by breast milk proteases are highly similar. Front Nutr. 2017;(4):54. https://doi.org/10.3389/fnut.2017.00054. PMID: 29164128; PMCID: PMC5673630.
7. Ballard O, Morrow AL. Human Milk composition: nutrients and bioactive factors. Pediatr Clin North Am [Internet]. 2013;60(1):49–74. Available from: https://www.ncbi.nlm.nih.gov/pmc/articles/PMC3586783/.
8. American Dietetic Association. Pediatric Nutrition Care Manual®. Breastfeeding & Lactation Support (2023) Nutrition care manual. https://www.nutritioncaremanual.org/. Accessed 6 Aug 2024.
9. Goday PS, Walia CLS. Chapter 5 infant nutrition. In: Pediatric nutrition for dietitians. Boca Raton: CDR Press; 2022. p. 65–78.
10. Cohen SS, Alexander DD, Krebs NF, Young BE, Cabana MD, Erdmann P, et al. Factors associated Breastfeeding initiation and continuation: a meta-analysis. J Pediatr [Internet]. 2018;203:190–196.e21. Available from: https://doi.org/10.1016/j.jpeds.2018.08.008.
11. Baby-Friendly USA. 10 steps and international code [internet]. Baby-Friendly USA; [cited 2024 Aug 30]. Available from: https://babyfriendlyusa.org/for-facilities/practice-guidelines/10-steps-and-international-code/.
12. Centers for Disease Control and Prevention. Breast Milk Storage and Preparation [Internet]. 2023 Nov. Centers for disease control and prevention; [cited 2024 Aug 30]. Available from: https://www.cdc.gov/breastfeeding/breast-milk-preparation-and-storage/handling-breastmilk.html.
13. Centers for Disease Control and Prevention. How to Clean, Sanitize, and Store Infant Feeding Items Frequently Asked Questions [Internet]. 2024 Centers for disease control and prevention; [cited 2024 Aug 30]. Available from: https://www.cdc.gov/hygiene/faq/index.html.
14. Moreira Denise H, et al. Human milk fortification and use of infant formulas to support growth in the neonatal intensive care unit. Nutr Clin Pract. 2023;38:S56–65.

15. Gatti L. Maternal perceptions of insufficient milk supply in breastfeeding. J Nurs Scholarsh. 2008;40(4):355–63. Sigma Theta Tau Int Honor Soc Nurs.
16. Centers for Disease Control and Prevention. Breastfeeding data [Internet]. 2024. Centers for disease control and prevention; [cited 2024 Aug 30]. Available from: https://www.cdc.gov/breastfeeding/data/facts.html.
17. Centers for Disease Control and Prevention. Contraindications to breastfeeding [Internet]. 2024 Feb. Centers for disease control and prevention; [cited 2024 Aug 30]. Available from: https://www.cdc.gov/breastfeeding-special-circumstances/hcp/contraindications/index.html.
18. Abrams SA, Landers S, Noble LM, Poindexter BB. Donor human milk for the high-risk infant: preparation, safety, and usage options in the United States. Pediatrics [Internet]. 2017;139(1):e20163440. Available from: https://doi.org/10.1542/peds.2016-3440.
19. U.S. Food and Drug Administration. Use of donor human milk [Internet]. 2018 Mar. U.S. Food and Drug Administration; [cited 2024 Aug 30]. Available from: https://www.fda.gov/science-research/pediatrics/use-donor-human-milk.
20. Drugs and lactation database (LactMed) [Internet]. PubMed. National Library of Medicine (US); 2006. Available from: https://www.ncbi.nlm.nih.gov/books/NBK501922/.
21. InfantRisk Center [Internet]. infantrisk.com. Available from: https://infantrisk.com/.
22. Hale's Medications & Mothers' Milk [Internet]. www.halesmeds.com. Available from: https://www.halesmeds.com/.
23. Eglash A, Leeper K. The little green book of breastfeeding management for physicians and other healthcare providers. 2020.
24. Breastfeeding practice tools for health professionals [internet]. Aaporg 2024 [cited 2024 Aug 30]. Available from: https://www.aap.org/en/patient-care/breastfeeding/breastfeeding-practice-tools-for-health-professionals/?srsltid=AfmBOorShSNJRfh6cXhlOM7kNx2WjlGmwXUWxWZh02hj8a84YQ3YLOaR.
25. Johnson B. PROTOCOLS [Internet]. Bfmed.org. 2019. Available from: https://www.bfmed.org/protocols.
26. Homepage | WIC Breastfeeding [Internet]. Usdagov 2000. Available from: https://wicbreastfeeding.fns.usda.gov/.
27. Home – The Institute for Breastfeeding and Lactation Education (IABLE) [Internet]. The Institute for Breastfeeding and Lactation Education (IABLE). 2018 [cited 2024 Aug 30]. Available from: https://lacted.org/.

4 Formulas Including Special Formulas

Margherita Shook

How to Choose Baby Formula

The FDA approves certain infant formulas to ensure these products have at least 30 different nutrients to meet the infant/child's needs. Based on the infant/child's needs, there are many different categories of formula to choose from. All formulas contain a carbohydrate, protein, and fat source to make the product complete, as infant formulas are the primary source of nutrition (Fuchs and Abrams [2]) (Table 4.1).

Disclaimer: *This information is purely for clinical use and does not favor any certain formula company. The American Academy of Pediatrics (AAP) recommends exclusive breastfeeding for approximately 6 months followed by continued breastfeeding with complementary foods for at least 2 years as desired and able. Human milk is the best source of nutrition for infants, though when not available, iron fortified formula is an appropriate alternative.*

M. Shook (✉)
Pediatric Nutrition Support, Division of Pediatric Gastroenterology, Hepatology, and Nutrition, Cleveland Clinic Children's Hospital, Cleveland, OH, USA
e-mail: SHOOKM2@ccf.org

K. Radhakrishnan (ed.), *Handbook of Clinical and Practical Pediatric Nutrition*, https://doi.org/10.1007/978-3-031-97759-6_4

Table 4.1 Types of infant formula

Preterm Infant Formula: contain increased amounts of specific macro and micro nutrients to meet the needs of rapidly growing premature infants (higher calcium and phosphorus, along with increased calorie per ounce concentrations). Premature formulas may also have high protein option to meet the needs of rapidly growing infants. Conversation with medical team advised when discussing and choosing the appropriate preterm formula for infant. Also note that patients should be transitioned to standard infant formula depending on prematurity and weight status, given increased nutrient amounts	Indications for use: Premature birth Low birth weight	Examples: Enfamil NeuroPro Enfacare Enfamil Premature Similac Neosure Enfamil Premature Similac Special Care
Human Milk fortifier: Mixed at a standard dilution of 5 mL fortifier +25 mL human milk	Indications for use: Premature infants who are taking breast milk	Examples: Enfamil and Similac human Milk fortifiers available
Cow's Milk-based formula (most common formula used): Milk-based formula made with lactose as the main source of carbohydrate and casein as the primary protein source	Indications for use: Full term (>37 weeks), healthy infants Hospitalized infants with no nutrient/tolerance concerns Breast-fed infants when supplementation is needed	Examples: Enfamil NeuroPro infant Similac 360 Total care Gerber good start gentle pro Parent's choice infant

Low lactose formula: Lactose reduced or lactose free in the form of cornstarch, tapioca dextrin, or tapioca starch	Indications for use: Mild GI symptoms such as flatulence, discomfort, diarrhea, and abdominal bloating Benefits shown for use in neonatal abstinence syndrome	Examples: Enfamil Gentlease Similac sensitive Gerber good start soothe pro
Extensively hydrolyzed formula: "Hypoallergenic" formulas containing MCT oil to aid in digestion. Lactose-free, containing free amino acids and peptides	Indications for use: Intact cow's milk protein allergy Soy allergy Feeding intolerance Severe GERD Malabsorption concerns	Examples: Similac Alimentum Similac Pregestimil Nutramigen Gerber good start extensive HA
Elemental formula: "Hypoallergenic" formulas, also containing MCT oil to aid in digestion. Lactose-free containing free amino acids	Indications for use: Severe malabsorption concerns and intolerance to intact protein and protein hydrolysates Infants with GI disorders (SBS, EOE) Multiple food allergy concerns	Examples: Elecare infant Neocate infant Puramino Alfamino infant
Soy formula: Lactose-free containing soy protein and either glucose or sucrose	Indications for use: Inability to digest lactose Galactosemia Vegetarian/vegan families	Examples: Enfamil ProSobee Similac soy Isomil Gerber good start gentle soy

(continued)

Table 4.1 (continued)

Anti-reflux formula: Contains added rice starch	Indications for use: Excessive spit ups GERD	Examples: Enfamil AR Similac for spit up
High MCT oil formula: Important to watch for essential fatty acid deficiency when formula is used for extended period of time	Indications for use: Infants with chylothorax or LCHAD deficiency	Examples: Enfaport
Renal formula: Additional iron may be needed from other sources given low amount in formula (low mineral formula)	Indications for use: Infants with impaired renal function or who would benefit from lowered mineral intake	Examples: Similac PM 60/40
Organic Formula	Indications for use: Preference for organic, GMO-free formula	Examples: Bobbie Burt's bees baby organic Bub's organic infant formula
High calorie formula: 1 kcal/mL OR 30 kcal/oz.; used for infants 0–18 months. Available as RTF product	Indications for use: For patients who are at risk for growth failure Increased energy needs Fluid restriction needs	Examples: Fortini

[a]*Disclaimer: Examples of formula are strictly examples, and not limited to the below. We do not favor one formula brand over another. Formula options may differ outside of the United States of America*

Transitioning Off of Infant Formula

Most infants are able to transition to whole cow's milk or a milk alternative at 12 months of age. Some children may warrant the need to transition to pediatric formula if solid food intake is not appropriate for age. Other indications for use may include patient's requiring enteral nutrition, infants who were on special infant formulas that require transition to the pediatric counterpart, and any acutely ill patient in a hospital setting that requires increased calorie and protein needs [3].

Milk and Milk Alternatives

- *Whole cow's milk*: Comprised of lactose, butter fat, and cow's milk (casein and whey).
- *Almond milk*: Almonds used as the source for carbohydrates, protein, and fat. Poor source of protein, calcium, and vitamin D when unfortified.
- *Coconut milk*: Coconut used as the source for carbohydrates, protein, and fat. Poor source of protein, calcium, and vitamin D when unfortified. May cause diarrhea due to high fat content.
- *Goat's milk*: Comprised of lactose, butter fat, and goat's milk. Clinical recommendation to purchase in pasteurized form.
- *Hemp milk*: Hemp seed used as the source for carbohydrates, protein, and fat. Poor source of protein, calcium, and vitamin D when unfortified.
- *Oat milk*: Comprised of oats and sunflower. Poor source of protein, calcium, and vitamin D when unfortified.
- *Soy milk*: Soybean and soybean oil used as the source for carbohydrates, protein, and fat. Poor source of calcium unless fortified. Typically recommended for infants with a lactose allergy given appropriate protein content, comparable to whole cow's milk [1] (Table 4.2).

Table 4.2 Types of pediatric formula

Standard Formula: made with intact proteins	Indications for use: Hospitalized infants with no nutrient/ tolerance concerns Slowed growth and/or delayed solid food intake	Examples: Pediasure Grow and Gain Pediasure 1.0 and 1.5 Nutren Junior Boost Kids Essentials
Extensively hydrolyzed formula: "Hypoallergenic" and lactose free, containing free amino acids and peptides	Indications for use: Intact cow's milk protein allergy Soy allergy Feeding intolerance Severe GERD Malabsorption concerns	Examples: Pediasure peptide Peptamen Jr Kate farms pediatric peptide
Elemental formula: "Hypoallergenic" and lactose free containing free amino acids	Indications for use: Severe malabsorption concerns and intolerance to intact protein and protein hydrolysates Infants with GI disorders (SBS, EOE) Multiple food allergy concerns	Examples: Elecare junior Neocate junior Neocate splash Alfamino junior
High MCT oil Formula	Indications for use: Pancreatitis	Examples: Vivonex pediatric.
Real food products	Indications for use: Used to add real food ingredients for tube fed patients	Examples: Nourish Pediasure harvest Kate farms blends Real food blends Compleat pediatric organic blends

[a]*Disclaimer: Examples of formula are strictly examples, and not limited to the below. We do not favor one formula brand over another. Formula options may differ outside of the United States of America*

Specialty Formulas

Some disease states and disorders require specific formulas that are formulated to aid in growth and digestion. Table 4.3 references common metabolic formulas used and indications [1] (Table 4.3).

Table 4.3 Types of specialty formula

Formula name	Indication for use
RCF, Abbott	Formula low in carbohydrate for those who are unable to tolerate carbohydrate amounts in standard formulas. RCF can also be used for patients who are requiring ketosis. This formula should not be used without an added carbohydrate source
KetoCal, Nutricia (comes in multiple ratios)	Formula used with a specific ratio for fat: Carbohydrate + protein for achievement of ketosis. These products are designed for children 1 year and older
PKU Periflex early years, Nutricia Phenyl free 2 powder, Mead Johnson Gylactin Bettermilk, Cambrooke therapeutics	Phenylketonuria (PKU)
BCAD 2, Mead Johnson MSUD Maxamum, Nutricia MSUD Anamix early years, Nutricia	Maple syrup urine disease (MSUD)
Essential amino acid supplement, Vitaflo (a blend of essential amino acids, carbohydrate, vitamins and minerals, for use where essential amino acids are required) Cyclinex-1, Abbott (nonessential amino acid-free to decrease the ingestion of waste nitrogen)	Urea cycle disorder (UCD)
Monogen, Nutricia (low in fat and high in medium chain triglycerides (MCT)) Liquigen, Nutricia (emulsified MCT oil)	Long-chain fatty acid disorders

[a]*Disclaimer: Examples of formula are strictly examples, and not limited to the below. We do not favor one formula brand over another. Formula options may differ outside of the United States of America*

References

1. Delgado NB, et al., editors. Pediatric Nutrition reference guide. 13th ed. Texas Children's Hospital; 2022.
2. Fuchs III, GJ, Abrams SA. Choosing a baby formula. n.d.. https://www.healthychildren.org/English/ages-stages/baby/formula-feeding/Pages/Choosing-an-Infant-Formula.aspx?ref=popsugar.com
3. Infant Nutrition and feeding – WIC works – USDA. 2019. https://wicworks.fns.usda.gov/sites/default/files/media/document/infant-feeding-guide.pdf

Enteral Nutrition Support

5

Sara Bewley, Christine Bowen,
Elizabeth Robinson,
and Senthilkumar Sankararaman

Enteral nutrition support should be considered when there is an inability to feed adequate nutrients by mouth.

- Enteral nutrition support should be initiated with the critically ill child within 48 h if medically feasible [1, 2].
- Evidence notes that enteral nutrition support is associated with reduction in length of hospital stay and decreased mortality.
- There are a few contraindications to enteral nutrition support such as hemodynamic instability, gastrointestinal (GI) bleeding, intestinal blockage, severe mucositis, and inability to safely place a tube [3–5]. For those children, parenteral nutrition support should be considered.
- The conversation with the families should include why enteral nutrition support is the gold standard over parenteral nutrition.
- Enteral nutrition support is preferred over parenteral nutrition for a variety of reasons including decreased cost, less risk of infections, preserves gut function, decreases liver insult, and reduces of the risk of hyperglycemia [2–5].

S. Bewley · C. Bowen · E. Robinson · S. Sankararaman (✉)
Division of Pediatric Gastroenterology, Hepatology and Nutrition, Cleveland Clinic Children's Hospital, Cleveland, OH, USA
e-mail: BEWLEYS@ccf.org; BOWENC@ccf.org; ROBINSE10@ccf.org; SANKARS6@ccf.org

K. Radhakrishnan (ed.), *Handbook of Clinical and Practical Pediatric Nutrition*, https://doi.org/10.1007/978-3-031-97759-6_5

Prior to discussion with the family, the medical provider should discuss what type of tube would be most appropriate for placement. Factors to consider would include medical diagnosis, anatomy of the patient, age, and intended length of use [3–5].

Considerations for Placement of a Feeding Tube

- Long term vs short term
  - Short term: <3 months
    - Failure to thrive
    - Respiratory distress/failure
    - Acute illness
    - Prematurity
  - Long term:
    - Failed swallow study—difficulty coordinating swallow or concern for aspiration
    - Ongoing failure to thrive with inability to wean off nasogastric (NG) tube
    - Global developmental delay and other neuromuscular disease
    - Chronic catabolic illnesses with inability to maintain optimal growth goals
- *Anatomy*: Most tubes are placed via nasal passage to either the stomach or into the small intestines. Post-pyloric feeds are sometimes required to help with feeding tolerance. The details of other tubes are discussed below.
- *Bridle considerations*: This is used to help prevent accidental removal/pulling of a NG/ND/NJ tubes. The tube is secured with tubing around septum.
  - Typically used for children age 2 and older.
  - Those who are at risk for self-pulling due to young age, developmental delay, and limited cognitive function.

Types of Enteral Tubes

- OG (orogastric) tube—inserted through the mouth into the stomach. Typically used for neonates <34 weeks gestational age
- NG (nasogastric) tube—inserted through the nose into the stomach (Fig. 5.1)
- ND (nasoduodenal) tube—inserted through the nose into the duodenum (Fig. 5.2)
  - Indicated when there is intolerance of gastric feedings
  - Generally will need feeds to be administered continuously
  - Potential for easy displacement into stomach
- NJ (nasojejunal) tube inserted through the nose into the jejunum
  - Indicated when there is intolerance of gastric feedings and frequent emesis. Less chances for gastric displacement when compared to ND tube.
  - Must be continuous feeds
- Gastrostomy tube or gastric tube (GT)—surgically or interventional (endoscopic) placement into the stomach (Fig. 5.3)
- Gastrojejunostomy or gastrojejunal tube (GJT)—surgically placed into the stomach with an extension that is fed into the jejunum (Fig. 5.4)
  - This tube is larger than standard tubes as it has two ports for gastric and jejunal access
- Jejunostomy or jejunal tube (JT)—surgically placed into the jejunum

Tube placements:

- Manually/bedside—for NG and possibly ND tubes
- Endoscopically—for ND/NJ tubes, G tube, and GJT
- Surgically—GT, GJT, and JT.
  - By interventional radiology using fluoroscopy—ND and NJ tubes, and replacement of GJT

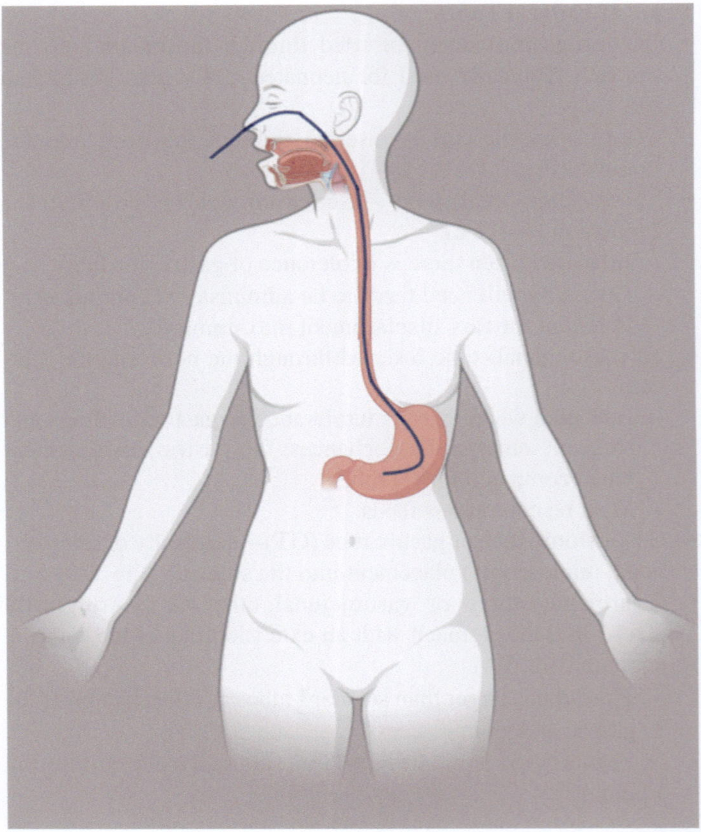

Fig. 5.1 NG tube

Verifying placement:

- Placement verification varies from institution to institution
- Can check pH if placed in the stomach
- X-ray to confirm position may be used (gold standard method of verification)

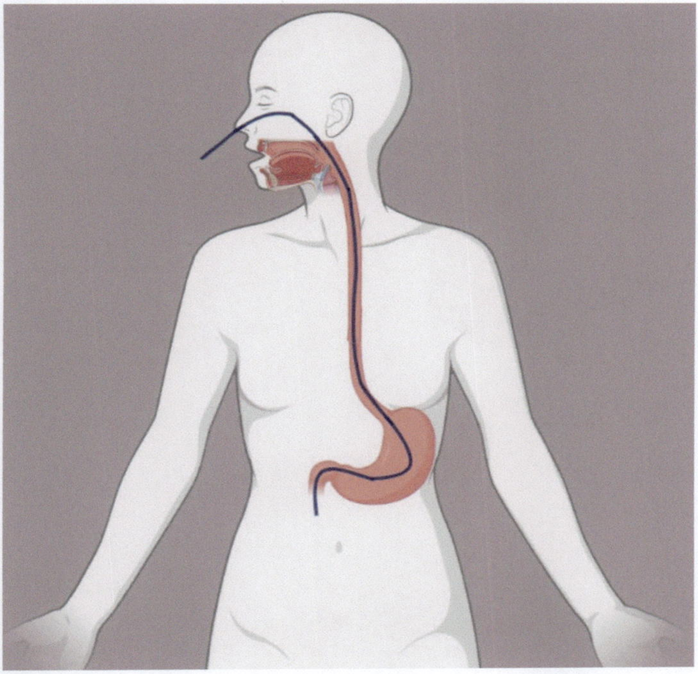

Fig. 5.2 ND/NJ tube

- Auscultation of the gastric area with administration of air boluses is less reliable
- Specialized equipment with tracking devises—particularly for ND/NJ tubes
- Enlisting input from radiology for injecting contrast to confirm placement may be needed, particularly when replacing GJT and JT

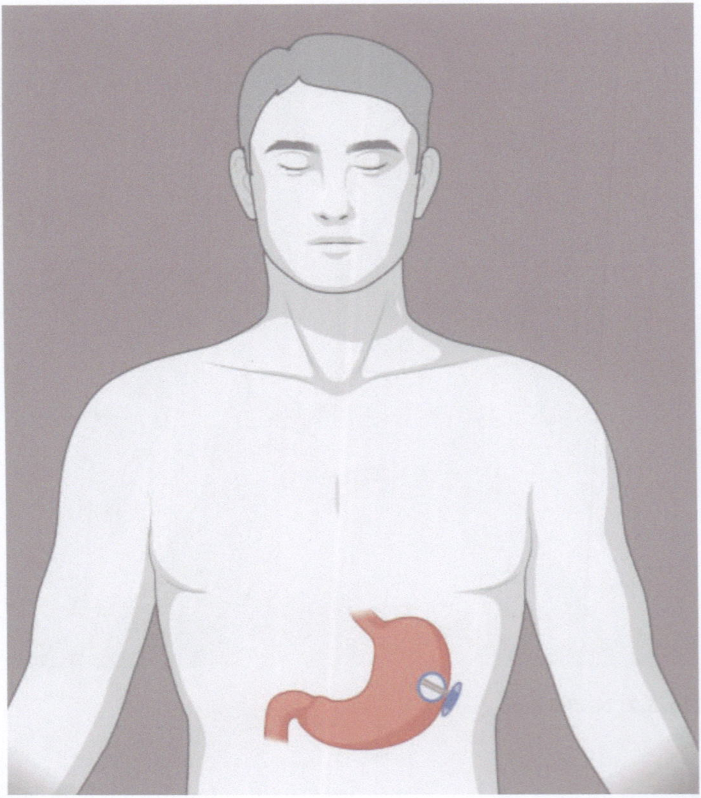

Fig. 5.3 G tube (gastric tube)

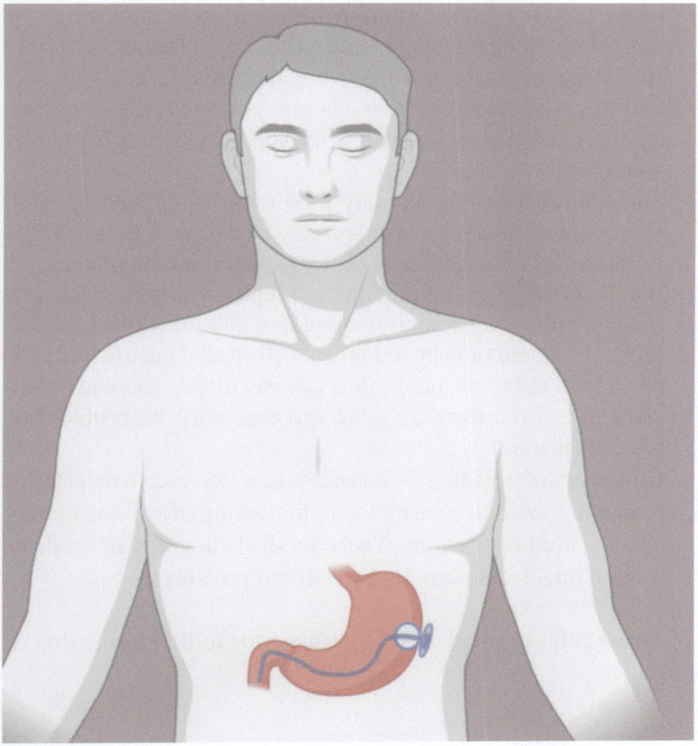

Fig. 5.4 Gastrojejunal tube

Formula Selection Considerations

Enteral products are commonly selected with considerations of the disease state, type of enteral tube, placement, and parent/guardian preferences. The caregiver may have strong preferences of type and source of formula, ingredient list of products, and cost associated with formula.

- Intact protein—most commonly used in gastric feedings for those with intact intestinal tracts. These are often more readily available and most cost-effective to the patient.
- Partially hydrolyzed protein—commonly used in post-pyloric feedings and those with feeding intolerances such as irritability and reflux.
- Free amino acids—commonly used with severe feeding intolerances, intestinal resections/surgery, and food allergies. These formulas are often the most costly products on the market.
- Blended feedings—commercially prepared or homemade real food blends are becoming more popular to request. These products should only be fed into a well-healed gastric tube. NG tubes tend to be too small, thus causing clogs. There are some concerns, for insurance, coverage that may be problematic once discharged.
- Concentrated feedings—consideration to use concentrated feedings should be considered in the setting of volume intolerance or fluid restrictions. These products are readily available in both intact and partially hydrolyzed proteins.

Please refer to Chap. 4 (on formulas) for further discussion on formula.

Formula Delivery Techniques

Feeding schedules should be reviewed and discussed with the multidisciplinary team as well as the caregiver. Considerations that should be discussed should include therapy services, nursing care, and medication administration. If the patient is going home with the enteral tube, the caregiver should be part of the long-term feeding plan to help increase compliance with considerations of the caregivers schedule.

- Bolus feedings—can be used with OG tube, NG tube, GT, and gastric portion of the GJT. Bolus feedings are contraindicated with any post-pyloric feedings. A rough guide for volume of initiation, advancement, and goal for bolus feed is noted in Table 5.1.

Table 5.1 Bolus feeds

Weight	Initiation	Advancement	Goal
2–15 kg	5–75 mL every 3–4 h	5–30 mL per feed every 3–12 h	50–200 mL every 3–4 h
16–30 kg	15–60 mL every 4 h	15–60 mL per feed every 4–12 h	150–350 mL every 4 h
>30 kg	30–60 mL every 4 h	30–60 mL per feed every 4–12 h	240–360 mL every 4 h

Table 5.2 Continuous feeds

Weight	Initiation	Advancement	Goal
2–15 kg	1–15 mL/h (0.5–1 mL/kg/h)	1–15 mL every 4–8 h (0.5–1 mL/kg/h)	15–55 mL/h
16–30 kg	8–30 mL/h (0.5–1 mL/kg/h)	8–15 mL every 4–8 h (0.5–1 mL/kg/h)	45–90 mL/h
30–50 kg	15–25 mL/h (0.5 mL/kg/h)	15–25 mL every 4–8 h (0.5–1 mL/kg/h)	70–130 mL/h
>50 kg	25 mL/h	10–25 mL every 4–8 h	90–125 mL/h

[a]The above tables are typical hospital-setting guidelines for the initiation and advancement of enteral nutrition support in pediatric patients [6]

- Intermittent feedings—volumes similar to bolus feeds are utilized using a pump for shorter duration. Typically run <24 h a day to allow time off the pump, therapies, encouragement of oral intake when applicable, and respiratory support such as BiPAP.
- Continuous feedings—most commonly used with the critically ill patient during initiation and advancement, those with volume intolerances. A rough guide for volume of initiation, advancement, and goal for continuous feed is noted in Table 5.2.

Initiation and Progression of Feeds

Long-Term Complications

- Granulation tissues—seen with gastrostomy tubes, when tissue forms around the feeding tube; often caused by pressure, moisture, and movement. Granulation tissue can be treated with topical steroid creams or with cauterization with silver nitrate [7].

- Oral feeding aversion
- Aspiration
- Dislodgement
- Track closure—occurs with GT and JT, if tubes are displaced or dislodged (as little as eight hours).
- Tube occlusion—more common in the small bore enteral tube and G-J tubes. Most common causes are crushed medications, inadequate flushing, and too thick of formula. When at all possible medications should be given a liquid elixirs, rather than crushed tablets.
  - Attempt to remove clog with warm flush
  - Clog Zapper a commercial product with acids, buffers, antimicrobial agents, and metal inhibitors
  - Pancreatic enzymes can used as well
- Leakage around site.
  - Skin breakdown from exposure to gastric/intestinal contents
- Risk of infection and cellulitis at G tube and J tube sites, as well as candida infection

EN Considerations/Monitoring

- Hypermetabolism: Often children have high energy needs at diagnosis of a new chronic medical condition. It is important to monitor weight trends closely and reestimate needs and enteral goals. It is important to monitor the intake of vitamins, minerals, and protein to prevent excessive intake.
- Hypometabolism: Assessment of vitamins, mineral, and protein intake from enteral feedings is imperative in the child with hypometabolism to ensure optimal growth.
- Refeeding syndrome:
  - Patients with rapid weight loss, ongoing poor weight gain, and malnutrition are at the greatest risk. Slow advancement

with close monitoring of electrolytes help decrease the risk [8, 9].

– Provide thiamin before starting nutrition support: 2 mg/kg/dose once daily up to a usual daily dose range of 100–200 mg/day; maximum reported daily dose: 300 mg/day; continue for 5–7 days; longer supplementation may be required in patients with severe starvation, other high risk for deficiency, and/or signs of thiamine deficiency [8, 9].
– Patients may also need phosphate supplementation.

Transitioning to Oral Feeds

If patient is started on oral feeds and expected to advance, calorie intake from enteral feeds can be decreased gradually to induce hunger and promote oral intake [10]. Recommend decreasing feeds 10–25% depending on patient's overall nutrition status (Table 5.3).

As oral intake progresses, enteral feeds should be gradually decreased to prevent overfeeding and wean from enteral nutrition.

Enteral feeds should not be discontinued until patient's oral intake is meeting 75% or greater of calorie and fluid needs for at least 48 h.

Table 5.3 Rought guide to wean enteral nutrition based on increase in oral feeding

No malnutrition	Mild/moderate malnutrition	Severe malnutrition
Can decrease EN by 20–25%	Recommend decrease EN 10–15%	Discuss with medical team—Typically maintain EN at 100% needs until appropriate weight gain trend is established

References

1. Musheng L, Lini C. Application of early enteral nutrition in critically ill children. Open J Pediatr [Internet]. 2021;11(04):543–50. Available from: https://doi.org/10.4236/ojped.2021.114050.
2. Nutrition Care Manual [Internet]. Nutritioncaremanual.org. [cited 2024 Aug 29]. Available from: https://www.nutritioncaremanual.org/topic.cfm?ncm_category_id=13&lv1=145089&lv2=145297&lv3=255500&ncm_toc_id=273800&ncm_heading=Nutrition%20Care%20home%20page.
3. Adeyinka A. Enteric feedings [Internet]. U.S. National Library of Medicine; 2022 [cited 2024 Aug 28]. Available from: https://www.ncbi.nlm.nih.gov/books/NBK532876/
4. Bechtold ML, Brown PM, Escuro A, Grenda B, Johnston T, Kozeniecki M, et al. When is enteral nutrition indicated? J Parenter Enter Nutr. 2022;46(7):1470–96. https://doi.org/10.1002/jpen.2364.
5. Boullata JI, Carrera AL, Harvey L, Escuro AA, Hudson L, Mays A, et al. ASPEN safe practices for enteral nutrition therapy. JPEN J Parenter Enteral Nutr [Internet]. 2017;41(1):15–103. Available from: https://doi.org/10.1177/0148607116673053.
6. Abad-Jorge A, Morris C, Perks P, Roman B. University of Virginia Children's Hospital Pediatric Nutrition Support Handbook. May 2010.
7. Philadelphia TCH of. Gastrostomy tubes (G-tube) [Internet] www-chopedu 2014. Available from: https://www.chop.edu/treatments/gastrostomy-tubes
8. Afzal NA, Addai S, et al. Refeeding syndrome with enteral nutrition in children: a case report, literature review and clinical guidelines. Clin Nutr. 2002;21(6):515–20.
9. da Silva JSV, Seres DS, Sabino K, Adams SC, Berdahl GJ, Citty SW, et al. ASPEN consensus recommendations for refeeding syndrome. Nutrition Clin Pract [Internet]. 2020;35(2):178–95. Available from: https://aspenjournals.onlinelibrary.wiley.com/doi/10.1002/ncp.10474.
10. Wright CM, Smith KH, Morrison J. Withdrawing feeds from children on long term enteral feeding: factors associated with success and failure. Arch Dis Child. 2011;96(5):433–9. https://doi.org/10.1136/adc.2009.179861. Epub 2010 Jul 23.

Parenteral Nutrition

6

Andrea Adler and Christina DeTallo

Introduction

Parenteral nutrition (PN) is an intravenous therapy comprised of macronutrients, electrolytes, vitamins, minerals, fluid, and additives [1]. It is delivered as a dextrose, amino acid, fluid, and electrolyte containing medication and is commonly referred as a 2-in-1 solution where lipids are administered separately. Another option is a total nutrient admixture where the solution is compounded with all nutrients combined. This solution is not typically recommended for neonatal and pediatric populations due to stability and compatibility concerns [2]. There are risks associated with PN prescribing that warrant trained clinician oversight to ensure appropriateness with initiation, advancement, monitoring, and weaning. Another clinician requirement is full understanding of the various growth and developmental needs of pediatric patients, including considerations for the premature, neonatal, and infant, as well as the disease state and clinical status across age ranges.

A. Adler (✉) · C. DeTallo
Pediatric Nutrition Support, Division of Pediatric Gastroenterology, Hepatology, and Nutrition, Cleveland Clinic Children's Hospital, Cleveland, OH, USA
e-mail: ADLERA@ccf.org; DETALLC@ccf.org

K. Radhakrishnan (ed.), *Handbook of Clinical and Practical Pediatric Nutrition*, https://doi.org/10.1007/978-3-031-97759-6_6

Routes of Administration

PN can be provided via peripheral or central lines [1, 3]

- Peripheral
  - Tip is in a small vein or not in the distal portion of the superior vena cava or at the junction of the superior vena cava and right atrium
  - Maximum osmolarity is 900 mOsm/L
  - Dextrose concentration limited to a maximum of 12.5%
- Central
  - Tip is in the distal portion of the superior vena cava or at the junction of the superior vena cava and the right atrium
  - No maximum osmolarity
  - Dextrose concentration is greater, up to 25% or higher
- Line types
  - Non-tunneled—used for short-term needs (up to 2 weeks)
  - PICC (peripherally inserted central catheters)
    - The tip of the catheter may be in a peripheral or central location
    - Caution with tip in a central location as it can become peripheral at any time
  - Tunneled—used for long-term needs and have lower infection rates
    - Broviac
    - Hickman
  - Port—central access but used for intermittent access and not intended for PN usage daily

Pediatric PN Indications

- Indications for PN vary and include acute clinical impact (short-term) to long-term clinical scenarios. These include prematurity, gastrointestinal issues, critical illness, extracorporeal membrane oxygenation (ECMO), graft-vs-host disease (GVHD), and organ failure.

- Medical diagnosis or disease state alone should not dictate PN therapy initiation.
- Malnutrition, organ failure, cancer, gastrointestinal anomalies, and critical illness could lead to the need for PN administration [4].
- Timing for PN therapy is dependent on overall nutritional status, nutrient requirements, and short- and long-term clinical consequences.
- When there is straightforward evidence for delayed enteral nutrition support, PN should be initiated within 1–3 days for infants and 4–5 days in children and adolescents [4].
- While early initiation of PN is advised for neonates, benefit has been demonstrated for delaying PN for 7 days in critically ill children in the intensive care unit (ICU).
- The delayed benefits may include improved infection rates, reduced time for mechanical ventilation, lower need for renal replacement therapy, and shorter length of stay, when compared with children who receive PN within 24-h of ICU admission [5, 6].

Considerations When Calculating PN Needs

- Nutritional needs vary across the age spectrum with increased demands per kilogram (kg) identified for those preterm and infants compared to pediatric and adolescents [7].
- Indirect calorimetry is the gold standard for calorie measurement in critically ill children; however, often not available.
- Predictive equations are used for calculating estimated calorie needs [8] and include Food and Agriculture Organization, World Health Organization, Schofield, and Institute of Medicine [9]. Please refer to Chap. 2 for equations.
- When estimating nutritional needs, clinicians further adjust for the losses with digestion, absorption, and synthesis associated with diet-induced thermogenesis. This accounts for about 10% of daily calorie needs [10].

PN Nutrient Composition

- PN is comprised of dextrose as the carbohydrate source, crystalline amino acids as the protein source, and various intravenous lipid emulsions (ILE) as the fat source.
- Dextrose provides 3.4 calories/g [1, 11].
- Crystalline amino acids provide 4 calories/g [1, 11]. Pediatric and adult protein solutions are commercially available. Pediatric solutions have lower pH levels to improve solubility and contain higher amounts of histidine and tyrosine and lower amounts of phenylalanine, methionine, and glycine in addition to glutamic and aspartic acid, taurine, and N-acetyl-L-tyrosine to mimic breast milk. These are routinely prescribed for individuals up to 1 year of age [1, 11].
- Intravenous lipid (ILE) calories vary depending on the percentage as 10%, 20%, or 30% compositions are available. 10% Intralipid ILE provides 1.1 calorie/mL (or 11 calories/g), 20% provides 2 calories/mL (or 10 calories/g), and 30% provides 3 calories/mL (or 10 calories/g) [1, 11]. ILE approved by the United States Food and Drug Administration (USFDA) for intravenous use include the oldest, soybean oil 20% [12], a multicomponent 20% ILE containing fish oil 10% ILE, soybean/olive oil 20% ILE have been approved by the USFDA [12, 13]. See Table 6.1 for dosing guidelines for dextrose, amino acid, and ILE. Table 6.2 lists the components of the USFDA approved ILE.

Table 6.1 Recommendations for dextrose, protein, and intravenous lipid emulsions [14]

Patient age	Initiation	Advancement	Goal
Recommended dextrose intake (mg/kg/min)			
Term infants <1 year	6–8	1–2	10–14 (maximum 14–18)
Children 1–10 years	3–6	1–2	8–10
Adolescents	2.5–3	1–2	5–6
Recommended protein intake (g/kg)			
Term infants <1 year	2.5–3	NA	2.5–3
Children 1–10 years	1.5–2.5	NA	1.5–2.5
Adolescents	0.8–2	NA	0.8–2
Recommended fat intake (g/kg)[a]			
Term infants <1 year	0.5–1	0.5–1	2.5–3
Children 1–10 years	1–2	0.5–1	2–2.5
Adolescents	1	1	1–2

[a]Based on 100% soybean oil emulsion

Table 6.2 Available pediatric intravenous lipid emulsions in the United States [13, 15–18]

Component	Soybean oil	Fish oil	Four-component oil	Soybean/olive oil
Soybean oil	100%	–	30%	20%
MCT oil	–	–	30%	NA
Olive oil	–	–	25%	80%
Fish oil	–	100%	15%	NA
Glycerol (g)	2.25	2.5	2.5	2.25
Egg phospholipid (g)	1.2	1.2	1.2	1.2
Calorie contribution	2 kcal/mL	1.1 kcal/mL	2 kcal/mL	2 kcal/mL
Dosing guidelines				
Birth to 1 year 1–10 years 11–17 years	2.5–3 g/kg 2.5 g/kg 2–2.5 g/kg	1 g/kg 1 g/kg 1 g/kg	3 g/kg 2.5–3 g/kg 2–2.5 g/kg	3 g/kg 3 g/kg 2.5 g/kg

MCT Medium chain triglycerides

Micronutrients

Electrolytes

- The American Society for Parenteral and Enteral Nutrition (ASPEN) has generalized recommendations on electrolyte dosages in PN. These guidelines are listed in Table 6.3.
- Clinical judgement should be used to adjust dosing based on patient's serum levels and medical diagnosis and status, along with knowledge of the medications the patient is receiving as some may be electrolyte wasting.

Vitamins

- Multivitamins (MVI) are added to the PN as a pediatric MVI for infants up to the age of 11 years and adult MVI for those over 11 years of age [1]. Dosing for the pediatric MVI is 2 mL/kg maximum 5 mL/day, while dosing for the adult MVI is 10 mL/day.
- Table 6.4 lists the vitamins provided in the pediatric and adult MVI product, noting that there is iron in the United States available products.

Trace Elements

- Trace elements, either as a multi-trace element product, or individually dosed, should be added to PN to prevent deficiencies. Adjustments should be made for clinical status.
- Patients with excessive stool output may require more zinc [21], while those with renal failure should have chromium removed [22].
- Additionally, trace element dosing should be adjusted based on the serum laboratory values, such as copper status should be assessed prior to decreasing the dosing if there is liver dysfunction [23].
- Manganese (Mn) is a known contaminant and for those requiring long-term PN support, it may be beneficial to remove Mn from the PN [24].

Table 6.3 Standard pediatric electrolyte doses [14]

Patient age	Sodium	Potassium	Calcium	Phosphorous	Magnesium	Chloride/acetate
Infants/children	2–5 mEq/kg	2–4 mEq/kg	0.5–4 mEq/kg	0.5–2 mmol/kg	0.3–0.5 mEq/kg	As needed to maintain acid–base balance
Adolescents and children >50 kg	1–2 mEq/kg	1–2 mEq/kg	10–20 mEq/day	10–40 mmol/day	10–30 mEq/day	As needed to maintain acid–base balance

mEq Milliequivalent, *mmol* millimole

Table 6.4 US commercially available multivitamin infusion (MVI) products [19, 20]

Vitamin	Adult MVI per 10 mL	Pediatric MVI per 5 mL
Vitamin A	3300 IU	2300 IU
Vitamin D	200 IU	400 IU
Vitamin E	10 IU	7 IU
Vitamin K 1 (phytonadione)	150 mcg	200 mcg
Vitamin C (ascorbic acid)	200 mg	80 mg
Vitamin B1 (thiamine)	6 mg	1.2 mg
Vitamin B2 (riboflavin)	3.6 mg	1.4 mg
Niacinamide	40 mg	17 mg
Folic acid	600 mcg	140 mcg
Vitamin B12 (cyanocobalamin)	5 mcg	1 mcg
Vitamin B6 (pyridoxine)	6 mg	1 mg
Biotin	60 mcg	20 mcg
Dexpanthenol	15 mg	5 mg

IU International Units, *mcg* micrograms, *mg* milligrams, *mL* milliliter

- ASPEN recommendations for trace element dosages are listed in Table 6.5. The available multi-trace element product composition is listed in Table 6.6.

Other Additives

- Carnitine—aids in the transport of long-chain fatty acids into mitochondria for beta oxidation, improved lipid tolerance, and improved weight gain
- Dosing: 10–15 mg/kg/day [1, 11]
- Cysteine—conditionally an essential amino acid for infants; decreases the pH of the mixture resulting in the ability to increase the calcium and phosphorous solubility
  - Dosing: 40 mg of cysteine per gram of amino acid [1, 11]
- Iron—specific forms of IV iron can be added to PN; however, there is concern for anaphylactic reactions [1] (Table 6.8).

Complications related to parenteral nutrition—please see Table 6.7.

Table 6.5 ASPEN recommendations for trace elements in PN [14]

Patient weight	Zinc (mcg/kg)	Copper (mcg/kg)	Manganese (mcg/kg)	Chromium (mcg/kg)	Selenium (mcg/kg)
3–10 kg	250	20	1	0.2	2
10–40 kg	50 (max 5000 mcg/day)	20 (max 500 mg/day)	1 (max 55 mcg/day)	0.2 (max 5 mcg/day)	2 (max 100 mcg/day)
	Zinc (mg/day)	Copper (mcg/day)	Manganese (mcg/day)	Chromium (mcg/day)	Selenium (mcg/day)
>40 kg	2–5	200–500	40–100	5–15	40–60

kg Kilogram, *mcg* micrograms, *mg* milligram

Table 6.6 Available trace element products in the United States [25, 26]

1 mL	Zinc	Copper	Manganese	Chromium	Selenium
Pediatric trace element product <10 kg	1000 mcg	60 mcg	3 mcg	NA	6 mcg
Adult and pediatric trace element product ≥10 kg	3 mg	0.3 mg	55 mcg	NA	60 mcg

kg Kilogram, *mcg* microgram, *mg* milligram, *mL* milliliter

Table 6.7 Parenteral nutrition associated complications [1, 24, 27–31]

Complications	Risks
Line migration	Phlebitis, infiltration including pericadial infiltration in neonates and young infants
Infection	Morbidity, venous/access loss
Metabolic	Glucose and lipid instability, fluid and electrolyte derangement, EFAD
Nutritional	Nutrient toxicity or deficiency, refeeding syndrome, contamination from trace mineral content (Cr, Mn, Al)
Intestinal failure-associated liver disease (IFALD)	Liver disease from long-term PN. Refer to short bowel chapter

Table 6.8 Monitoring, evaluation, and clinical considerations [1, 32]

Monitoring	Evaluation	Clinical consideration
Weight	Prior to PN initiation for baseline assessment	Increased frequency with neonates/infants, clinical and nutritional status
Length/height	Prior to PN initiation for baseline assessment	Weekly, with neonates/infants, clinical and nutritional status
Weight/length, BMI/age	Prior to PN initiation for baseline assessment	Monthly with neonates/infants, clinical and nutritional status
Electrolytes	Na^+, K^+, Cl, CO_2, Ca, Mg, Phos, BUN, Cr, glucose, ALT, AST, Alk Phos, Bilirubin (total, conjugated, and direct), TG	Daily until stable, decreased frequency based on clinical and nutritional status Need for cycling for liver preservation and glucose stability [33]
Nutritional indices	Carnitine, Vitamins A, D, E, B12, Traces Zn, Se, Cu, Cr, Mn, iron studies, EFA profile, thyroid function	Surveillance every 3 months for individuals on home PN therapy including thyroid function due to US PN formulation without iodine [34]

Calculations

1. Calculating intakes
   (a) Total calories
      (i) Calculating calories from dextrose: volume (mL) × dextrose (percentage as a decimal) × 3.4 calories/g = calories dextrose
      (ii) Calculating calories from protein: total grams protein × 4 calories/g = calories protein
      (iii) Calculating calories from fat: volume of lipids (mL) × 2 calories/mL (if using 20% ILE) = calories from fat
         1. If 10% or 30% fat, substitute the calories/mL for appropriate product into above.
         2. Calculating calories from fat if ordered in grams: each 1 g/kg is equal to 5 mL/kg. Take the grams fat/kg × 5 mL/kg to get the volume/kg, then multiply by the kg to get the mL total volume. Then follow the above calculation.

(iv) Calculating total calories from PN: (dextrose calories + protein calories + fat calories) = total calories (then convert to calories/kg)

(b) Percentage of calories from fat: calories from fat/total calories = % calories from fat

2. Glucose infusion rate:
   (a) {[(Actual volume) × (dextrose percentage as a decimal)] / kg} × 1000 / 1440 = mg/kg/min
3. Cysteine:
   (a) Total grams protein × 40 mg cysteine/total gram = mg cysteine
4. Maximum lipid infusion rate: (grams fat/kg)/number of hours for the infusion
   (a) Maximum infusion rates depend on the lipid product; however, most are infused at <0.15 g/kg/h [13, 16–18]
5. Nonprotein calorie:nitrogen ratio (NPC:N) goal is >150–250:1
   (a) (calories dextrose + calories lipid)/(g protein/6.25) [6.25 is a constant]
6. Calcium correction (with low serum albumin):
   (a) Goal albumin level = 4 (standard)
   (b) 4 − serum albumin level × 0.8 = Ca correction value (1 g albumin adds 0.8 to Ca)
   (c) Ca correction value + serum Ca = corrected Ca level
7. Na correction (with elevated glucose levels) [35]
   (a) Corrected sodium = measured sodium + [1.6 (glucose—100) / 100]
8. Mg sulfate infusions: 1 g Mg sulfate = 8.12 mEq Mg
9. Ca gluconate infusion: 1 gram Ca gluconate = 4.5 mEq Ca

Lock Therapy

There are different ways to prevent central line-associated bloodstream infections (CLABSI) and preserve central line access. One option is for patients to receive time off PN, often referred to as PN cycling [33]. During this time, individuals receive a solution added to the catheter to prevent microbial growth [1, 36]. Types of lock therapies are identified below.

- Ethanol locks (70%)—no longer available; may be available in 2025
- Antibiotic lock therapy (vancomycin or gentamicin)
- Sodium bicarbonate 8.4%
- Other lock therapies are available, outside of the United States such as KiteLock 4% and TauroLock

References

1. Gura K, Crill C. Parenteral nutrition. In: Corkins M, Bobo E, Christensen M, Larson-Nath C, Nuse Tome R, Plogsted S, editors. ASPEN Pediatric Nutrition Support Care Curriculum. 3rd ed. Silver Springs: American Society for Parenteral and Enteral Nutrition; 2025. p. 689–713.
2. Blackmer AB, Partipilo ML. Three-in-one parenteral nutrition in neonates and Pediatric patients. Nutr Clin Pract. 2015;30(3):337–43.
3. Abdelhadi RA, Barakat AR, Lyman B. Enteral and parenteral devices. In: Goday P, Walia C, editors. Pediatric nutrition for dietitians. Boca Raton: CRC Press; 2022. p. 89–99.
4. Worthington P, Balint J, Bechtold M, Bingham A, Chan L, Durfee S, et al. When is parenteral nutrition appropriate? J Parenter Enter Nutr. 2017;41(3):324–77.
5. Jacobs A, Verlinden I, Vanhorebeek I, Van den Berghe G. Early supplemental parenteral nutrition in critically ill children: an update. J Clin Med. 2019;8(6):830.
6. Fivez T, Kerklaan D, Mesotten D, Verbruggen S, Wouters PJ, Vanhorebeek I, et al. Early versus late parenteral nutrition in critically ill children. N Engl J Med. 2016;374(12):1111–22.
7. ESPGHAN and ESPEN guidelines Paediatric parenteral nutrition – annex: list of products. J Pediatr Gastroenterol Nutr. 2005;41(S2):685.
8. Mehta NM, Skillman HE, Irving SY, Coss-Bu JA, Vermilyea S, Farrington EA, et al. Guidelines for the provision and assessment of nutrition support therapy in the Pediatric critically ill patient: Society of Critical Care Medicine and American Society for Parenteral and Enteral Nutrition. J Parenter Enter Nutr. 2017;41(5):706–42.
9. Fuentes-Servín J, Avila-Nava A, González-Salazar LE, Pérez-González OA, Servín-Rodas MDC, Serralde-Zuñiga AE, et al. Resting energy expenditure prediction equations in the Pediatric population: a systematic review. Front Pediatr. 2021;6:9.
10. 2. Energy. J Pediatr Gastroenterol Nutr. 2005;41(S2):S5–11.
11. Jain AK, Nilson J. Parenteral nutrition. In: Goday P, Walia C, editors. Pediatric nutrition for dietitians. Boca Raton: CRC Press; 2022. p. 111–25.

12. Teitelbaum DH, Guenter P, Griebel D, Abrams SA, Bark S, Baker M, et al. Proceedings from FDA/a.S.P.E.N. Public workshop. J Parenter Enter Nutr. 2015;39(7):768–86.
13. Clinolipid [package Insert] [Internet]. Baxter International Inc; 2024 [cited 2024 Apr 28]. Available from: https://www.accessdata.fda.gov/drugsatfda_docs/label/2024/204508s022lbl.pdf#xd_co_f=NDE2MjlmMmYtZWI3My00ZDk3LTgzM2EtYjQxOGQxYjgxYTQ5~.
14. ASPEN. ASPEN recommendations on appropriate parenteral nutrition dosing for neonatal and pediatric patients. [Internet]. 2020 [cited 2024 Apr 28]. Available from: https://www.nutritioncare.org/uploadedFiles/Documents/Guidelines_and_Clinical_Resources/PNDosing 1-Sheet-Nov 2020-FINAL.pdf.
15. ASPEN. ASPEN Lipid Injectable Emulsion Safety Recommendations: Neonates and Pediatric Considerations [Internet]. 2022 [cited 2024 Mar 7]. Available from: https://www.nutritioncare.org/uploadedFiles/Documents/Guidelines_and_Clinical_Resources/Pediatric ILE Factsheet.pdf.
16. Intralipid [package insert] [Internet]. Fresenius Kabi; 2022 [cited 2024 Apr 28]. Available from: https://www.accessdata.fda.gov/drugsatfda_docs/label/2022/020248s026lbl.pdf.
17. Omegaven [package insert] [Internet]. Fresenius Kabi USA; 2018 [cited 2024 Apr 28]. Available from: https://www.accessdata.fda.gov/drugsatfda_docs/label/2018/0210589s000lbledt.pdf.
18. SMOF lipid [package insert] [Internet]. Fresenius Kabi; 2022 [cited 2024 Apr 28]. Available from: https://www.accessdata.fda.gov/drugsatfda_docs/label/2022/207648s005lbl.pdf.
19. Infuvite Adult MVI [package insert] [Internet]. 2012 [cited 2024 Apr 28]. Available from: https://www.accessdata.fda.gov/drugsatfda_docs/label/2012/021559s015lbl.pdf.
20. Infuvite Pediatric MVI [package insert] [Internet]. 2014 [cited 2024 Apr 28]. Available from: https://www.accessdata.fda.gov/drugsatfda_docs/label/2014/021646s014lbl.pdf.
21. Jeejeebhoy K. Zinc: an essential trace element for parenteral nutrition. Gastroenterology. 2009 Nov;137(5 Suppl):S7–12.
22. Moukarzel A. Chromium in parenteral nutrition: too little or too much? Gastroenterology. 2009 Nov;137(5):S18–28.
23. Blackmer AB, Bailey E. Management of copper deficiency in Cholestatic infants. Nutr Clin Pract. 2013;28(1):75–86.
24. Olson LM, Wieruszewski PM, Jannetto PJ, Abbott JC, McMahon MM, Nystrom EM. Quantitative assessment of trace-element contamination in parenteral nutrition components. J Parenter Enter Nutr. 2019;43(8):970–6.
25. Multrys [package insert] [Internet]. 2021 [cited 2024 Apr 28]. Available from: https://www.fda.gov/media/151047/download.

26. Tralement [package insert] [Internet]. 2020 [cited 2024 Apr 28]. Available from: https://www.accessdata.fda.gov/drugsatfda_docs/label/2020/209376s000lbl.pdf.
27. Berlana D. Parenteral nutrition overview. Nutrients. 2022;14(21):4480.
28. Smith BS, Kothari H, Hayes BD, Tataronis G, Hudlin M, Doole J, et al. Effect of additive selection on calculated aluminum content of parenteral nutrient solutions. Am J Heal Pharm. 2007;64(7):730–9.
29. Gramlich L, Ireton-Jones C, Miles JM, Morrison M, Pontes-Arruda A. Essential fatty acid requirements and intravenous lipid emulsions. J Parenter Enter Nutr. 2019;43(6):697–707.
30. Vanek VW, Seidner DL, Allen P, Bistrian B, Collier S, Gura K, et al. A.S.P.E.N. Position paper: clinical role for alternative intravenous fat emulsions. Nutr Clin Pract. 2012;27(2):150–92.
31. Food and Drug Administration. Amendment of regulations on parenteral nutrition; delay of effective date. Fed Regist. 2003;68:32979–81.
32. Szeszycki E, Cruse W, McLauglin C. Evaluation and monitoring of Pediatric patients receiving specialized nutrition support. In: Corkins M, Bobo E, Christensen M, Larson-Nath C, Nuse Tome R, Plogsted S, editors. ASPEN Pediatric nutrition support Core curriculum. 3rd ed. Silver Spring Md: American Society for Parenteral and Enteral Nutrition; 2025. p. 715–42.
33. Surgery KA. In: Corkins M, Bobo E, Christensen M, Larson-Nath C, Nuse Tome R, Plogsted S, editors. ASPEN Pediatric nutrition support Core curriculum. 3rd ed. Silver Springs Md: American Society for Parenteral and Enteral Nutrition; 2025. p. 591–614.
34. Zimmermann MB. Iodine: it's important in patients that require parenteral nutrition. Gastroenterology. 2009 Nov;137(5):S36–46.
35. Hillier TA, Abbott RD, Barrett EJ. Hyponatremia: evaluating the correction factor for hyperglycemia. Am J Med. 1999 Apr;106(4):399–403.
36. Josyabhatla R, Naik M, Liu Y, Speer AL, Imseis EM. Sodium bicarbonate locks may be a safe and effective alternative in Pediatric intestinal failure: a pilot study. J Pediatr Gastroenterol Nutr 202275(3):304–7.

Part II

Macronuttrients

Fat

7

Kritika Sukumar, Kyleigh Rodriguez,
and Kadakkal Radhakrishnan

Introduction

- The third and final macronutrient that contributes energy (measured as calories or kilojoules). Fats are the highest energy density macronutrient, providing 9 kcal/g [1, 2].
- Fats work to enhance the taste, palatability, and texture of foods, as well as promote growth in infants and keep us warm [1].

Types of Fat

- Triglycerides are the main dietary form of fats, consisting of three fatty acids (joined by a glycerol backbone) [2]—free fatty acids are absorbed readily by the body either directly or

K. Sukumar · K. Radhakrishnan (✉)
Division of Pediatric Gastroenterology, Hepatology and Nutrition, Cleveland Clinic Children's Hospital, Cleveland, OH, USA
e-mail: RADHAKK@ccf.org

K. Rodriguez
Pediatric Nutrition Support, Division of Pediatric Gastroenterology, Hepatology and Nutrition, Cleveland Clinic Children's Hospital, Cleveland, OH, USA
e-mail: RODRIGK20@ccf.org

K. Radhakrishnan (ed.), *Handbook of Clinical and Practical Pediatric Nutrition*, https://doi.org/10.1007/978-3-031-97759-6_7

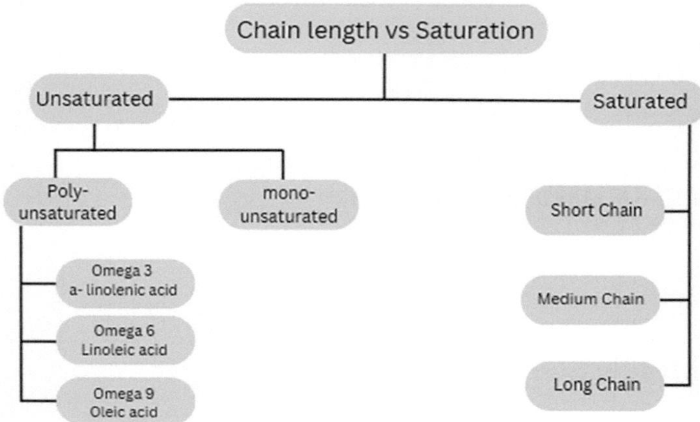

Fig. 7.1 Classifications of fats [2]

in lymph [3]. Fatty acids can range in chain length and contain various substituents (Fig. 7.1 and Table 7.1).

- Saturated fatty acids contain no double bonds in the molecule, usually present in dairy foods/animal sources such as animal fat and manufactured meat products, ice cream, cheese, butter, palm oil, etc. [1–4]
- Monounsaturated fatty acids contain one double bond on the molecule [1–3] (usually found in olive oil, avocado, nuts, flaxseed) [1, 3] polyunsaturated fatty acids (PUFAs) have two or more double bonds on the molecule [1].

  There are two essential fatty acids (PUFAs) (Table 7.2) that cannot be synthesized by the human body and therefore need to be incorporated in the diet, as many physiological body processes depend on these fatty acids [2]:

  - linoleic acid (18:2 ω6)
  - α-linolenic acid (18:3 ω3)
    - Without proper intake of essential PUFAs; findings suggestive of deficiency can include dermatitis, alopecia, liver dysfunction related to mitochondrial dysfunction, and increased susceptibility to infections.

Table 7.1 Fat types

	Names	Type of fat	Food sources	Function
Short-chain FA	Acetic acid, propionic acid, and butyric acid	<6 carbon chain, saturated	Dietary fibers	Short-chain FA (SCFA) have many properties in the human body, including immunoregulatory, anti-inflammatory effects, with some preventative and therapeutic effects on diseases, such as obesity, cardiovascular disease, liver disease, diabetes, cancers, IBD, neurodegenerative disease, etc.
Medium chain FA	Caproic acid, caprylic acid, capric acid, and lauric acid	6–14 carbon chain (saturated)	Coconut oil, palm kern oil, and milk fat	MCT is readily absorbed and can serve as an immediate energy source, especially for athletes/sports people. Because of their nature, they are directly transported via the hepatic portal vein to the liver, resulting in quick metabolism. MCT is beneficial for diagnoses such as chylothorax, epilepsy, and obesity
Long-chain FA	Linoleic acid (LA), arachidonic acid (AA), α-linolenic acid (ALA), eicosapentaenoic acid (EPA), docosahexaenoic acid (DHA), stearidonic acid (SDA), γ-linolenic acid, dihomo-γ-linolenic acid, and docosapentaenoic acid	18–21 carbon chain (polyunsaturated or saturated)	Fish, crustaceans, mollusks, meat, eggs, milk, plant sources, fruits, herb, seeds, etc	Can play an important role in the immune system regulation, cholesterol metabolism, neurotransmitters, normal vision and brain function, blood clotting, and prevention of CVD, cancer, CHD, among others

Table 7.2 Essential fatty acids [2]

Essential PUFAs	Type of FA	Food sources
α-Linolenic acid (omega-3)	Polyunsaturated (essential fatty acid)	Found in foods such as flaxseed, fish, fish oils, walnuts, and seeds
Linoleic acid (omega-6)	Polyunsaturated (essential fatty acid)	Found in fish/fish oils and cooking oils

Table 7.3 Fat requirements across ages—this table represents adequate intake, DRI table

	Fat (total)	α-Linolenic acid (omega-3)	Linoleic acid (omega-6)
Infants:			
0–6 months	31 g/day	0.5 g/day	4.4 g/day
6–12 months	30 g/day	0.5 g/day	4.6 g/day
Children:			
1–3 years	ND	0.7 g/day	7 g/day
4–8 years	ND	0.9 g/day	10 g/day
Adolescents:			
Males 9–13 years	ND	1.2 g/day	12 g/day
Males 14–18 years	ND	1.6 g/day	16 g/day
Females 9–13 years	ND	1.0 g/day	10 g/day
Females 14–18 years	ND	1.1 g/day	11 g/day

  - People on a regular diet usually get enough; populations to worry about EFAD are fat-free parenteral nutrition and fat malabsorption populations.
- Typically, the suggestion is that 25–30% of daily calories come from fat, with saturated fat being no more than 10% (Table 7.3).

Essential Fatty Acids

- **Linoleic acid (LA)**: omega-6 fatty acid and **alpha-linolenic acid (ALA)**: omega-3 fatty acid

- Cannot be synthesized by the body
- Must be obtained through diet
- They are precursors to longer-chain fatty acids

Essential Fatty Acids Synthesis

- A series of enzymatic reactions, primarily through the desaturase and elongase systems to synthesize longer-chain fatty acids from LA and ALA
  - **Desaturases:**
    Enzymes that introduce double bonds into fatty acid chains
    Converts LA and ALA into their longer-chain counterparts
  - **Elongases:**
    Enzymes that lengthen fatty acid chains by adding two carbon units
  - **Pathways:**
    LA (omega-6) → GLA → AA → (via elongation) to EPA
    ALA (omega-3) → SDA → EPA → DHA
- LA and ALA compete for these enzymes: when dietary intake of omega-6 fatty acids is high, LA competes with ALA for these enzymes, which leads to reduced conversion of ALA into EPA and DHA
- The desaturase enzymes show preference for the different series of fatty acids in the following order: omega-3 > omega-6 > omega-9 (oleic acid—not an essential fatty acid)
- Oleic acid to mead acid (Fig. 7.2) occurs when dietary intake of omega-3 and omega-6 are low

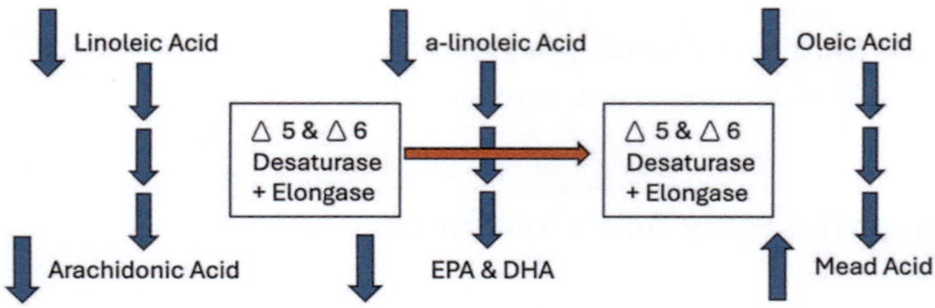

Fig. 7.2 Desaturase enzymes show preference for the different series of fatty acids in the following order: omega-3 > omega-6 > omega-9 (red arrow)

Essential Fatty Acids (EFA) Deficiency

- **Causes:**
  - Inadequate dietary intake of omega-6 and omega-3; malabsorptive disorders such as inflammatory bowel disease, pancreatitis and pancreatic insufficiency; body's increased demand during certain states (illnesses, pregnancy)
  - In neonates, insufficient maternal EFA intake or exclusive parenteral nutrition can lead to EFA deficiency
  - Premature infants are at a higher risk for EFA deficiency
  - Children with short bowel syndrome have higher nutrient and energy needs in the setting of decreased surface area for absorption posing a higher risk for EFA deficiency
- **Symptoms:**
  - Dry scaly skin, fatigue, poor night vision, cognitive impairments, growth delays, developmental issues, menstrual irregularities, and immune dysfunction
- **Diagnosis:**
  - Biochemical evaluation:

    Fatty acid profile omega-3 (ALA, EPA, DHA) and omega-6 (LA, GLA, AA)

    Lipid panel

    Mead acid (Fig. 7.1)

    A plasma eicosatrienoic acid:arachidonic acid (triene:tetraene) ratio greater than 0.2

- **Treatment:**
  - Increasing dietary intake of deficient fatty acid or making adjustments in parenteral nutrition
  - Supplementation of diet rich in LA and ALA, as well as EPA and DHA.
  - Control/treatment of underlying malabsorptive disorder

Digestion and Absorption of Fats

1. **Digestion:**
   - Mouth:
     - Mastication + action of salivary enzymes (lingual lipase secreted from von Ebner's glands) emulsify triglycerides into a food bolus that subsequently travels through the GI tract
   - Stomach:
     - Gastric lipase, which is secreted from chief cells of the fundus, breaks down triglycerides into diglycerides and free fatty acids.
   - Small intestine:
     - The complex interplay between the process of peristalsis and secretion of bile and pancreatic juice allows for the majority of digestion and absorption of fat to occur here

       Emulsification:
       - Bile is a complex fluid composed of bile salts, bilirubin, phospholipids, cholesterol and water.
         - Produced in the liver, stored in the gallbladder and secreted in the duodenum
         - Released into the duodenum in response to cholecystokinin (CCK), which is a hormone secreted by enterocytes in response to presence of fats and proteins in the small intestine
       - Bile salts break down large fat globules into small spherical structures called micelles. Micelles increase the surface area for enzymatic digestion to occur by pancreatic lipase micelles that eventu-

ally transport free fatty acids and monoglycerides to the enterocytes for absorption

Enzymatic digestion:

- Pancreatic lipase is also secreted in response to CCK
- Pancreatic lipase hydrolyzes triglycerides into monoglycerides, free fatty acids, and glycerol by acting on the surface of emulsified fat droplets
- Colipase is an essential cofactor for pancreatic lipase, which is activated by a protease enzyme (trypsin).
  - Binds to fat droplets, allowing for appropriate positioning of the lipid–water interface to allow enzymatic digestion of fats by pancreatic lipase

2. **Absorption and Transport:**
   - Micelles containing monoglycerides and free fatty acids are transported across the apical membrane of enterocytes via passive diffusion or by protein mediated transport mechanisms
   - Monoglycerides, free fatty acids, and glycerol then recombine by enzymatic action to form triglycerides, and are extruded at the basal membrane of the enterocytes to form large lipoprotein particles called chylomicrons
   - Chylomicrons are then transported through the lymphatic system and subsequently released into the blood stream where they can be delivered to tissues
   - Lipoprotein lipase, which is found on the surface of capillaries, hydrolyzes triglycerides into fatty acids and glycerol, allowing for passage through the capillary wall into tissues
   - Fatty acids are either oxidized and serve as energy sources for various cellular functions or reesterized for storage in adipose tissue

Disorders of Digestion and Absorption

- Common disorders of digestion and absorption of fat include:
  - Pancreatic disorders: insufficient pancreatic enzyme release

Pancreatic insufficiency (some relatively common causes—please refer to Chap. 43 for more details)
  - Cystic fibrosis
  - Schwachman–Diamond syndrome
  - Autoimmune pancreatitis
  - Johanson–Blizzard syndrome
  - Transiently, post-pancreatitis
  - Post-pancreatectomy
- Biliary disorders—anatomic abnormalities contributing to bile flow obstruction
  - Biliary obstruction
  - Primary sclerosing cholangitis
  - Biliary atresia
  - Disorders of bile acid secretion (progressive familial intrahepatic cholestasis—PFIC) or synthesis
- Luminal disorders—any condition affecting absorption ability of enterocytes

  Short bowel syndrome (reduced surface area for nutrient absorption)

  Celiac disease (blunting of surface villi)

  Inflammatory bowel disease (mucosal inflammation)

  Intestinal lymphangiectasia

  Zollinger–Ellison syndrome (gastric acid hypersecretion leading to altered pH and secondary malabsorption)

  Infections (leading to superficial damage to small intestinal villi)—chronic giardiasis (in IgA deficiency) and Whipple Disease

Unique Situations of Fat Malabsorption

- Lipase and colipase deficiency
  - Low levels of lipase and colipase due to a mutation in the PNLIP (pancreatic lipase) gene on chromosome 10q25
  - Infants will have poor growth and steatorrhea since birth
  - Treatment: pancreatic enzyme replacement therapy

- Diacylglycerol (DAG) deficiency
  - Deficiency of DAG, which is a precursor for triglycerides and fatty acids, involved in biochemical signaling
  - Glyceride consisting of two fatty acid chains liked by glycerol backbone
  - Present with diarrhea and malabsorption
  - Diagnosis: DAG assay
- Hypobetalipoproteinemia
  - Disorder where there are substantially low levels of apo B lipoprotein and LDL cholesterol
  - Due to mutations in APOB gene or secondary causes such as liver disease or luminal malabsorption
  - Diagnosis: low levels of LDL and apolipoprotein B
  - Management—high MCT diet and supplementation of fat soluble vitamins, particularly vitamin E
- Abetalipoproteinemia
  - Disorder affecting the metabolism of lipids
  - Autosomal recessive inheritance—mutation in the MTTP gene

    Affects the synthesis and secretion of lipoproteins

    Clinically, patients will have steatorrhea, failure to thrive, fat soluble vitamin deficiency, particularly vitamin E.

    Diagnosis: low levels on serum VLDL, LDL, absent apolipoprotein B, and genetic testing for MTTP gene mutations

    Management—high MCT diet and supplementation of fat soluble vitamins, particularly vitamin E. Vitamin E deficiency can be severe.
- Chylomicron retention disorder
  - Disorder of secretion of chylomicrons in the intestine
  - Present with malabsorption, poor weight gain, and fat soluble vitamin deficiency
  - Due to mutations in the SAR1B gene
  - Diagnosis: low or absent chylomicrons and genetic testing for SAR1B gene mutations
  - Management—high MCT diet and supplementation of fat soluble vitamins, particularly vitamin E.

References

1. Xu E, Chen C, Fu J, et al. Dietary fatty acids in gut health: absorption, metabolism and function. Anim Nutr. 2021;7(4):1337–44. https://doi.org/10.1016/j.aninu.2021.09.010.
2. Omer E, Chiodi C. Fat digestion and absorption: normal physiology and pathophysiology of malabsorption, including diagnostic testing. Nutr Clin Pract. 2024;39:S6–S16.
3. Van Tilbeurgh H, Bezzine S, Cambillau C, Verger R, Carrière F. Colipase: structure and interaction with pancreatic lipase. Biochimica et Biophysica Acta (BBA) – Mol Cell Biol Lipids. 1999;1441(2–3) https://doi.org/10.1016/S1388-1981(99)00149-3.
4. Higdon J, Drake VJ, Angelo G, Delage B. Title of the document or article. Linus Pauling Institute, Oregon State University. 2003, 2005, 2009, 2014, 2019. Reviewed by Donald B. Jump. Copyright 2003–2024 Linus Pauling Institute.

Proteins and Amino Acids

8

Meenal Karuvannur, Kristina Pytlak, and Kadakkal Radhakrishnan

Protein

- Protein functions as building blocks for bones, muscles, cartilage, skin, and blood, and they play a vital role in the function of the nervous system [1, 5]
- Protein provides 4 calories/g
- Protein consists of many chains of amino acids to form primary structure [1]
  - Primary structure is formed by sequences of amino acids
  - Secondary structure of a protein occurs when nearby amino acids chains are bonded by disulfide bonds to form alpha helices and beta pleated structures [3]
  - Tertiary structure is the complete 3D structure of a polypeptide [3]

M. Karuvannur · K. Radhakrishnan (✉)
Division of Pediatric Gastroenterology, Hepatology and Nutrition, Cleveland Clinic Children's Hospital, Cleveland, OH, USA
e-mail: KARUVAM@ccf.org; radhakk@ccf.org

K. Pytlak
Pediatric Nutrition Support, Division of Pediatric Gastroenterology, Hepatology and Nutrition, Cleveland Clinic Children's Hospital, Cleveland, OH, USA
e-mail: pyllakk@ccf.org

K. Radhakrishnan (ed.), *Handbook of Clinical and Practical Pediatric Nutrition*, https://doi.org/10.1007/978-3-031-97759-6_8

  - Quaternary structure is the three-dimensional arrangement of protein subunits. All proteins do not have quaternary structure.
- A food is considered a "complete" protein when it contains all nine essential amino acids, while "incomplete" protein do not contain all nine of the essential amino acids [1]
  - Complete proteins are found in fish, poultry, eggs, beefs, pork, dairy, and soy
  - Incomplete proteins are found in legumes, nuts, seeds, whole grains, and vegetables

    Combining incomplete proteins together can make a complete protein, also called complimentary proteins [2]
    - Nuts or seeds with whole grains
    - Beans with whole grains
    - Beans with nuts or seeds

    Limiting amino acids are any of the essential amino acids that are in the shortest supply (relative to need). For example, lysine is the limiting amino acid in rice and wheat and methionine in legumes [4].
- A reference protein is a protein that contains all indispensable amino acids at the required level per gram of protein, based on 100% digestibility [5]

Amino acids are addressed in Tables 8.1, 8.2, and 8.3.

Table 8.1 Essential amino acids [1, 6–8]

Essential amino acids	Body does not produce: must get them from the food you eat
Histidine	Makes histamine (neurotransmitter). Involved in body's immune function, digestion, and sleep. **Essential for infants**
Isoleucine	Muscle metabolism and immune function. Helps make hemoglobin and regulate energy
Leucine	Helps make protein and growth hormone, grow and repair muscle tissue, heal wounds, regulate blood sugar levels

(continued)

Table 8.1 (continued)

Essential amino acids	Body does not produce: must get them from the food you eat
Lysine	Involved in the production of hormones and energy and important for calcium and immune function
Methionine	Tissue growth, metabolism, detoxification, and absorption of essential minerals (Zn, se)
Phenylalanine	Needed for production of your brain's chemical messengers (dopamine, epinephrine, norepinephrine) and production of other amino acids
Threonine	Collagen, elastin, and fat metabolism—Helps form blood clots
Tryptophan	Maintains correct nitrogen balance and helps make neurotransmitter (serotonin)
Valine	Muscle growth, tissue regeneration, and making energy

Table 8.2 Nonessential amino acids [6–8]

Nonessential amino acids	Produced by the body
Alanine	Used for synthesis of proteins and as an energy fuel
Arginine	Used for protein synthesis, nitric oxide production, and has an energy fuel. **Premature infants cannot synthesize—Therefore essential for infants**
Asparagine	Used for synthesis of proteins
Aspartic acid	Used for synthesis of proteins and as an energy fuel
Cysteine	Used for protein synthesis and as an energy fuel. Lowers the pH. **Becomes essential for premature infants**
Glutamic acid	Used for synthesis of proteins and as a neurotransmitter
Glutamine	Used for protein synthesis, neurotransmitters, nucleotides, glycoproteins, and glycans. Precursor for glucose metabolism
Glycine	Inhibitory neurotransmitter
Proline	Used for protein synthesis and as an energy fuel
Serine	Used for protein synthesis and as an energy fuel
Tyrosine	Used for protein, catecholamine, and thyroid hormone synthesis. **Becomes essential for premature infants**

Table 8.3 Conditionally essential amino acids [6–8]

Conditionally essential amino acids	Only essential when you are ill or stressed
Arginine	Used for protein synthesis, nitric oxide production, and has an energy fuel. **Premature infants cannot synthesize—Therefore essential for infants**
Cysteine	Used for protein synthesis and stimulates production of collagen and keratin. Lowers the pH. **Becomes essential for premature infants**
Glutamine	Used for protein synthesis, neurotransmitters, nucleotides, glycoproteins, and glycans. Precursor for glucose metabolism
Glycine	Inhibitory neurotransmitter
Proline	Used for protein synthesis and as an energy fuel
Serine	Used for protein synthesis and as an energy fuel
Tyrosine	Used for protein, catecholamine, and thyroid hormone synthesis. **Becomes essential for premature infants**

Table 8.4 DRI for protein

Age	g/kg/day
0–6 months	1.52
6–12 months	1.2
12–36 months	1.05
4–13 years	0.95
14–18 years	0.85
>18 years	0.8

- Basic protein requirements [9]
  - 10–30% of total calories from protein
- Dietary Reference Intake (DRI) for protein [10] (Table 8.4):
- ASPEN protein recommendations for critically ill patients [11] (Table 8.5):

Table 8.5 Protein recommendations for critically ill patients

Age	g/kg/day
0–2 years	2–3
2–13 years	1.5–2
13–18 years	1.5

Assessing Optimal Protein Intake

- Clinical assessment (Chap. 2).
- The Recommended Dietary Allowance (RDA)—see above and Chap. 1.
- Protein turnover is a process that includes the continuous production and degradation of protein—a process known as proteostasis, which is essential to ensure that aged or damaged proteins are removed while healthy proteins continue to circulate and get absorbed.
- Markers of protein turnover include albumin, transferrin, prealbumin, and retinol binding protein. These markers should be interpreted in the appropriate clinical situations.
- Digestible Indispensable Amino Acid Score (DIAAS) is a method used to determine the digestibility or quality of ingested protein. DIAAS value of 100 or greater indicates excellent quality, 75–100 indicates good quality, and below 75 indicates no quality. These quality estimates are based on ileal digestibility.

Protein Digestion

Proteins consumed from foods get broken down into di- and tripeptides and amino acids, which are then taken up by cells to be subsequently used for anabolic processes. When proteins are consumed, the body's digestive system breaks them down into amino acids using two stages: mechanical digestion and chemical digestion—each of which occur at separate anatomical locations as outlined below.

Oral Digestion

- The first step of mechanical digestion consists of teeth mechanically breaking down food during the process of chewing.
- Once the food is broken down into pieces small enough to swallow, the mouth's salivary glands secrete saliva to lubricate food boluses, allowing them to easily pass from the oropharynx through the esophagus and subsequently into the stomach.

Gastric Digestion

- Once in the stomach, gastric peristalsis further breaks down the protein before passing into the small intestine.
- In the stomach, pepsinogen is released by gastric chief cells and converted to the enzyme pepsin by the acidic pH of the stomach (pH below 5). Pepsin is an endopeptidase.
- Pepsin and hydrochloric acid together help break down protein. The acidic pH of the stomach allows proteins to be denatured and further broken down into fragments. This chemical digestion in addition to the mechanical contractions of the stomach transform the protein consumed into a mixture called chyme. Chyme is then propelled into the small intestine where most of the protein digestion takes place.

Pancreatic and Duodenal Digestion

- In the duodenum, pancreatic enzymes (predominantly chymotrypsin and trypsin) secreted from the pancreas further break down the protein fragments into polypeptides, tripeptides, and dipeptides.
- Enterokinase, a protease found in the brush border of intestinal enterocytes, is responsible for converting trypsinogen into its active form, trypsin. Trypsin is an endopeptidase, specifically targeting peptide bonds, breaking apart arginine and lysine carboxyl segments, thus breaking down proteins into peptides [12].

- Trypsin is also responsible for activating other pancreatic enzymes needed for chemical digestion of all macronutrients.
- Chymotrypsin further breaks down proteins into smaller peptides and amino acids by targeting peptide bonds between the carboxy group of amino acids. In addition, chymotrypsin acts on peptide bonds between leucine, glutamine, and methionine.
- The brush border of the small intestine is located on the apical side of the cell membrane. Located here are brush border enzymes, specifically, carboxypeptidase, aminopeptidase N, tripeptidase, and dipeptidase [13]. These enzymes are responsible for fully breaking down proteins into tripeptides, dipeptides, and amino acids for absorption to begin.

Jejunal and Ileal Digestion

- Muscular contractions continue through the small intestine propelling nutrients toward the areas of absorption—jejunum and ileum, which occur in the small intestine with minimal protein making it to the colon.
- Protein digestion is completed in the jejunum and ileum by both the microbiome and brush border enzymes.
- Proteins and amino acids are taken up by the microbiome and subsequently either used to make components of the bacterial cells or are catabolized. In addition, the microbiome releases proteinases and peptidases to aid in the breakdown of protein as well.

Absorption

After chemical and mechanical digestion occur, majority of protein absorption occurs in the small intestine, beginning in the duodenum.

- Amino acids and di/tripeptides are transported from the intestinal lumen into enterocytes by specific transporters and subsequently into the blood through amino acid transport proteins at the base.

- Once amino acids reach the blood, they are transported to the liver/body for anabolic needs.
- The liver/body metabolizes some of the amino acids, releasing ammonia, which is then converted in the liver to urea and excreted through urine.
- Nonessential amino acids can be synthesized from tricyclic acid cycle (TCA) intermediates.

Amino Acid Transporters

Amino acids and di/tripeptides are absorbed through specific mucosal transporters:

- Amino acid transport proteins that span the small intestinal cell membrane are required for protein absorption, as amino acids are not readily absorbed across the cell membrane.
- Na^+/K^+ ATPase pumps located at the basolateral membrane of small intestinal epithelial cells create a Na^+ and H^+ electrochemical gradient, which then allow for the transport of amino acids across basolateral cell membranes and into the blood.
- There are specific transporters for neutral, basic, acidic, and imino acids, as well as di/tripeptides (Table 8.6).

Table 8.6 Amino acid transporters

Type of amino acid transporter	Name of transporter	Amino acids transported
Neutral	Alanine, serine, cysteine transporter 2 (ASCT2)	Alanine, serine, cysteine, glutamine, threonine, methionine, valine, leucine
Neutral	Large neutral amino acid transporter 1 (LAT1)	Leucine, isoleucine, valine, phenylalanine, methionine, tryptophan, tyrosine, histidine, glutamine, asparagine
Neutral	Cystine/glutamate transporter (xCT)	Cystine, glutamate

(continued)

Table 8.6 (continued)

Type of amino acid transporter	Name of transporter	Amino acids transported
Neutral	Sodium-coupled amino acid transporter 1 and 2 (SNAT1/2)	Alanine, glutamine, asparagine, serine, cysteine, methionine, glycine, histidine
Neutral	Proton-coupled amino acid transporter 1 (PAT1)	Proline, alanine, glycine, GABA amino acids
Di/tripeptides	Solute carrier family 15 member 1 (SLC15A1)	Dipeptides and tripeptides
Cationic/basic	Solute carrier family 7 member 1 (SLC7A1)	Arginine, lysine, ornithine
Cationic/basic	Solute carrier family 7 member 2 (SLC7A2)	Arginine, lysine, ornithine, L-Homoarginine
Cationic/basic	Solute carrier family 7 member 3 (SLC7A3)	Arginine, lysine, ornithine
Cationic/basic	Solute carrier family 7 member 4 (SLC7A4)	Arginine, lysine, ornithine
Cationic/basic	Solute carrier family 7 member 14 (SLC7A14)	GABA, arginine
Anionic/acidic	Excitatory amino acid transporter 1 (EAAT1)	Cystine, glutamate
Anionic/acidic	Excitatory amino acid transporter 2 (EAAT2)	Cystine, glutamate
Anionic/acidic	Excitatory amino acid transporter 3 (EAAT3)	Cystine, glutamate
Anionic/acidic	Alpha-glucoside transporter 1 (AGT1)	Aspartate, glutamate

Disorders of Protein Digestion

For a description of additional exocrine pancreatic insufficiency, please refer to chapter on “Exocrine Pancreatic Disorders.”

Specific Enzyme Deficiencies

Enterokinase Deficiency

- An autosomal recessive genetic disorder known as congenital enterokinase deficiency leads to a decrease in protease enzyme activity with resultant lack of activation of trypsinogen.
- The gene responsible for this deficiency is the pro-enteropeptidase gene (TMPRSS15), which codes for the serine protease in the small intestine responsible for activating trypsinogen.
- In the absence of trypsinogen, trypsin is not formed, and other pancreatic enzymes needed for the chemical digestion of protein are unable to be activated, leading to the absence of protein breakdown and subsequent absorption. Without trypsin, a key portion of protein digestion does not occur.
- The absence of protein breakdown clinically presents in infants as diarrhea, poor weight gain, anemia, hypoalbuminemia, and edema.
- Treated by pancreatic enzyme supplementation.

Trypsin Deficiency

- Deficiency of trypsin leads to the inability to activate pancreatic enzymes necessary in the digestion and subsequent absorption of protein.
- Symptoms of this deficiency reflect those of pancreatic insufficiency and include malnutrition, steatorrhea, fat soluble vitamin deficiencies, abdominal pain, and failure to thrive.

- Diagnosis is made by direct pancreatic function testing using endoscopic pancreatic function testing with pancreatic fluid revealing isolated trypsin deficiency.
- The diagnosis is also supported by abnormal fecal elastase testing and fat soluble vitamin deficiencies.
- Condition is treated with pancreatic enzyme supplementation.

Disorders of Amino Acid Transport

Hartnup Disorder

- Is an inherited disorder leading to the reduction in intestinal absorption of neutral amino acids.
- It is caused by a mutation in the amino acid transporter responsible for the transport of neutral amino acids, known as SLC6A19 [14].
- Clinical symptoms typically occur in the pediatric population and are a result of decreased plasma amino acid concentrations.
- These symptoms include cerebellar ataxia and photosensitive skin. In addition, as a result of disruption in tryptophan uptake, individuals with this disorder may experience a skin rash resembling pellagra secondary to niacin deficiency given that niacin is typically made from tryptophan.
- Long-term management of Hartnup disorder includes a protein-rich diet and niacin supplementation with resultant resolution of clinical symptoms.

Blue Diaper Syndrome

- Is a rare inherited disorder thought to be caused by a defect in intestinal tryptophan absorption [15].
- Clinical symptoms include diarrhea, poor weight gain, and a blue discoloration of urine.
- Hypercalcemia and nephrocalcinosis occur in some children.

- Whole genome sequencing performed on an infant with clinical symptoms of blue diaper syndrome suggested that mutations in PCSK1, a gene that encodes enzymes needed for peptide hormone processing and activation, may play a role [15].
  - It is thought that a deficiency in PCSK1 is associated with a disruption of the leptin–melanocortin signaling pathway, which is theorized to lead to a disruption in the transport of tryptophan across intestinal cell membranes and has also been implicated in hormone deficiencies and malabsorptive diarrhea.
  - Mutations in genes LAT2 and TAT1 have also recently been linked to blue diaper syndrome—X-linked inheritance.
- This condition is managed with a lower protein, low calcium, and low vitamin D diet in addition to limiting foods high in tryptophan.

Cystinuria

- Is an inherited disorder that leads to the impairment of intestinal absorption of cysteine and cationic amino acids [14].
- This disorder is caused by mutations of the amino acid transporters rBAT or b0,+AT.
- The main clinical symptom of this disorder is kidney damage secondary to kidney stones composed of cysteine.
- Management includes increased fluid intake to reduce the concentration of cystine in the urine and close follow-up to evaluate for signs and symptoms of kidney stones.

Lysinuric Protein Intolerance

- Lysinuric protein intolerance (LPI) is an inborn error of metabolism inherited in an autosomal recessive manner.
- It is caused by an abnormal variant of a gene known as *SLC7A7*, which is a gene known to encode a system responsible for the transport of amino acids across cell membranes of enterocytes [16].

- This leads to alterations in the absorption of cationic amino acids.
- This disorder typically presents in infants after they are weaned off of breast milk or formula.
- Clinical symptoms consist of feeding difficulties, vomiting, diarrhea, poor weight gain, and hepatosplenomegaly.
- Multisystemic involvement can occur, including:
  - Progressive interstitial changes in the lungs,
  - Renal disease (progressive glomerular or proximal tubular disease), and
  - Hematologic disease (anemia, thrombocytopenia, or leukopenia)—risk for macrophage activation syndrome.
- Laboratory values suggestive of LPI include:
  - An elevated 24-h urine cationic amino acids, elevated blood ammonia level (specifically following a protein rich meal),
  - Increased urinary orotic acid,
  - Increased blood levels of certain amino acids (serine, glycine, citrulline, proline, alanine, and glutamine), and
  - Hyperammonemia due to loss of urea cycle intermediates—ornithine and citrulline.
- Diagnosis of this disorder is confirmed with genetic testing identifying biallelic *SLC7A7* pathogenic variants.
- Long-term management typically consists of a careful protein-restricted diet and citrulline, lysine, and carnitine supplementation and monitoring for complications.

References

1. Cleveland Clinic. Amino acids [Internet]. Cleveland Clinic. 2021. Available from: https://my.clevelandclinic.org/health/articles/22243-amino-acids.
2. American Society for Nutrition. Protein complementation [internet]. American society for nutrition. 2011. Available from: https://nutrition.org/protein-complementation/.
3. 3.9: Proteins - Protein Structure [Internet]. Biology LibreTexts 2018. Available from: https://bio.libretexts.org/Bookshelves/Introductory_and_General_Biology/General_Biology_(Boundless)/03%3A_Biological_Macromolecules/3.09%3A_Proteins_-_Protein_Structure.

4. 8.3: The proteins in our food [internet]. Chemistry LibreTexts 2023. Available from: https://chem.libretexts.org/Courses/Whitworth_University/Science_of_Food_(Russel)/08%3A_Proteins/8.03%3A_The_Proteins_.
5. Adhikari S, Schop M, de Boer IJM, Huppertz T. Protein quality in perspective: a review of protein quality metrics and their applications. Nutrients. 2022;14(5):947.
6. Corkins MR, Balint J. American society for parenteral and enteral nutrition. A.S.P.E.N. Pediatric nutrition support core curriculum. Silver Spring: American Society For Parenteral And Enteral Nutrition; 2015.
7. MedlinePlus. Amino acids: MedlinePlus medical encyclopedia [internet]. Medlineplusgov. 2017. Available from: https://medlineplus.gov/ency/article/002222.htm.
8. Kubala J. Essential amino acids: definition, benefits and food sources [internet]. Healthline. 2018; Available from: https://www.healthline.com/nutrition/essential-amino-acids
9. USDA Dietary guidelines for Americans 2020-2025 [Internet]. USDA; 2020 Dec. Available from: https://www.dietaryguidelines.gov/sites/default/files/2020-12/Dietary_Guidelines_for_Americans_2020-2025.pdf.
10. National Academy of Sciences, Institute of Medicine, food and nutrition board. Dietary reference intakes for energy, carbohydrate, fiber, fat, fatty acids, cholesterol, protein, and amino acids. Washington, DC: National Academies Press; 2005.
11. A.S.P.E.N. Clinical Guidelines: Nutrition Support of the Critically Ill Child Mehta NM, Compher C; A.S.P.E.N. Board of Directors. A.S.P.E.N. Clinical guidelines: nutrition support of the critically ill child. JPEN J Parenter Enteral Nutr 2009;33(3):260–276.
12. Liu X, Lyu W, Liu L, et al. Comparison of digestive enzyme activities and expression of small intestinal transporter genes in Jinhua and landrace pigs. Front Physiol. 2021;12:669238. Published 2021 Jun 14. https://doi.org/10.3389/fphys.2021.669238.
13. Jochems PGM, Garssen J, van Keulen AM, Masereeuw R, Jeurink PV. Evaluating human intestinal cell lines for studying dietary protein absorption. Nutrients. 2018;10(3):322. Published 2018 Mar 7. https://doi.org/10.3390/nu10030322.
14. Bröer S, Fairweather SJ. Amino acid transport across the mammalian intestine. Compr Physiol. 2018;9(1):343–73.
15. Distelmaier F, Herebian D, Atasever C, et al. Blue diaper syndrome and *PCSK1* mutations. Pediatrics. 2018;141(Suppl 5):S501–5. https://doi.org/10.1542/peds.2017-0548.
16. Nunes V, Niinikoski H. Lysinuric protein intolerance. 2006 Dec 21 [updated 2018 Apr 12]. In: Adam MP, Feldman J, Mirzaa GM, et al., editors. GeneReviews® [internet]. Seattle (WA): University of Washington, Seattle; 1993–2024. Available from: https://www.ncbi.nlm.nih.gov/books/NBK1361/.

Carbohydrates

9

Mira Younis, Kristina Pytlak, and Kadakkal Radhakrishnan

Basics of Carbohydrates

- Carbohydrates are your body's main source of fuel. They provide 4 calories/g. Carbohydrates include both simple sugars and complex carbohydrates, which are differentiated by how quickly the body digests it [1]. The three main groups are simple carbohydrates (monosaccharides), disaccharides (which consist of two monosaccharides), and complex carbohydrates (starch, glycogen, glycolipids, and fiber).
  - **Simple sugars** are often smaller in structure and break down quickly for a more immediate source of energy causing spikes in your blood sugar [1].

M. Younis · K. Radhakrishnan (✉)
Division of Pediatric Gastroenterology, Hepatology & Nutrition, Cleveland Clinic Children's Hospital, Cleveland, OH, USA
e-mail: YOUNISM@ccf.org; RADHAKK@ccf.org

K. Pytlak
Pediatric Nutrition Support, Division of Pediatric Gastroenterology, Hepatology and Nutrition, Cleveland Clinic Children's Hospital, Cleveland, OH, USA
e-mail: pyllakk@ccf.org

K. Radhakrishnan (ed.), *Handbook of Clinical and Practical Pediatric Nutrition*, https://doi.org/10.1007/978-3-031-97759-6_9

  - Naturally occurring sugar, which are found in milk and fresh fruits or added sugars in sweets, desserts, juice, soda.
- The common monosaccharides include glucose, fructose, galactose, xylose, and ribose (Table 9.1).

Disaccharides consist of two monosaccharides and require breakdown to monosaccharides for absorption. The common ones we consume on a daily basis are sucrose and lactose.

Complex carbohydrates take longer for your body to digest and thus provides a steadier release of energy and do not spike blood sugar as quickly [1].

Table 9.1 Classification of carbohydrates: [3–5]

Monosaccharides	Single molecule
	Glucose (sugar) Fructose (fruit sugar) Galactose (component of milk) Xylose (fruits and vegetables) Ribose (mushrooms, plant, and animal sources)
Disaccharides	Two monosaccharides
	Sucrose = glucose + fructose (table sugar) Lactose = galactose + glucose (milk sugar) Maltose = glucose + glucose
Oligosaccharides	Made up of 3–10 glucose molecules: Act as prebiotics
	Maltodextrin (common component of infant formula) Fructo-oligosaccharides
Polysaccharides	12+ chains of smaller glucose molecules
	Starch = amylose and amylopectin Glycogen = complex storage form of glucose through straight and branched chains of glucose Cellulose = structural component of cell wall of plants (insoluble) Beta-glucan = naturally occurring in cell wall of cereal, bacteria, and fungi (soluble) Pectin = soluble fiber found in fruits Xanthan = used as thickening agent and stabilizer Carrageenan = used as thickening agent and stabilizer Agar = used as thickening agent and stabilizer, vegetarian gelatin substitute Inulin = type of prebiotic fiber

- **Fiber** is an important complex carbohydrate that is needed to regulate blood sugar and bowel movements and aids in lowering cholesterol [1].

  There are two types of fiber:

  - **Soluble fiber** dissolves in water and forms a gel to help slow down digestion
    - Examples include oats, barley, nuts, seeds, beans, lentils, fruits, and vegetables
  - **Insoluble fiber** helps bulk the stool to help food pass through the intestine quicker
    - Examples include whole wheat and skin on fruits/vegetables
- **Starches** are complex carbohydrates and starch-containing foods also give us important vitamins and minerals [1].

  Examples include beans, legumes, fruits, vegetables, and whole grains such as brown rice, wheat bread, and oatmeal

  Resistant starch is a carbohydrate that resists digestion in the small intestine and ferments in the large intestine acting as a prebiotic [2]

Basic carbohydrate requirements across all ages [6]:

- 45–65% of total calories from carbohydrate
  - Recommended <10% of total calories from added sugar

Dietary Reference Intake (DRI) for fiber [7] (Please refer to Chap. 1):

- 1–3 years = 19 g/day
- 4–8 years = 25 g/day
- Females 9–18 years = 26 g/day
- Males 9–13 years = 31 g/day
- Males 14–18 years = 38 g/day

Digestions of Carbohydrates Fig. 9.1)

Digestion of carbohydrates from complex carbohydrates to oligosaccharides and then to monosaccharides is required for absorption.

- Initial digestion of complex carbohydrates begins in the mouth by salivary α-amylase, which is released from salivary serous cells by the process of chewing. Amylase targets the α-1,4 glycosidic bonds of complex carbohydrates and accordingly digests starch into maltose and polysaccharides, namely, maltotriose (isomaltose), trisaccharides, larger oligosaccharides, and α-limit dextrins [8].
- α-Amylase is inactivated by acidic pH, thereby limited digestion of carbohydrates occurs in the stomach [8].
- Salivary amylase is responsible for about 5% of total starch breakdown. It plays a more significant role in two groups: infants who have reduced pancreatic amylase production in the first 9 months and children suffering from pancreatic insuffi-

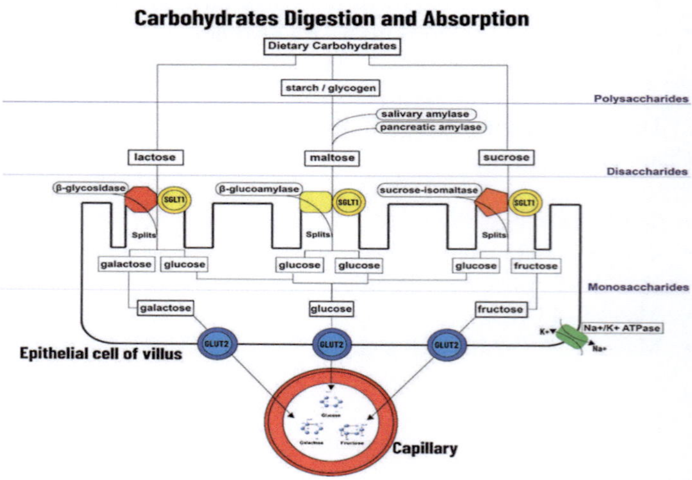

Fig. 9.1 Overview of carbohydrate digestion and absorption

ciency due to cystic fibrosis or other causes pancreatic insufficiency [9].

- As the food bolus enters the small intestine, pancreatic juice containing high bicarbonate concentration neutralizes the stomach acid. Pancreatic α-amylase secretion from the acinar cells into the duodenum is stimulated by secretin and cholecystokinin (CCK).
- Pancreatic amylase is unable to break terminal bonds or α-1,6 bonds [8].
- Oligosaccharides and disaccharides are digested by brush border enzymes, including [9]:
  - Maltase digests maltose to glucose and glucose.
  - Sucrase digests sucrose to fructose and glucose.
  - Lactase digests lactose to galactose and glucose.
  - β-Glucoamylase digests amylopectin and amylose to glucose, targeting α-1,4 and α-1,6 bonds.
  - Isomaltase is a de-branching enzyme that digests α-1,6 bonds of limit dextrin to produce glucose.
- Sucrose-isomaltase levels have been found to increase with high carbohydrate intake, indicating a transcriptional regulation process [9].

Absorption of Simple Sugars (Transporters) (Fig. 9.2)

- Glucose and galactose are actively transported by the sodium-glucose cotransporter (SGLT-1) on the brush border of the small intestine, mostly located in the duodenum and jejunum [8].
- Active transport is driven by the Na + K + -ATPase pump on the basal side of the small intestine creating a low intracellular sodium concentration by transporting three Na + ions out of the cell and tow K+ ions. This negative gradient facilitates the absorption of Na + ions and the SGLT-1 cotransporter, then transports two Na + ions with one glucose molecule [9].

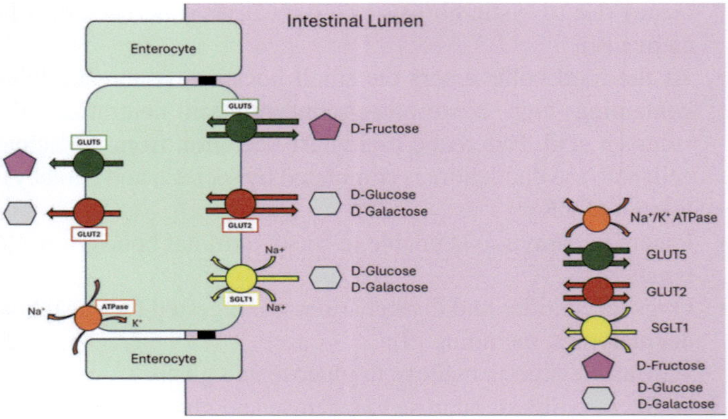

Fig. 9.2 Enterocyte monosaccharide transporters

- Glucose is then transported from the intestine cell to the blood stream by facilitated diffusion via GLUT-2 [9].
- Fructose absorption is completed via the GLUT-5 transporter by facilitated diffusion, by utilizing a carrier protein to achieve transport at rates greater than simple diffusion and does not rely on concentration gradients [9].
- GLUT-5 is found throughout the small intestine, mostly located in the duodenum and proximal ileum.
- Fructose is then transported to the bloodstream via GLUT-2 and GLUT-5.
- Absence of SGLT1 results in glucose–galactose malabsorption, leading to a severe osmotic diarrhea, failure to thrive and malnutrition presenting in the neonatal period, requiring aggressive hydration and avoidance of glucose and galactose while providing fructose-containing formula [10].

Disorders of Carbohydrate Digestion and Absorption

Disorders of Carbohydrate Digestion

Disorders of carbohydrate digestion and absorption can be divided into primary and secondary categories. Primary disorders are typically caused by congenital defects in brush-border enzymes or the transport enzymes [11]. Primary disorders include:

- Congenital lactase deficiency and primary hypolactasia deficiency
- Congenital sucrase–isomaltase deficiency
- Maltase–glucoamylase deficiency
- Trehalase deficiency
- Sodium/glucose cotransporter (SGLT1) deficiency

Secondary disorders are caused by conditions that disrupt the structure or function of the pancreas and small intestine. These disorders include:

- Pancreatic insufficiency
- Mucosal disease as in celiac disease, giardiasis, and Crohn's disease
- Loss of mucosal surface area as in intestinal resection
- Small intestinal bacterial overgrowth (SIBO)

Clinical manifestations of carbohydrate maldigestion and malabsorption generally include abdominal pain, cramping, flatulence, bloating, and altered bowel movements, namely diarrhea. This is caused by increased osmotic load caused by unabsorbed carbohydrates and short-chain fatty acids (SCFA), which is then followed by their metabolism by colonic bacteria leading to the formation of hydrogen, methane, and carbon dioxide [11].

Lactose Malabsorption and Intolerance

- Lactose malabsorption is caused by lactase downregulation that occurs after infancy. Lactase levels decrease with age, which is known as lactase nonpersistence and is mostly seen in African Americans, Asians, and Native Americans. Lactase persistence, where lactase activity remains at the infantile level, is observed in people of Northern European ancestry and certain small population groups around the world [8].
- Undigested lactose in the small intestine moves into the large intestine, where it is broken down by colonic bacteria. This process produces SCFA such as acetate, propionate, and butyrate as well as methane. SCFA in normal levels are rapidly absorbed by the colon and provide an important source of energy for the colonocytes and support concomitant absorption of water and electrolytes. Diarrhea can result from osmotic overload of lactose if fermentation rate is less than the rate of lactose arrival to the colon [8, 12].
- Symptoms typically arise after greater than 50% of lactase activity is lost, as well as the balance between the production and elimination of fermentation products.
- Lactose intolerance as opposed to lactose malabsorption refers to the onset of gastrointestinal symptoms of bloating, flatulence, abdominal pain, and diarrhea in patients with lactose malabsorption [12]. Generally, lactose intolerance is not seen under the age of 5 and if suspected should prompt looking for secondary causes (see below).
- Congenital lactase deficiency is extremely rare (only few infants have been reported worldwide) and seen when lactase enzyme is absent from birth due to genetic inactivation of the protein. Neonates manifest with osmotic diarrhea when exposed to lactose-containing feeds including breast milk, with significant symptoms.
- *Secondary lactose intolerance*: This is seen due to decreased expression of lactase enzyme in the intestinal mucosa due to intestinal mucosal disorders. This would include viral gastro-

enteritis, celiac disease, Crohn's disease, autoimmune enteropathy, and so on to quote some examples. Symptoms improve when the triggering process resolves or is treated.

Sucrase–Isomaltase Deficiency

- Sucrase–isomaltase enzyme deficiency can be congenital or acquired. Congenital sucrase–isomaltase deficiency (CSID) is rare, and symptoms arise with the introduction of sucrose-containing formulas or fruit in the diet from sucrose malabsorption, leading to severe watery diarrhea with abdominal pain, bloating, and growth retardation [12].
- Symptoms in adulthood are similar to irritable bowel syndrome (IBS), including bloating, abdominal pain, and diarrhea, with a longstanding history of gastrointestinal symptoms [12].
- Acquired forms of sucrase–isomaltase deficiency are due to chronic conditions leading to intestinal villous atrophy including enteric infections, celiac disease, and Crohn's disease [12].
- Isomaltose is a result of starch digestion. Due to its low osmotic power, symptoms are mild and mostly tolerated well [12].
- Diagnosis is confirmed with a disaccharidase assay using a small bowel tissue biopsy, genetic testing, or sucrose breath testing [13].
- Recent studies have shown that evaluation of disaccharidase activity in small bowel samples identified deficiency with functional sucrose–isomaltase genetic variants in patients with IBS. This provides evidence that screening for sucrose–isomaltase mutations in patients with IBS can help guide management with a restrictive diet or enzyme replacement therapy [14, 15].
- Dietary manipulation required by patients with CSID is stricter in childhood than adulthood. The degree of restriction typically achieved by trial-and-error trials guided by resolution of symptoms [12].

- Use of enzyme replacement with sacrosidase (Sucraid®) has been shown to be superior to placebo in prevention of symptoms in double bling studies [12, 16].

Dietary Fructose Malabsorption

- Fructose malabsorption is mainly due to the insufficient uptake of fructose into enterocytes relative to the amount of luminal fructose [12].
- In humans, fructose absorption capacity is much lower than glucose absorption capacity: increasing in life in response to dietary fructose. The capacity for fructose absorption increases in combination with glucose due to the additional fructose uptake associated with Na + -glucose cotransport (Fig. 9.1). Glucose stimulates fructose absorption in a dose-dependent manner, and malabsorption occurs when fructose is present in excess of glucose.
- Unabsorbed fructose then passes into the colon and is fermented similar to lactose in patients who have lactase nonpersistence [12].
- Hydrogen breath tests have been used to assess fructose malabsorption. However, the clinical utility is debated given the wide variations in the ability to absorb fructose in healthy adults, as well variations on the dose, and solution concentration that can affect test results. Neither is it clear whether fructose administration alone is truly reflective of dietary fructose ingestion. Ingestion of fructose with solid food delays gastric emptying as opposed to the aqueous solution administered as part of breath testing.
- Patients with functional gastrointestinal disorders are more symptomatic to same quantity of fructose ingestion compared to those without.
- Management includes fructose-restricted diet to control symptoms.

- Xylose isomerase has been proposed as a potential treatment, given its ability to convert fructose to glucose. Studies have shown significant improvement as compared to placebo; however, further research is required to study long-term health effects of xylose isomerase [12].

Glucose–Galactose Malabsorption

- Glucose–galactose malabsorption is a rare genetic disorder, where intestinal D-glucose and D-galactose absorption are defective due to multiple mutations in SGLT1 [17].
- It presents as neonatal onset of severe, watery diarrhea (osmotic diarrhea), which can result in significant morbidity and death unless fluid and electrolyte balance is quickly restored [17].
- Diagnosis is confirmed with genetic testing.
- Complete removal of glucose, galactose, and lactose from the diet leads to resolution of symptoms [17]. Special carbohydrate formulas are required in this setting, with addition of fructose for carbohydrate source and needs input from a dietician with experience with this disorder.

Trehalose Deficiency

- Trehalose is a disaccharide (two glucose molecules) that is found in mushrooms, algae, and insect hemolymph. It is responsible for cryptobiotic plants' ability to undergo cycles of desiccation and rehydration without injury, leading to the interest of the food industry to improve the quality of dried food activity [18].
- Isolated trehalase deficiency is an autosomal dominant disorder, mostly found in the Greenland population [18].
- Patients present with generalized abdominal pain, increased bloating, diarrhea, and sometimes vomiting.

- Diagnosis by measuring trehalase activity in intestinal mucosa during upper endoscopy. Treatment involves avoidance of food containing trehalose.

Pancreatic Insufficiency[1]

- Exocrine pancreatic insufficiency (EPI) refers to decreased pancreatic enzyme activity (mainly pancreatic lipase) in the intestinal lumen below the threshold required for digestion, which leads to an inadequate absorption of fat, proteins, and carbohydrates [19, 20].
- Malabsorption of fat precedes malabsorption of proteins and carbohydrates and is clinically more apparent [20].
- The increased presence of lipids and other nutrients in the distal small bowel leads to changes in gut motility and accelerated gastric emptying and intestinal transit. Decreased time available for digestion and absorption of nutrients further contributes to malabsorption [20].
- Symptoms include voluminous, fatty stools, flatulence, weight loss, and chronic abdominal pain [19].
- Management starts with pancreatic enzyme replacement therapy (PERT). In addition, management of EPI should include dietary counselling to improve digestion tailored by a dietician to fat intake, as best control of symptoms is achieved by self-dosing of pancreatic enzymes according to fat intake, compared with a fixed-dose regimen [20].

Mucosal Disorders

Celiac Disease[2]

- Celiac disease is an immune-mediated enteropathy affecting the small intestine caused by a permanent sensitivity to gluten

[1] Please refer to Chap. 43 for further information

[2] Please refer to Chap. 44 for further information.

in genetically susceptible individuals. Gluten is found in wheat, rye, barley, among other grains [21].

- Mucosal injury to the small intestine leads to malabsorption of carbohydrates, fats, iron, folate, calcium, and vitamin D, as well as fat-soluble vitamins (A, D, E, and K) [21].
- The mainstay of treatment for celiac disease is dietary gluten elimination. Therefore, dietitians' role is pivotal to patient care.

Inflammatory Bowel Disease (IBD)

- IBD-caused inflammation can lead to decreased mucosal disaccharidases, with little data on the actual rate of sucrose/lactose intolerance in IBD patients [22].
- The possibility of carbohydrate intolerance (i.e., lactose, sucrose, and fructose) should always be considered in IBD patients when managing symptoms [22].
- Symptoms should therefore improve with good mucosal healing.

Autoimmune Enteropathy

- Autoimmune enteropathy is an extremely rare condition, which is identified by an abnormal intestinal immune response manifesting as severe, intractable diarrhea that does not respond to dietary modification in early infancy, typically between 2 and 4 weeks of age [23].
- This diagnosis often may have an underlying genetic disorder as the underlying etiology. The classic example if IPEX (Immune Dysfunction, Polyendocrinopathy, Enteropathy, X chromosome-linked disorder), a disorder that affects males and is due to *FOXP3* gene that affects regulatory T cells.
- The diagnosis is achieved through clinical symptoms that include laboratory studies, and histological features on small bowel biopsy. Hallmark features include significant malabsorption, growth failure, and electrolyte abnormalities [23].
- Concurrent, additional autoimmune gastrointestinal conditions include autoimmune atrophic gastritis and lymphocytic colitis.
- Extraintestinal conditions may include hypothyroidism, autoimmune hepatitis, arthritis, eczema, nephrotic syndrome, and rheumatoid arthritis [23, 24].

References

1. Cleveland Clinic. Carbohydrates [internet]. Cleveland Clinic. Cleveland Clinic; 2021. Available from: https://my.clevelandclinic.org/health/articles/15416-carbohydrates.
2. What is Resistant Starch? [Internet]. The Johns Hopkins Patient Guide to Diabetes. 2018. Available from: https://hopkinsdiabetesinfo.org/what-is-resistant-starch/
3. Corkins MR, Balint J. American society for parenteral and enteral nutrition. A.S.P.E.N. Pediatric nutrition support core curriculum. Silver Spring: American Society For Parenteral And Enteral Nutrition; 2015.
4. Lovegrove A, Edwards CH, De Noni I, Patel H, El SN, Grassby T, et al. Role of polysaccharides in food, digestion, and health. Critical Rev Food Sci Nutr [Internet]. 2015;57(2):237–53. Available from: https://www.ncbi.nlm.nih.gov/pmc/articles/PMC5152545/
5. Oligosaccharide – an overview | ScienceDirect Topics [Internet]. www.sciencedirect.com. Available from: https://www.sciencedirect.com/topics/agricultural-and-biological-sciences/oligosaccharide.
6. USDA Dietary guidelines for Americans 2020-2025 [internet]. USDA; 2020 Dec. Available from: https://www.dietaryguidelines.gov/sites/default/files/2020-12/Dietary_Guidelines_for_Americans_2020-2025.pdf.
7. Children Need Carbohydrates [Internet]. www.eatright.org. Available from: https://www.eatright.org/health/essential-nutrients/carbohydrates/children-need-carbohydrates
8. Barrett K. Carbohydrate, protein and water-soluble vitamin assimilation. In: GI physiology. 2nd ed. New York: NY. McGraw Hill; 2013. p. 256–84.
9. Goodman BE. Staying current insights into digestion and absorption of major nutrients in humans Goodman BE. Insights into digestion and absorption of major nutrients in humans. Adv Physiol Educ. 2010;34:44–53. https://doi.org/10.1152/advan.00094.2009.-Nutrient.
10. Russo P. Enteropathies of infancy and childhood. Adv Pediatric. 2013;60(1):217–61. https://doi.org/10.1016/j.yapd.2013.04.010.
11. Omer A, et al. Carbohydrate maldigestion and malabsorption. Clin Gastroenterol Hepatol. 16(8):1197–9.
12. Fernández-Bañares F. Carbohydrate Maldigestion and intolerance. Nutrients. 2022;14(9):1923. https://doi.org/10.3390/nu14091923. PMID: 35565890; PMCID: PMC9099680.
13. Burke M. Carbohydrate intolerance and Disaccharidase measurement—a mini-review. Clin Biochem Rev. 2019;40:167–74. https://doi.org/10.33176/AACB-19-00025.
14. Henström M, Diekmann L, Bonfiglio F, Hadizadeh F, Kuech EM, von Köckritz-Blickwede M, Thingholm LB, Zheng T, Assadi G, Dierks C, et al. Functional variants in the sucrase-isomaltase gene associate with

increased risk of irritable bowel syndrome. Gut. 2018;67:263–70. https://doi.org/10.1136/gutjnl-2016-312456.
15. Garcia-Etxebarria K, Zheng T, Bonfiglio F, Bujanda L, Dlugosz A, Lindberg G, Schmidt PT, Karling P, Ohlsson B, Simren M, et al. Increased prevalence of rare Sucrase-isomaltase pathogenic variants in irritable bowel syndrome patients. Clin Gastroenterol Hepatol. 2018;16:1673–6. https://doi.org/10.1016/j.cgh.2018.01.047.
16. Treem WR, McAdams L, Stanford L, Kastoff G, Justinich C, Hyams J. Sacrosidase therapy for congenital sucrase-isomaltase deficiency. J Pediatr Gastroenterol Nutr. 1999;28:137–42. https://doi.org/10.1097/00005176-199902000-00008.
17. Goodman BE. Insights into digestion and absorption of major nutrients in humans. Adv Physiol Educ. 2010;34(2):44–53.
18. Montalto M, Gallo A, Ojetti V, Gasbarrini A. Fructose, trehalose and sorbitol malabsorption. Eur Rev Med Pharmacol Sci. 2013;17(Suppl 2):26–9. PMID: 24443064
19. Ghodeif AO, Azer SA. Pancreatic Insufficiency. [Updated 2023 Jan 16]. In: StatPearls [Internet]. Treasure Island (FL): StatPearls Publishing; 2025. Available from: https://www.ncbi.nlm.nih.gov/books/NBK555926/
20. Sikkens ECM, Cahen DL, Kuipers EJ, Bruno MJ. Pancreatic enzyme replacement therapy in chronic pancreatitis, best Practice & Research Clinical. Gastroenterology. 2010;24(3):337–47. ISSN 1521, 6918. https://doi.org/10.1016/j.bpg.2010.03.006.
21. Holtmeier W, Caspary WF. Celiac disease. Orphanet J Rare Dis. 2006;1:3. https://doi.org/10.1186/1750-1172-1-3. PMID: 16722573; PMCID: PMC1435993.
22. Barros LL, Farias AQ, Rezaie A. Gastrointestinal motility and absorptive disorders in patients with inflammatory bowel diseases: prevalence, diagnosis and treatment. World J Gastroenterol. 2019;25(31):4414–26. https://doi.org/10.3748/wjg.v25.i31.4414. PMID: 31496621; PMCID: PMC6710178
23. Chen CB, Tahboub F, Plesec T, et al. A review of autoimmune enteropathy and its associated syndromes. Dig Dis Sci. 2020;65:3079–90. https://doi.org/10.1007/s10620-020-06540-8.
24. Montalto M, D'Onofrio F, Santoro L, Gallo A, Gasbarrini A, Gasbarrini G. Autoimmune enteropathy in children and adults. Scand J Gastroenterol. 2009;44:1029–36.

Part III

Micronutrients

Iron

10

Haig Manougian and Ravi Talati

Iron Sources and Bioavailability

- Iron is available in the human diet as food or supplementation present in either heme or nonheme form [1, 2].
- Heme iron is available from animal food sources, makes up a smaller percentage of total iron intake (10–15%), and represents a disproportionately larger percentage (25–40%) of total absorbed iron due to its easily absorbed ferrous (Fe^{2+}) ionic state [2, 3].
- Nonheme iron is available from both plant and animal sources, and is less well absorbed due to its highly insoluble oxidized ferric (Fe^{3+}) nature, which is influenced by common dietary factors.
- The limitations of physiologic iron absorption result in approximately 1 mg of absorbed iron from a diet containing 10–20 mg of iron per day [3, 4].
- Higher iron intake is required for plant-based diets (vegetarianism, veganism), as compared to animal-based diets, due to this differing effectiveness of absorption.

H. Manougian · R. Talati (✉)
Division of Pediatric Hematology/Oncology and Bone Marrow Transplantation, Cleveland Clinic Children's Hospital, Cleveland, OH, USA
e-mail: MANOUGH@ccf.org; TALATIR@ccf.org

K. Radhakrishnan (ed.), *Handbook of Clinical and Practical Pediatric Nutrition*, https://doi.org/10.1007/978-3-031-97759-6_10

Iron needs vary depending on stage of growth through childhood. In pediatrics, periods of rapid growth (infancy, toddlerhood, adolescence) require increased iron intake to account for elevated physiologic consumption/loss.

- *Infancy*: Low bioavailability of iron in breast milk prompts supplementation in exclusively breastfed infants, as compared to iron inclusion in formula fed infants [5].
- *Toddlerhood*: Cow's milk consumption impacts iron bioavailability, while goat's milk consumption is iron poor, prompting supplementation during this age [4].
- *Adolescence*: Consumption during growth spurts and iron losses for adolescent females at the onset of menstruation may reach as high as 2 mg/day (average of 14 mg/menstrual period), making up the highest dietary replacement group in pediatrics [4, 6].
- The recommended dietary allowance (RDA) of iron—i.e., the average daily level of iron intake sufficient to meet the nutrient requirements of nearly all healthy individuals (as described by the Food and Nutrition Board at the Institute of Medicine of the National Academies), is shown in Appendix Table 10.1 [7].
- Animal products such as lean meat and seafood contain the greatest quantity of heme iron. Nonheme iron is found in a variety of foods including vegetables, grains, legumes and nuts. Fortification of food products (with ferrous sulfate, ferrous fumarate, ferric sodium EDTA, or electrolytic iron) has become common practice in Western nations over the last few decades, providing an additional source of nonheme iron to supplement the diet of a growing child [9].
- Infant dietary iron intake presents a unique challenge. The American Association of Pediatrics (AAP) recommends exclusive breastfeeding for approximately 6 months, due to a multitude of well-documented benefits, prior to the introduction of complementary food [5]. Infant iron stores gained during the fetal third trimester wane throughout this period however,

while iron availability remains one of the few nutritional scarcities in breast milk.

- Thus, several strategies may be implemented to ensure adequate iron intake.
- Complementary table foods with sources of heme-iron can be introduced in a timely fashion at 6 months of age [4].
- By adopting the strategy of iron fortification to readily available foods, iron-fortified formulas are designed to provide sufficient micronutrient amounts [4, 5, 10].
- Recent studies have shown the benefit of low-dose iron supplementation with variable dosing schedules through infancy [11].
- Pregnant and lactating patients present another unique population. Adequate maternal iron intake is essential for fetal growth and development (expanding fetal iron storage), assisted by physiologically increased capacity of iron absorption by the maternal intestine [12].
- After a term birth, neonatal iron stores are estimated to total approximately 270 mg, obtained in totality from the mother's diet. Iron store deficiencies in early infancy may serve as a reflection of maternal deficiency during pregnancy. Thus, iron stores at conception are a strong predictor of maternal iron status and predict the risk of developing anemia later during the pregnancy course [12, 13].
- Adolescent pregnancies should be monitored carefully during routine care due to this population's increased risk for insufficient iron stores and for fetal/birth complications [14].
- Multiple births further increase the risk of iron deficiencies of mothers and infants alike [14].
- After delivery and during lactation, iron needs significantly decrease (as shown in Appendix Table 10.1). Despite iron's low concentration in breast milk, it is not influenced by maternal iron status changes, making supplementation less effective as compared to during pregnancy [12, 13].
- Common sources of heme and nonheme iron in the pediatric diet is provided in Appendix Table 10.2 [15].

Iron's Role and Function

Iron's capacity to accept and donate electrons allows it to partake in many enzymatic reactions, essential for the function of a variety of cellular processes.

- *DNA metabolism*: Iron is required for the appropriate function and stability of synthetic enzyme complexes (DNA polymerase, ribonucleotide reductase) in addition to being a vital cofactor for DNA repair enzymes (helicases, glycosylases, nucleases, demethylases). Iron's implication in genomic stability and DNA damage repair has led to ongoing investigations in this mineral's role for understanding DNA-related disorders, aging, and their association with cancer [16, 17].
- *Cellular respiration*: Interconversion between Fe^{2+} and Fe^{3+} oxidation states by iron–sulfur cytochrome cofactors in the electron transport chain is vital in the production of redox energy and the conversion of this energy into the cross-membrane proton gradient mediated ATP synthesis [16, 18].
- *Oxygen transportation*: Iron is important for hemoglobin/myoglobin formation for erythrocyte oxygen transport [19]. Hemoglobin is a tetrameric protein made up of two α and two β globin peptide chains/units, each unit incorporated with a heme moiety. Heme is composed of a protoporphyrin ring with a central iron ion in the reduced ferrous state (Fe^{2+}).
  - Heme synthesis is a complex process, involving eight constructive steps, the final one of which is the addition of Fe^{2+} to the constructed protoporphyrin IX ring by ferrochelotase [20]. This iron atom forms a covalent bond with oxygen, allowing the carriage and transport of oxygen throughout the body [21].
  - Differences in vascular modulatory factors such as temperature, carbon dioxide concentration, and pH, all influence hemoglobin's affinity for oxygen, allowing appropriate oxygen loading in the lung, and offloading in the periphery [21, 22].

Fenton Reaction

$$Fe^{3+} + \cdot O_2^- \rightarrow Fe^{2+} + O_2$$
$$Fe^{2+} + H_2O_2 \rightarrow Fe^{3+} + OH^- + \cdot OH$$

Haber-Weiss Reaction

Reaction Net:

$$\cdot O_2^- + H_2O_2 \xrightarrow{Fe^{3+}} O_2 + OH^- + \cdot OH$$

Fig. 10.1 The Fenton/Haber–Weiss reaction [16, 23]

  - Other: A small percentage of body iron is utilized for the synthesis of collagen, neurotransmitters, and for appropriate immune function [19].
- Despite these essential functions, it is important to note that iron in excess is directly toxic at the cellular level due to hydroxyl radical generation, demonstrated by the Haber–Weiss reaction (as shown in Fig. 10.1) [16, 23]. Reactive oxygen species such as hydroxide anions and radicals can be produced at an accelerated rate secondary to catalysis by the interconversion of free redox ferrous (Fe^{2+}) and ferric (Fe^{3+}) iron forms. The resulting radicals cause nonspecific cellular damage (affecting lipids, protein, DNA), leading to apoptosis [16, 23, 24].

Iron Metabolism

Overview

Iron metabolism and homeostasis is tightly regulated due to its conservation, recycling, and lack of physiologic excretion pathways by the human body.

- Of the approximate 10–20 mg of iron contained in the daily diet, about 1–2 mg is absorbed in the intestine and then circulated via transferrin, the primary iron transport protein [3, 16]
- The majority (~65–75%) of absorbed iron is incorporated into the mitochondria for hemoglobin synthesis during erythropoi-

esis to support systemic oxygenation. About 5–15% is incorporated into metalloproteins for the cellular processes described above. The remaining 10–20% is incorporated into cytosolic ferritin in the liver and heart for excess iron storage [19].

- Despite no physiologic route of iron excretion, about 1–2 mg of iron per day is shed via epithelial desquamation (skin, GI, GU tract) [25].
- Iron is otherwise eliminated via bleeding and menstruation, hence placing adolescent females at higher risk for iron deficiency compared to other pediatric populations [2, 4, 19, 25].

Iron Absorption

After ingestion, the stomach's acidic environment allows the solubilization of ferrous iron (by amino acids, sugars, and amines/amides) for absorption in the small intestine.

- In the setting of gastric achlorhydria where pH cannot be lowered less than 3, downstream iron absorption cannot occur, as iron remains in the insoluble ferric state [26].
- In heme iron, the high absorption rate by intestinal enterocytes is secondary to the natural enterocyte uptake of the ferrous protoporphyrin formation [3, 25, 27].

Dietary factors may inhibit and enhance iron absorption.

- Significant inhibitors of both heme and nonheme iron found in vegetal diets include phytates, polyphenols, phosphate, and oxalate, forming complexes with ferrous iron, reducing its enterocyte uptake [27, 28].
- Calcium is a significant inhibitor of absorption of iron, thought to be via iron receptor (DMT1) internalization and interference of iron transfer within the enterocyte [29]. This inhibition, however, appears to be limited over a longer period, likely due to physiologic adaptation to varied dietary intake [30].

- Animal source inhibitors include milk protein (casein and whey), egg protein, and albumin—forming high affinity complexes with iron, preventing its uptake [27, 31].
- Ascorbic acid (Vitamin C) is the most significant enhancer of iron absorption secondary to its effect on ferric iron conversion to ferrous form for more efficient uptake [28, 30, 32].

The primary site of absorption of iron in the small intestine is the duodenum and proximal jejunum.

- Disease/inflammatory states affecting this region (e.g., Celiac disease, Crohn's disease/inflammatory bowel disease, etc.) may negatively impact iron absorption locally [33]. In contrast, due to the human body's lack of physiological iron excretion, regulation at the level of absorption is essential to prevent iron overloaded states.
- Ferrous iron is absorbed by the enterocyte by a membrane transport protein—divalent metal transporter 1 (DMT1), while ferric iron must first be reduced to ferrous state via apical brush border ferric reductase cytochrome B [25–27].
- Enterocyte intracellular iron is then exported into systemic circulation via ferroportin, the only known cellular exporter of iron.
- Ferroportin is also found on iron storage tissues, such as the liver and systemic macrophages (spleen, liver), to regulate iron storage export via its interaction with hepcidin, a hepatic hormone [25, 34].
- Hepcidin is an inhibitor of iron absorption (and iron storage release) by one of two mechanisms: (1) changing ferroportin's conformation (a rapidly reversible qualitative effect), or (2) inducing ferroportin endocytosis and degradation by the enterocyte (a quantitative effect) [34, 35].
- Hepatocyte hepcidin production is complex, inhibited by erythropoietic requirements, and promoted by excess iron stores and inflammation [35, 36]

Iron Transport, Distribution, and Storage

- Following exocytosis by ferroportin, iron is oxidized from the absorbed ferrous state, back to ferric state by membrane-bound hephaestin (or ceruloplasmin, when concerning iron storage export), to allow binding to transferrin, the main iron transport protein [37].
- Although circulating iron can exist in a non-transferrin bound form, transferrin is vital to prevent iron induced free radical damage as described above, transporting iron in a redox-inactive form [38].
- Upon reaching a target cell, the iron-loaded transferrin undergoes receptor-mediated endocytosis (via ubiquitous transferrin receptor 1 and 2). Iron is released from transferrin through endosomal acidification and exits into the cytosol once again by the DMT1 transporter.
- Iron is then again reduced from the transported ferric state to ferrous for cellular utilization (via six-transmembrane epithelial antigen of the prostate 3 (STEAP3) ferric reductase) [39]. Ferrous iron may then be utilized by the cell for synthetic function.
- The remaining transferrin-receptor complex is recycled upon return to the cell surface to repeat iron circulation from the intestine or macrophage storage [25, 39].
- The level of transferrin receptor expression on the cell surface corresponds to that cell's rate of proliferation. For example, erythroid bone marrow progenitor cells have increased transferrin receptor concentration given their higher proliferation rate [38–40].
- More recently identified functions of transferrin include antimicrobial activity by free iron sequestration (making it less available to pathogenic bacteria), growth and differentiating activity, as well as cytoprotective effects [38, 41].
- Concerning storage, hepatic/macrophage ferritin is the primary intracellular iron storage protein, limiting the labile iron pool. The heavy chain subunit of ferritin oxidizes ferrous iron back to ferric state for storage. The light chain subunit of fer-

ritin promotes iron nuclei formation, capable of storing up to 4500 iron atoms [42].

Iron Regulation

Iron availability is tightly controlled at the systemic and cellular levels, due to the harmful nature of both iron excess and its deficiency.

- Hepcidin (as mentioned above) is the main regulator of *systemic* iron, often referred to as the hepcidin–ferroportin axis, given its main inhibitory effect on ferroportin [42, 43]. Hepcidin expression is influenced by serum/systemic iron concentrations, inflammation, hypoxia, and degree of erythropoiesis, in promotion or inhibition of enterocyte iron absorption [34–36, 42, 43].
- *Cellular* iron homeostasis is regulated by iron regulatory proteins (IRP1 and IRP2). On a posttranscriptional level, IRPs regulate iron transport elements (including ferroportin, transferrin receptors, DMT1, and ferritin), via iron-responsive element (IRE) interaction [42–44].
- In iron-deficient states, IRPs bind to IRE on transferrin receptor, DMT1, ferritin, and ferroportin mRNA transcripts, stabilizing the transcript, thus increasing protein translation and cellular expression. In iron overloaded states, IRPs are blocked from IRE binding, resulting in repressed protein expression [43, 45].

Iron Recycling

- Senescent and damaged red blood cells undergo erythrophagocytosis by macrophages of the reticuloendothelial system.
- Within the phagolysosome, iron is released from heme via digestion by heme oxygenase 1 (HO-1) and then transported into the cytosol via the NRAMP1 transporter (similar function to DMT1).

- Iron can then enter systemic circulation via export into the plasma [46, 47]. Thus, the major iron pool within red blood cells once again becomes available for new erythropoiesis or to be stored as ferritin as described above [48].

Iron's Implication in Health and Disease

Iron Deficiency and Anemia

- Iron deficiency and its complications occur due to an inadequate supply to meet age-specific demands, estimated to affect approximately 25–30% of the world's population, and contributing to significant healthcare burden in the United States [49, 50].
- Pediatric populations at particular risk include older infants, children less than 5 years old (rapid growth and potential for absorption interference by milk protein), adolescent females with iron loss from menstrual bleeding, patients with chronic bleeding in the setting of inherited bleeding disorders, vegetarian/vegan diets, and those with food insecurity/low dietary diversity [51, 52].
- "Functional" iron deficiency may occur with chronic inflammation (e.g., inflammatory bowel disease, congestive heart failure, chronic kidney disease, obesity, malignancy)—due to withholding of iron from the plasma by elevated systemic hepcidin, and lack of availability for erythropoiesis [49, 51].

Iron deficiency occurs in three stages based on erythropoiesis: (1) deficiency of iron storage, (2) iron-deficient erythropoiesis (with symptom development), and (3) iron-deficiency anemia [53].

- Iron deficiency is most commonly an *acquired* disorder but may rarely present as an *inherited* disease due to hepcidin dysregulation.

- This entity is called iron refractory iron deficiency anemia (IRIDA), due to a recessive defect in the transmembrane protease, serine 6 (*TMPRSS6*) gene, coding for Matripase-2 [54].
- Patients with iron deficiency due to inadequate intake portray suppressed hepcidin levels, while patients with IRIDA have abnormally elevated hepcidin, inappropriately preventing iron absorption, a state resistant to enteral iron therapy [55, 56].

Iron deficiency may present with a variety of signs/symptom or may be asymptomatic altogether.

- Patients may present with fatigue/lethargy, dizziness, lightheadedness, headaches, palpitations, and pallor; or may be more behavioral in younger children, with irritability, pica, poor feeding/appetite, exercise intolerance, breath-holding spells, sleep disorders, or restless leg syndrome [57].
- Cutaneous signs include hair thinning/alopecia, koilonychia, angular cheilitis, or atrophic glossitis.
- When severe, iron deficiency may present with hemodynamic instability and organ dysfunction (ischemic stroke and hypoperfusion injuries) [56–58]. Chronic conditions (e.g., heart failure) may be exacerbated by the development of iron deficiency and anemia [51].
- Routine screening via CBC for iron-deficiency anemia is recommended by the AAP at 12 months of age, and for all children/adolescents portraying signs and symptoms of anemia or iron deficiency [58]. Gold standard evaluation of absent stainable iron on bone marrow evaluation is no longer performed due to the invasive nature of this procedure [49].
- Hemoglobin confirms the presence of anemia if below the reference value for age (Hgb <11 g/dL in children <10 years old or < 12 g/dL in children >10 years old).
- Aberrant red blood cell indices include ↓ RBC count, MCV, MCH, and MCHC, and ↑ RDW.
- The Mentzer index [(MCV/RBC count)] is therefore elevated (>13) to distinguish from other forms of anemia such as thalassemia, which may present with similar blood count findings.

- Reticulocyte count will be inappropriately low, indicating a hypo-proliferative state [58, 59].
- Serum ferritin is the most sensitive, specific, and cost-effective test to detect iron deficiency, levels <30 ug/L being highly suggestive, and levels <15 ug/L being confirmatory [56–59].
- Serum iron is expected to be low with decreased plasma iron content.
- Transferrin/total iron binding capacity (TIBC) can both be elevated as the body's compensatory response to transfer minimally saturated iron complexes. Transferrin saturation can reflexively be expected to be decreased [58, 59].
  - Note that ferritin and transferrin are acute phase reactants, and may be falsely elevated in states of inflammation, patients therefore benefitting from evaluation of inflammatory markers such as ESR or CRP [59–61].
- Supplementary lab parameters include ↓ serum soluble transferrin receptor, ↑ zinc protoporphyrin (zinc absorption increases with iron depletion), and ↓ reticulocyte hemoglobin content [56, 58, 62]. Labs should be interpreted along with the patient's history, as information on dietary intake may assist with lab interpretation, when provided with incongruent results.

Management of Iron-Deficiency Anemia

- Management should first address insufficiencies in iron intake and concurrent absorption enhancers/inhibitors, reducing risk of recurrence after resolution [52, 59].
- Second, active repletion of deficient stores should be performed with oral or parenteral iron supplementation [63].
- Third, underlying diseases that may contribute to excess iron loss should be addressed (e.g., bleeding disorders, inflammatory GI disorders, chronic conditions, etc.) [63, 64].
- Oral iron supplementation (with many available formulations) is the mainstay of therapy, including iron salts (ferrous sulfate, ferrous fumarate, ferrous gluconate), iron–polysaccharide complex, ferric citrate, and heme iron polypeptide.

- Weight-based replacement doses for children are 3–6 mg/kg/day of elemental iron, divided 2–3 times daily [65].
- Newer evidence suggests lower doses (max 60 mg compared to traditional 100–200 mg), dosed every other day may be more effective for absorption and treatment tolerance. This phenomenon may be associated with upregulation of hepcidin with frequent iron availability in the GI tract, limiting enteral absorption to <25% of the administered dose [63–65].
- There is no significant difference between the tolerability among oral iron formulations, though they do differ in elemental iron content and absorption efficacy, depending on ferrous vs. ferric preparations [64].
- Anticipatory guidance should be offered regarding potential adverse effects of oral iron, including dyspepsia (gastrointestinal mucosal injury), constipation, diarrhea, nausea, and vomiting. Such symptoms may threaten compliance and result in treatment failure, mitigated with dose reduction or decreasing dose frequency [64, 66].
- Parenteral iron therapy may be required where enteral iron absorption is limited, such as due to IBD, short gut syndrome, chronic inflammation, or IRIDA [55, 66, 67].
- Patients with severe/life-threatening anemia and hemodynamic compromise may benefit from urgent parental iron or emergent blood transfusion prior to transitioning to oral therapy.
- Prompt improvement of erythropoiesis and anemia-associated symptoms can be expected.
- Available IV iron formulations include iron sucrose, ferric carboxymaltose, ferric gluconate, ferumoxytol, iron isomaltoside, and low molecular weight iron dextran [59, 63, 67]. Many formulas exist to guide IV iron therapy (supplemented over a period of weeks), the most studied of which is the Ganzoni formula, described as follows (units in *italics*): [67, 68]

$$\begin{aligned}\text{Total iron deficit}(\text{mg}) &= \text{Patient Weight}(\text{kg}) \\ &\times(\text{target Hgb} - \text{actual Hgb})(\text{g/dL}) \\ &\times 2.4 + \text{storage iron}(\text{mg})\end{aligned}$$

- Where storage iron is 15 mg/kg for patients <35 kg in weight, or 500 mg for patients >35 kg.
- Where the constant factor 2.4 is derived from the percentage of body weight making up blood volume, and iron content of hemoglobin.
- Patients receiving IV iron therapy require monitoring for mild to moderate infusion reactions, including hypophosphatemia, mild allergic reactions, early complement activation-related pseudo-allergic reactions, and oxidative/cardiovascular stress [69, 70]. Severe anaphylaxis is now extremely rare following removal of high molecular weight iron dextran availability [69].

Iron Overload

- The tight regulation of bodily iron content prevents nonspecific free-radical injury from iron excess [16, 53]. Iron deposition can occur in many organs, driving organ-specific pathology: cardiac dysfunction, liver dysfunction, endocrinopathies (diabetes mellitus, hypopituitarism), skin pigmentation change, and musculoskeletal impairment (joint/articular deposition) [71, 72].
- Hemochromatosis is a disease state of primary iron overload due to genetic defects of the *HFE* gene, resulting in decreased hepcidin production, and therefore lacking negative inhibition on iron absorption.
- Other rare mutations can involve hemojuvelin, hepcidin protein itself, transferrin receptor 2, and ferroportin, with various phenotypes and ranges in age and presentation [73].
- Secondary iron overload is most often a result of hematologic disorders, primarily chronic hemolytic anemias and disorders of ineffective erythropoiesis. Common disorders include severe thalassemia phenotypes (Hemoglobin H disease and Cooley's anemia), sickle cell disease, glucose-6-phosphate dehydrogenase deficiency, hereditary spherocytosis, pyruvate-kinase deficiency, and recurrent/refractory autoimmune hemolytic anemia [73, 74]. Disorders of erythropoiesis are rare,

including congenital dyserythropoietic anemias, sideroblastic anemia, myelodysplastic syndromes, Diamond Blackfan anemia, and aplastic anemia [74].

- Resultant iron overload is multifactorial. Transfusion-dependent patients receive 200–250 mg of iron from every unit of transfused blood compounding over time [71, 75]. Despite a state of iron overload, erythropoietic drive and increased marrow iron utilization may suppress hepcidin, promoting further enterocyte iron absorption [25, 74]. Other contributory mechanisms include oxidative stress and hypoxia-inducible factors [71, 76].

The standard of care for iron overload is with iron chelation, via three available formulations:

- Deferoxamine—short half-life, via continuous intravenous or subcutaneous administration.
- Deferasirox—intermediate half-life, via oral administration three times daily.
- Deferiprone—long half-life, via oral administration once daily [77].
- Chelated iron in this manner is excreted via biliary/fecal and urinary routes. Due to improved compliance and ease of administration, oral therapy has largely replaced IV therapy, treatment tailored according to magnetic resonance imaging of a patient's degree of iron overload [77–79].
- Adverse effect profiles differ among chelator formulation, which may result in switching to alternative agents. Deferoxamine is associated with injection site reactions, ocular and auditory toxicity, and slowing of bone growth, implying careful monitoring if used for pediatric patients [77, 80]. Defirasirox is commonly associated with dyspepsia, nausea, vomiting, and liver dysfunction. Deferiprone is associated with similar gastrointestinal symptoms and neutropenia/leukopenia [80].
- For iron overload *without* concern for anemia, induction and maintenance courses of phlebotomy remain the gold standard [72, 80].

Other Iron-Associated Disease States

- *Lead Poisoning*: Lead intake may predispose a patient to iron deficiency, through competitive inhibition of iron absorption. Lead may also exacerbate iron-deficient states by interfering with metabolic heme synthesis [81, 82]. Prevention of lead poisoning with early childhood screening is paramount. Low levels of poisoning should prompt environmental investigation into sources, while utilizing chelation therapy for high/life-threatening toxicity [83].
- *Atransferrinemia*: An extremely rare autosomal recessive deficiency of serum transferrin, atransferrinemia results in severe iron-deficiency anemia and iron overload in non-hematopoietic tissue. Life-threatening complications occur because of iron overloaded organ toxicity [84]. Treatment is via plasma infusions (as a source of transferrin), iron chelation therapy, with ongoing clinical trials assessing replacement therapy with apotransferrin [84, 85]
- *Aceruloplasminemia*: This is an extremely rare dysfunction of ceruloplasmin, required for iron efflux from macrophage stores. Patients develop microcytic anemia, with manifestations of iron overload, in addition to neuropsychiatric symptoms [84]. Treatment is via iron chelation and ongoing investigation into plasma infusions (as a source of ceruloplasmin) [86].

Appendix

Table 10.1 Recommended dietary allowance and tolerable upper intake levels for iron dependent on age and pregnancy/lactation

Age	Male (mg)	Female (mg)	Tolerable upper intake level (mg)
Birth–6 months old	0.27	0.27	40
7–12 months old	11	11	40
1–3 years old	7	7	40
4–8 years old	10	10	40
9–13 years old	8	8	40
14–18 years old	11	15	45
14–18 years old (pregnancy)		27	45
14–18 years old (lactation)		10	45
19–50 years old	8	18	45
19–50 years old (pregnancy)		27	45
19–50 years old (lactation)		9	45
51+ years old	8	8	45

Note: In the "birth to 6 month old" age range, current evidence is insufficient to develop an RDA, thus values are described as adequate intake (AI) [7]
Note: For vegetarians/vegans who do not have access to heme iron, the RDA values are multiplied by a factor of 1.8. This accounts for the lower bioavailability of nonheme iron (5–12%) as compared to heme-iron (14–18%) [3, 7, 8]

Table 10.2 Common sources of heme and nonheme iron in the pediatric diet [15]

Heme iron	Milligrams/ serving	Nonheme iron	Milligrams/ serving
Beef	2–3 mg (3 ounces)	Apricots, dried	1 mg (5 apricots)
Chicken, dark	1 mg (3 ounces)	Asparagus, cooked	1 mg (4 spears)
Chicken, white	1 mg (3 ounces)	Avocado	1–2 mg (1 avocado)
Clams	2–3 mg (3 ounces)	Bagel	3 mg (4 ounces)
Fish	0.2–2.5 mg (3 ounces)	Black-eyed peas	2 mg (1/2 cup)
Lamb	2 mg (3 ounces)	Bread, white	1 mg (1 slice)
Liver, beef	5 mg (3 ounces)	Bread, whole wheat	1 mg (1 slice)
Liver, chicken	10 mg (3 ounces)	Broccoli	1 mg (1/2 cup)
Oysters	8 mg (3 ounces)	Cashew nuts	2 mg (18 nuts)
Pork/ham	1 mg (3 ounces)	Chickpeas	2 mg (1/2 cup)
Sardines	2 mg (3 ounces)	Chocolate, dark (45–70%)	2 mg (1 ounce)
Shrimp	3 mg (3 ounces)	Egg, hard boiled	1 mg (1 large egg)
Tuna, canned	1 mg (3 ounces)	Fortified breakfast cereals	4–18 mg (1 cup)
Turkey	1–2 mg (3 ounces)	Garbanzo beans	2 mg (1/2 cup)
Veal	1 mg (3 ounces)	Green peas	1 mg (1/2 cup)
		Lentils	3 mg (1/2 cup)
		Macaroni, enriched, cooked	1–2 mg (1/2 cup)
		Molasses	1–3 mg (1 tbsp)
		Pistachio nuts	1 mg (49 nuts)
		Potato, baked with skin	2 mg (1 potato)
		Prune juice	3 mg (8 ounces)
		Pumpkin seeds	3 mg (1 ounce)
		Raisins, seedless	1 mg (1/4 cup)
		Red kidney beans	3 mg (1/2 cup)

Table 10.2 (continued)

Heme iron	Milligrams/ serving	Nonheme iron	Milligrams/ serving
		Rice, brown	1 mg (1 cup)
		Rice, enriched	1 mg (1/2 cup)
		Soy beans, cooked	5 mg (1/2 cup)
		Spaghetti, whole wheat	1 mg (1 cup)
		Spinach, boiled	3 mg (1/2 cup)
		Tofu, extra firm	2–3 mg (3 ounces)
		Tomatoes	2 mg (1/2 cup)
		Wheat germ, toasted	1 mg (2 tbsp)
		White beans	8 mg (1 cup)

References

1. Moscheo C, Licciardello M, Samperi P, La Spina M, Di Cataldo A, Russo G. New insights into iron deficiency anemia in children: a practical review. Meta. 2022;12(4):289.
2. Chifman J, Laubenbacher R, Torti SV. A systems biology approach to iron metabolism. Adv Exp Med Biol. 2014;844:201–25.
3. Hurrell R, Egli I. Iron bioavailability and dietary reference values. Am J Clin Nutr. 2010;91(5):1461S–7S.
4. Tong S, Vichinsky E. Iron deficiency: implications before anemia. Pediatr Rev. 2021;42(1):11–20.
5. DiMaggio DM, Cox A, Porto AF. Updates in infant nutrition. Pediatr Rev. 2017;38(10):449–62.
6. Petkus DL, Murray-Kolb LE, Scott SP, Southmayd EA, De Souza MJ. Iron status at opposite ends of the menstrual function spectrum. J Trace Elem Med Biol. 2019;51:169–75.
7. Trumbo P, Yates AA, Schliker S, Poos M. Dietary reference intakes: vitamin a, vitamin K, arsenic, boron, chromium, copper, iodine, iron, manganese, molybdenum, nickel, silicon, vanadium, and zinc. J Am Diet Assoc. 2001;101(3):294–301.
8. Pawlak R, Berger J, Hines I. Iron status of vegetarian adults: a review of literature. Am J Lifestyle Med. 2018;12(6):486–98.
9. Hurrell RF. Ensuring the efficacious iron fortification of foods: a tale of two barriers. Nutrients. 2022;14(8):1609.

10. Abrams SA, Hampton JC, Finn KL. A substantial proportion of 6- to 12-month-old infants have calculated daily absorbed iron below recommendations, especially those who are breastfed. J Pediatr. 2021;231:36–42.
11. Varea A, Disalvo L, Fasano MV, Sala M, Avico AJ, Azrack MA, Padula G, Gonzalez HF. Effectiveness of weekly and daily iron administration for the prevention of iron deficiency in infants. Arch Argent Pediatr. 2023;121(4):e202202815.
12. Khayat S, Fanaei H, Ghanbarzehi A. Minerals in pregnancy and lactation: a review article. J Clin Diagn Res. 2017;11(9):QE01–5.
13. Lindsay A. Multiple micronutrients in pregnancy and lactation: an overview. Am J Clin Nutr. 2005;81(5):1206S–12S.
14. Cao C, O'Brien KO. Pregnancy and iron homeostasis: an update. Nutr Rev. 2013 Jan;71(1):35–51.
15. U.S. Department of Agriculture, Agricultural Research Service, Beltsville Human Nutrition Research Center. Food Data Central. [Internet]. [cited 5/2024]. Available from https://fdc.nal.usda.gov/
16. Abbasi U, Abbina S, Gill A, Takuechi LE, Kizhakkedathu JN. Role of iron in the molecular pathogenesis of diseases and therapeutic opportunities. ACS Chem Biol. 2021;16(6):945–72.
17. Puig S, Ramos-Alonso L, Romero AM, Martinez-Pastor MT. The elemental role of iron in DNA synthesis and repair. Metallomics. 2017;9(11):1483–500.
18. Martin DR, Matyushov DV. Electron-transfer chain in respiratory complex I. Sci Rep. 2017;7(1):5495.
19. Abbaspour N, Hurrell R, Kelishadi R. Review on iron and its importance for human health. J Res Med Sci. 2014;19(2):164–74.
20. Chaibrando D, Mercurio S, Tolosano E. Heme and erythropoiesis: more than a structural role. Haematologica. 2014;99(6):973–83.
21. Gell DA. Structure and function of haemoglobins. Blood Cells Mol Dis. 2018;70:13–42.
22. Webb KL, Dominelli PB, Baker SE, Klassen SA, Joyner MJ, Senefeld JW, Wiggins CC. Influence of high hemoglobin-oxygen affinity on humans during hypoxia. Front Physiol. 2022;12:763933.
23. Kehrer JP. The Haber-Weiss reaction and mechanisms of toxicity. Toxicology. 2000;149(1):43–50.
24. Kaminskyy VO, Zhivotovsky B. Free radicals in cross talk between autophagy and apoptosis. Antioxid Redox Signal. 2014;21(1):86–102.
25. Wallace DF. The regulation of iron absorption and homeostasis. Clin Biochem Rev. 2016;37(2):51–62.
26. Conrad ME, Umbreit JN. Iron absorption and transport – an update. Am J Hematol. 2000;64(4):287–98.
27. Piskin E, Cianciosi D, Gulec S, Tomas M, Capanoglu E. Iron absorption: factors, limitations, and improvement methods. ACS Omega. 2022;7(24):20441–56.

28. Damian MT, Vulturar R, Login CC, Damian L, Chis A, Bojan A. Anemia in sports: a narrative review. Life (Basel). 2021;11(9):987.
29. Abioye AI, Okuneye TA, Odesanya O, et al. Calcium intake and iron status in human studies: a systematic review and dose-response meta-analysis of randomized trials and crossover studies. J Nutr. 2021;151(5):1084–101.
30. Saunders AV, Craig WJ, Baines SK, Posen JS. Iron and vegetarian diets. Med J Aust. 2013;199(S4):S11–6.
31. Kibangou IB, Bouhallab S, Henry G, Bureau F, Allouche S, Blais A, Guerin P, Arhan P, Bougle DL. Milk proteins and iron absorption: contrasting effects of different case in phosphopeptides. Pediatr Res. 2005;58(4):731–4.
32. Dosedel M, Jirkovsky EJ, Macakova K, Krcmova LK, Javorska L, Pourova J, Mercolini L, Remiao F, Novakova L, Mladenka P. Vitamin C – sources, physiological role, kinetics, deficiency, use, toxicity, and determination. Nutrients. 2021;13(2):615.
33. Owen DR, Owen DA. Celiac disease and other causes of Duodenitis. Arch Pathol Lab Med. 2018;142(1):35–43.
34. Nemeth E, Ganz T. Hepcidin-Ferroportin interaction controls systemic iron homeostasis. Int J Mol Sci. 2021;22(12):6493.
35. Agarwal AK, Yee J. Hepcidin. Adv Chronic Kidney Dis. 2019;26(4):298–305.
36. Rana S, Prabhakar N. Iron disorders and hepcidin. Clin Chim Acta. 2021;523:454–68.
37. Anderson GJ, Frazer DM, McKie AT, Vulpe CD. The ceruloplasmin homolog hephaestin and the control of intestinal iron absorption. Blood Cells Mol Dis. 2002;29(3):367–75.
38. Gomme PT, McCann KB, Bertolini J. Transferrin: structure, function and potential therapeutic actions. Drug Discov Today. 2005;10(4):267–73.
39. Yanatori I, Kishi F. DMT1 and iron transport. Free Radic Biol Med. 2019;133:55–63.
40. Brandsma MR, Jevnikar AM, Ma S. Recombinant human transferrin: beyond iron binding and transport. Biotechnol Adv. 2011;29(2):230–8.
41. Lesnikov V, Lesnikova M, Deeg HJ. Pro-apoptotic and anti-apoptotic effects of transferrin and transferrin-derived glycans on hematopoietic cells and lymphocytes. Exp Hematol. 2001;29(4):477–89.
42. Gao G, Li J, Zhang Y, Chang YZ. Cellular iron metabolism and regulation. Adv Exp Med Biol. 2019;1173:21–32.
43. Galy B, Conrad M, Muckenthaler M. Mechanisms controlling cellular and systemic iron homeostasis. Nat Rev Mol Cell Biol. 2024;25(2):133–55.
44. Rupani DN, Connell GJ. Transferrin receptor mRNA interactions contributing to iron homeostasis. RNA. 2016;22(8):1271–82.
45. Wang J, Pantopoulos K. Regulation of cellular iron metabolism. Biochem J. 2011;434(3):365–81.

46. Slusarczyk P, Mleczko-Sanecka K. The multiple facets of iron recycling. Genes (Basel). 2021;12(9):1364.
47. Beaumont C, Delaby C. Recycling of iron in normal and pathological states. Semin Hematol. 2009;46(4):328–38.
48. Kurz T, Eaton JW, Brunk UT. The role of lysosomes in iron metabolism and recycling. Int J Biochem Cell Biol. 2011;43(12):1686–97.
49. Pasricha SR, Tye-Din J, Muckenthaler MU, Swinkels DW. Iron deficiency. Lancet. 2021;397(10270):233–48.
50. World Health Organization. Haemoglobin concentrations for the diagnosis of anaemia and assessment of severity. Vitamin and Mineral Nutrition Information System; 2011. https://www.who.int/vmnis/indicators/haemoglobin.pdf
51. Kumar A, Sharma E, Marley A, Samaan MA, Brookes MJ. Iron deficiency anaemia: pathophysiology, assessment, practical management. BMJ Open Gastroenterol. 2022;9(1):e000759.
52. VanderMeulen H, Sholzberg M. Iron deficiency and anemia in patients with inherited bleeding disorders. Transfus Apher Sci. 2018;57(6):735–8.
53. Gattermann N, Muckenthaler MU, Kulozik AE, Metzgeroth G, Hastka J. The evaluation of iron deficiency and iron overload. Dtsch Arztebl Int. 2021;118(49):847–56.
54. De Falco L, Sanchez M, Silvestri L, Kannengiesser C, Muckenthaler MU, Iolascon A, Gouya L, Camaschella C, Beaumont C. Iron refractory iron deficiency anemia. Haematologica. 2013;98(6):845–53.
55. Keskin EY, Yenicesu I. Iron-refractory iron deficiency anemia. Turk J Haematol. 2015;32(1):1–14.
56. Cappellini MD, Musallam KM, Taher AT. Iron deficiency anaemia revisited. J Intern Med. 2020;287(2):153–70.
57. Leung AKC, Lam JM, Wong AHC, Hon KL, Li X. Iron deficiency anemia: an updated review. Curr Pediatr Rev. 2024;20(3):339–56.
58. Mattiello V, Schmugge M, Hengartner H, von der Weid N, Renella R. SPOG pediatric hematology working group. Diagnosis and management of iron deficiency in children with or without anemia: consensus recommendations of the SPOG pediatric hematology working group. Eur J Pediatr. 2020;179(4):527–45.
59. Camaschella C. Iron deficiency: new insights into diagnosis and treatment. Hematology Am Soc Hematol Educ Program. 2015;2015:8–13.
60. Plays M, Muller S, Rodriguez R. Chemistry and biology of ferritin. Metallomics. 2021;13(5):mfab021.
61. Elsayed ME, Sharif MU, Stack AG. Transferrin saturation: a body iron biomarker. Adv Clin Chem. 2016;75:71–97.
62. Pfeiffer CM, Looker AC. Laboratory methodologies for indicators of iron status: strengths, limitations, and analytical challenges. Am J Clin Nutri. 2017;106(Suppl 6):1606S–14S.
63. DeLoughery TG. Safety of Oral and intravenous iron. Acta Haematol. 2019;142(1):8–12.

64. Ning S, Zeller MP. Management of iron deficiency. Hematology Am Soc Hematol Educ Program. 2019;2019(1):315–22.
65. Richardson M. Microcytic anemia. Pediatr Rev. 2007;28(1):5–14.
66. Taylor S, Rampton D. Treatment of iron deficiency anemia: practical considerations. Pol Arch Med Wewn. 2015;125(6):452–60.
67. Koch TA, Myers J, Goodnough LT. Intravenous iron therapy in patients with iron deficiency anemia: dosing considerations. Anemia. 2015;2015:763576.
68. Ganzoni AM. Intravenous iron-dextran: therapeutic and experimental possibilities. Schweiz Med Wochenschr. 1970;100(7):301–3.
69. Blumenstein I, Shanbhag S, Langguth P, Kalra PA, Zoller H, Lim W. Newer formulations of intravenous iron: a review of their chemistry and key safety aspects – hypersensitivity, hypophosphatemia, and cardiovascular safety. Expert Opin Drug Saf. 2021;20(7):757–69.
70. Mcdougall IC, Vernon K. Complement activation-related pseudo-allergy: a fresh look at hypersensitivity reactions to intravenous iron. Am J Nephrol. 2017;45(1):60–2.
71. Fibach E, Rachmileqitz EA. Iron overload in hematological disorders. Presse Med. 2017;46(12 Pt 2):e296–305.
72. Bring P, Partovi N, Ford JAE, Yoshida EM. Iron overload disorders: treatment options for patients refractory to or intolerant of phlebotomy. Pharmacotherapy. 2008;28(3):331–42.
73. Brissot P, Pietrangelo A, Adams PC, de Graaff B, McLaren CE, Loreal O. Haemochromatosis. Nat Rev Dis Primers. 2018;4:18016.
74. Hsu CC, Senussi NH, Fertrin KY, Kowdley KV. Iron overload disorders. Hepatol Commun. 2022;6(8):1842–54.
75. Saliba A, Taher A. Iron overload in transfusion-dependent thalassemia. Hematology. 2015;20(5):311–2.
76. Xu M, Wang J, Xie J. Regulation of iron metabolism by hypoxia-inducible factors. Sheng Li Xue Bao. 2017;69(5):598–610.
77. Brissot P. Optimizing the diagnosis and the treatment of iron overload diseases. Expert Rev Gastroenterol Hepatol. 2016;10(3):359–70.
78. Borgna-Pignatti C, Marsella M. Iron chelation in thalassemia major. Clin Ther. 2015;37(12):2866–77.
79. Bruzzese A, Martino EA, Mendicino F, Lucia E, Olivito V, Bova C, Filippelli G, Capodanno I, Neri A, Morabito F, Gentile M, Vigna E. Iron chelation therapy. Eur J Haematol. 2023;110(5):490–7.
80. Entezari S, Haghi SM, Norouzkhani N, Sahebnazar B, Vosoughian F, Akbarzadeh D, Islampanah M, Naghsh N, Abbasalizadeh M, Deravi N. Iron Chelators in treatment of iron overload. J Toxicol. 2022;2022:1.
81. Kwong WT, Friello P, Semba RD. Interactions between iron deficiency and lead poisoning: epidemiology and pathogenesis. Sci Total Environ. 2004;330(1–3):21–37.

82. Hegazy AA, Zaher MM, El-Hafez MAA, Morsy AA, Saleh RA. Relation between anemia and blood levels of lead, copper, zinc and iron among children. BMC Res Notes. 2010;3:133.
83. Mayans L. Lead poisoning in children. Am Fam Physician. 2019;100(1):24–30.
84. Piperno A, Pelucchi S, Mariani R. Inherited iron overload disorders. Transl Gastroenterol Hepatol. 2020;5:25.
85. Hayashi A, Wada Y, Suzuki T, Shimizu A. Studies on familial hypotransferrinemia: unique clinical course and molecular pathology. Am J Hum Genet. 1993;53(1):201–13.
86. Piperno A, Alessio M. Aceruloplasminemia: waiting for an efficient therapy. Front Neurosci. 2018;12:903.

Calcium

11

Andrea Mucci

Calcium levels are tightly regulated both extracellularly, where it plays a central role in bone formation and turnover, and intracellularly, given its numerous roles in intracellular signaling (i.e., involved in hormone secretion, neuronal activation and muscular contraction) [1]. Serum calcium (Ca^{2+}) levels are tightly controlled along with inorganic phosphate (P_i) and magnesium (Mg) by a network of hormone regulators (parathyroid hormone (PTH), calcitriol, calcitonin, and FGF23). Meeting adequate dietary requirements of calcium is imperative for maintaining adequate calcium homeostasis and optimizing bone health. This is particularly important in medical conditions that impact calcium absorption or losses.

Dietary Calcium Intake

- Recommended daily allowance (RDA) for older children (>1 year) and adolescents are based on intakes associated with adequate bone accumulation and positive calcium balance.

A. Mucci (✉)
Section of Pediatric Endocrinology, Cleveland Clinic Children's Hospital, Cleveland, OH, USA
e-mail: MUCCIA@ccf.org

K. Radhakrishnan (ed.), *Handbook of Clinical and Practical Pediatric Nutrition*, https://doi.org/10.1007/978-3-031-97759-6_11

- Calcium RDA increases throughout childhood, and are maximal during adolescence (ages 9–18 years old) to allow for optimal bone accrual (Table 11.1).
- A wide range of foods contain calcium
  - Milk products are the major contributor in most diets but there are many nondairy-based foods that can also be calcium-fortified (cf) (Table 11.2, right column).
  - Diets not meeting the RDA are not uncommon, especially in low-income households, developing countries, or restrictive dietary practices.

Table 11.1 RDA calcium by age as recommended by the NIH [2]

Age	RDA calcium (mg)
0–6 months	200
7–12 months	260
1–3 years	700
4–8 years	1000
9–13 years	1300
14–18 years	1300
18–70 years	1000

Table 11.2 Calcium content and percent daily value (DV) including calcium-fortified (cf) [2]

Dairy-based food	mg/ serving	DV%	Non-dairy-based food	mg/ serving	DV%
Milk (1 cup)			Vegetables (1/2 cup)		
Whole (2.5% fat)	276	21	Spinach (boiled)	123	9
Nonfat	299	21	Broccoli (raw)	21	2
Yogurt (8 oz)			Canned fish with bones (3 oz)		
Low fat (plain)	415	32	Sardines	325	25
Low fat (fruit)	344	27	Salmon	181	14
Mozzarella (part skim) (1.5 oz)	333	26	Soymilk (1cup) (cf)	299	23
Cottage cheese (1 cup)			Breakfast cereals (cf)	130	10
Frozen yogurt (1/2 cup)	103	8	Orange juice (1 cup) (cf)	349	27

Dietary Calcium Absorption and Storage

- 30–80% of ingested calcium is absorbed.
  - Calcium is mostly absorbed in the upper portion of the small intestine, with lesser amounts form the middle and lower small intestine [3]
  - Passive paracellular absorption through tight junctions in intestinal epithelia is concentration and voltage dependent
    - Large role when there is adequate dietary calcium
  - Transcellular absorption in the apical epithelium or brush border of the enterocyte is facilitated through transient receptor potential (TRP) proteins, TRPV5 and TRPV6 [4]
    - Calbindins facilitate both the paracellular calcium transport, as well as binding to the Ca^{2+} on the apical aspect of the enterocyte [4]
    - Ca^{2+} pumps and $Na+/Ca^{2+}$ exchangers are responsible for active release of Ca^{2+} from the enterocytes to the lamina propria [4]
  - Calcitriol helps to align the intestinal absorption of calcium to the body's needs:
    - Calcium absorption is facilitated by protein, citrus, and leafy green vegetables
    - Calcium absorption is inhibited by phosphates and oxalates [3]
  - Low Ca^{2+} diets increase the intestinal Ca^{2+} absorption ratio by altering the role of vitamin D and the lipid composition (i.e., the fluidity of intestinal membranes) [4]
- Almost all the calcium in the initial glomerular filtrate is reabsorbed by the renal tubules.
  - Approximately 65% calcium in the glomerular filtrate is reabsorbed by transcellular mechanisms in the proximal convoluted and straight tubules (passively due to transepithelial voltage gradient); this is independent of PTH [1]

    - Low Ca^{2+} can promote renal calcium reabsorption by its reduced action on CaSR in the thick ascending loop in the distal convoluted tubule (DCT), as well as in the collecting duct [1]
- Total body calcium is mostly (98–99%) stored as mineral salts in the bone and is used as a reservoir for homeostasis [5]
  - Remainder of body calcium (900–100 mg) are circulating and in constant flux [6]
- Serum calcium circulates in three main fractions: free (or ionized) Ca^{2+} (30–50%), protein bound (30–50%), and complexes to with anions (5–15%), such as phosphate, citrate, or bicarbonate [5]
  - 70% of protein-bound calcium is bound to albumin; the degree of binding is pH dependent
    - For every 50% reduction in plasma albumin, the total calcium concentration decreases by 20% [5]

Calcium Physiology and Homeostasis

- Three hormones (PTH, calcitonin, and calcitriol (1α,25 $(OH)_2D_3$) and their interactions with target organs (mainly bone, gut, and kidney) are mostly responsible for regulating the extracellular homeostasis of calcium, phosphorus (and to lesser extent magnesium)
  - FGF23 is another important hormone in bone metabolism but is beyond the scope of this chapter since it does not have a direct impact on calcium but tightly regulates phosphorus (so discussed in more detail in Chapter "Phosphorus") (Table 11.3)

Table 11.3 Hormone regulation of calcium and phosphorus

	Bone	Intestine	Kidney	Overall impact
PTH Peptide hormone secreted in acute response to ionized calcium levels detected by the calcium sensing receptors (CaSR) in the parathyroid glands (inverse sigmoid relationship between extracellular Ca^{2+} and PTH secretion)	Enhances osteoclastic bone absorption resulting in calcium mobilization	Minimal direct effects (mostly via impact of PTH on kidney hydroxylation of 25(OH)vit D to calcitriol (see below)	Promotes calcium reabsorption from distal renal tubule, including the cortical thick ascending look of Henle (TAL) where its PTH binds to PTHR1, increasing Na/K/2Cl-transporter activity, resulting in reabsorption of calcium, sodium, chloride, and magnesium [1] Inhibits phosphorus reabsorption, mostly proximal tubules with fine tuning in TAL)	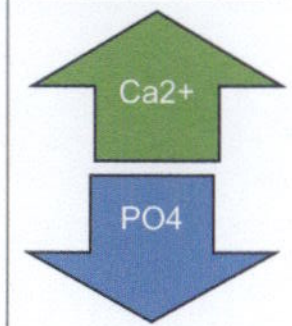
Calcitriol (1α,25 $(OH)_2D_3$) Activated form of vitamin D released in low calcium states PTHR1 in proximal renal tubule increases hydroxylation of 25-OH-vit D to 1α,25 $(OH)_2D_3$ Actions via gene transcription via nuclear vitamin D receptor (VDR)		Activates VDR in the intestine to facilitating active transcellular calcium reabsorption in the small intestine via TRPV6, followed by intracellular calcium transport and extrusion	Renal tubular calcium reabsorption (mainly driven by PTH via reduced CaSR stimulation as noted above) is also enhanced by calcitonin-stimulated expression of calbindin-D28K in the distal tubules	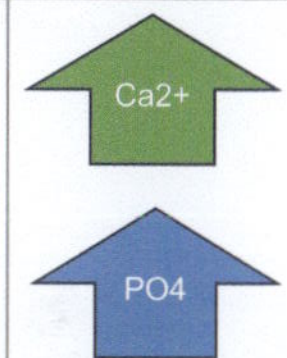

(continued)

Table 11.3 (continued)

	Bone	Intestine	Kidney	Overall impact
Calcitonin Polypeptide that is secreted by parafollicular cells of thyroid in linear response to calcium levels -gastrin is a potent stimulator of calcitonin Overall physiological role remains uncertain	Directly inhibits bone reabsorption leading to decrease in serum calcium		Increases calcium excretion in urine	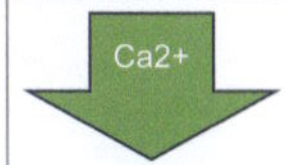

Hypocalcemia: Common Pediatric Causes and Management

Neonatal Hypocalcemia

Neonatal hypocalcemia is relatively common and most commonly transient [6].

- Early onset (<3–4 days of life): typically seen in infants born to mothers with diabetes mellitus or prematurity mainly attributable to functional hypoparathyroidism
  - Treatment indicated if the total serum Ca <8 mg/dL in term infants or premature infants <1500 g or < 7.5 mg/dL in premature infants <1500 g
    - Supplement calcium carbonate while ensuring overall ratio of calcium:phosphate intake of 4:1. May consider a low phosphate formula (e.g., SimilacPM 60/40) [7]
    - Maintain urinary calcium: creatinine ratio <0.2 to minimize risk of nephrocalcinosis and other complications [7]
- Late onset (5–10 days of life): mostly seen in term infants due to excessive phosphate intake in infants who are fed cow's milk or cow's milk-based infant formulas
  - Immature kidney function and/or transiently low PTH may also contribute
  - Maternal factors (hyperparathyroidism, phenytoin, or phenobarbital use) may also contribute
  - Iatrogenic causes include use of citrated blood products and lipid infusions
- Usually self resolves after 2–4 weeks and does not need treatment
- If severe or requiring acute treatment, maintenance of oral calcium supplementation can be considered with or without calcitriol, but is typically only needed for a short period
  - For details about calcium supplementation in TPN-dependent infants, see Chap. 6
- If a non-transient cause may require ongoing treatment, as noted below

Hypocalcemia of Infancy and Childhood

Broadly speaking, in most cases, hypocalcemia can be considered as being related to hypoparathyroidism

- Vitamin D deficiency
  - Hypocalcemia is the most feared side effect of severe vitamin D deficiency
  - In addition to considering maternal vitamin D in infancy, inadequate intake (i.e., lack of supplementation in exclusively breastfed infants) should be considered
    - If adequate vitamin D intake is confirmed, consider malabsorption etiology
    - Other risk factors include lack of sunlight exposure and dark pigmentation to skin
  - In severe deficiency (25(OH)vit D < 10 ng/dL), stoss therapy is typically used before transitioning to daily maintenance (see Chap. 32)
- Hypoparathyroidism
  - Common causes include genetics (i.e., DiGeorge or 22q11 deletion syndrome) or post-thyroidectomy
  - Oral supplementation with calcium, calcitriol, and vitamin D supplementation are the mainstays of chronic management
    - Elemental calcium: 30–75 mg/kg/day divided in four daily doses with meals [7]
      - Typically, calcium carbonate (such as that found in TUMS) is used

        calcium carbonate contains 40% elemental calcium
    - Calcitriol: initial dose is typically 20–100 ng/kg/g
      - Some suggest starting 0.25 μg per day and raising the dose in increments of 0.25 μg every 3 days until targets are reached [6]
    - Vitamin D: due to inability of PTH to activate vitamin D, supplementation is indicated

    - Monitoring: since there is high risk for calcium–phosphate precipitation, once calcium is normalized, calcium × phosphate product should be kept <55 to minimize deposition in kidney, basal ganglia, and optic lens [6, 7]
- Other causes of hypocalcemia may have specific treatments including magnesium supplementation if low (see Chap. 13)
    - Recombinant human PTH (rh-PTH) is approved for treatment of various hypoparathyroid states in adults but is not FDA-approved for use in children (Table 11.4)

Table 11.4 Causes of hypocalcemia throughout infancy, childhood, and adolescence

Neonatal hypocalcemia	Hypocalcemia in childhood and adolescence
Early (1–4 days of age) Prematurity Maternal diabetes Perinatal stress IUGR Maternal hyperparathyroidism or anticonvulsants	**High PTH** Pseudohypoparathyroidism Vitamin D deficiency Calcipenic rickets
Late (5–15 days of age) Maternal vitamin D deficiency Alkalosis Pseudohypoparathyroidism Genetic (1α-OHD or VDR mutations)	**Low PTH** Hypoparathyroidism 22q11 deletion syndrome Post-thyroidectomy Hypomagnesemia
	Increased urinary calcium Hypercalciuric hypocalcemia Fanconi syndrome
	Chronic diseases Malabsorption Liver disease Nephrotic syndrome, renal failure

Hypercalcemia

- Causes of hypercalcemia in children can be contributed to a wide array of factors including genetic, vitamin D toxicity, hyperparathyroidism, and malignancy among other causes.
- Treatment of the underlying cause whenever possible is first line
- In infants with hypercalcemia (such as in Williams syndrome), low-calcium formula such as Calcilo should be considered, and in older patients a calcium-restricted diet
- In severe or symptomatic hypercalcemia (Table 11.5), various measures including bisphosphonates, glucocorticoids, or diuretics can be considered depending on the cause

Table 11.5 Causes of hypercalcemia in childhood

Hypercalcemia
High PTH/inappropriately "normal"
Hyperparathyroidism
MEN1, MEN2
Familial hypocalciuric hypercalcemia
Low PTH
Vitamin D or A excess
Hypophosphatasia
Malignancy
Granulomatous disease
Genetic (Williams-Beuren, down syndrome)
Iatrogenic
Immobilization
Adrenal insufficiency
Hyperthyroidism
Renal failure

References

1. Bilezikian JP, Walker MD, Binkley N, Goltzman D, Mannstadt M. Hormones and disorders of mineral metabolism. In: Schlomo M, Auchus RJ, Goldfine AB, Rosen CJ, Kopp PA, editors. Williams textbook of endocrinology. 15th ed. Elsevier; 2025. p. 1171–226.
2. National Institutes of Health (NIH) Office of Dietary Supplements (ODS). Calcium: Fact sheet for Health Professionals [Internet]. 2024 [cited 2024 Jul 31]. Available from: https://ods.od.nih.gov/factsheets/Calcium-HealthProfessional/.
3. Barrett KE, Barman SM, Brooks HL, Yuan JX-J. Digestion & absorption of nutrients. In: Ganong's review of medical physiology, 26e [internet]. McGraw-Hill Education: New York; 2019. Available from: https://accessmedicine.mhmedical.com/content.aspx?aid=1159054070
4. Pérez AV, Picotto G, Carpentieri AR, Rivoira MA, Peralta López ME, Tolosa De Talamoni NG. Minireview on regulation of intestinal calcium absorption: emphasis on molecular mechanisms of transcellular pathway. Digestion. 2008;77(1):22–34.
5. Diaz R. Calcium disorders in children and adolescents. In: Lifshitz F, editor. Pediatric endocrinology: growth, adrenal, sexual, thyroid, calcium, and fluid balance disorders. 5th ed. CRC Press; 2017.
6. Ward LM, Konji VN, Ma J, Munns CF, Petryk A, Polgreen LE, et al. Disorders of calcium, phosphate, and bone metabolism. In: Sarafoglou K, Hoffmann GF, Roth KS, editors. Pediatric endocrinology and inborn errors of metabolism, 2e [internet]. New York: McGraw-Hill Education; 2017. Available from: accesspediatrics.mhmedical.com/content.aspx?aid=1140322197.
7. Root AW, Levine MA, Disorders of Mineral Metabolism II. Abnormalities of mineral homeostasis in the newborn, infant, child, and adolescent. In: Sperling M, Majzoub JA, Menon RK, Stratakis CA, editors. Sperling pediatric endocrinology. 5th ed. Philadelphia: Elsevier; 2021.

Phosphorus

12

Anuradha Viswanathan

Introduction

Phosphorus is present in human body in both organic and inorganic forms. Organic forms are bound to fats, sugars, and proteins and inorganic forms are complexed with sodium, calcium, and magnesium. It is an essential component of DNA, RNA nucleotides, critical for generation, utilization, and storage of energy in the form of ATP, is part of cell membranes, cell signaling pathways, and is a component of bone mineral [1].

Distribution Within the Body

- 85% in bone as hydroxyapatite
- 14% intracellular
- 1% interstitial fluids and serum.

A. Viswanathan (✉)
Section of Pediatric Endocrinology, Cleveland Clinic Children's Hospital, Cleveland Clinic Learner College of Medicine, Case Western Reserve University, Cleveland, OH, USA
e-mail: viswana2@ccf.org

K. Radhakrishnan (ed.), *Handbook of Clinical and Practical Pediatric Nutrition*, https://doi.org/10.1007/978-3-031-97759-6_12

Table 12.1 Normal serum concentrations of phosphate (measured as phosphorus) by age [2]

Age	Phosphate levels (mg/dL)
Neonate	4.8–8.2
1–3 years	3.8–6.5
4–11 years	3.7–5.6
12–15 years	2.9–5.4
16–19 years	2.7–4.7
Adults	2.5–4.5

Serum concentration is affected by balance between intake and excretion and dynamic shifts between intra- and extracellular spaces and formation and resorption of hydroxyapatite in bone. Normal serum levels are noted as in Table 12.1.

Dietary Sources of Phosphate and Recommended Daily Allowances (Tables 12.2 and 12.3)

- Phosphorus is almost ubiquitously available through dietary sources.
- Main sources include dairy, meat, grains, and food additives.
- It is more readily absorbed from animal products.
- Phosphate in plant-based sources is available as phytates and is less bioavailable as human gut lacks phytases.

Table 12.2 Dietary sources [3]

Food	Milligrams (mg) per serving	Percent DV[a]
Yogurt, plain, low fat, 6-ounce container	245	20
Milk, 2% milkfat, 1 cup	226	18
Salmon, Atlantic, farmed, cooked, 3 ounces	214	17
Scallops, breaded and fried, 3 ounces	201	16
Cheese, mozzarella, part skim, 1.5 ounces	197	16
Chicken, breast meat, roasted, 3 ounces	182	15
Lentils, boiled, ½ cup	178	14
Beef patty, ground, 90% lean meat, broiled, 3 ounces	172	14
Cashew nuts, dry roasted, 1 ounce	139	11
Potatoes, russet, flesh and skin, baked, 1 medium	123	10
Kidney beans, canned, ½ cup	115	9
Rice, brown, long grain, cooked, ½ cup	102	8
Peas, green, boiled, ½ cup	94	8
Oatmeal, cooked with water, ½ cup	90	7
Egg, hard boiled, 1 large	86	7
Tortillas, corn, 1 medium	82	7
Bread, whole wheat, 1 slice	60	5
Sesame seeds, 1 tablespoon	57	5
Bread, pita, whole wheat, 4-inch pita	50	4
Asparagus, boiled, ½ cup	49	4
Tomatoes, ripe, chopped, ½ cup	22	2
Apple, 1 medium	20	2
Cauliflower, boiled, 1″ pieces, ½ cup	20	2
Beverages, carbonated, cola, 1 cup	18	1
Clementine, 1 medium	16	1
Tea, green, brewed, 1 cup	0	0

[a]DV = daily value for phosphorus is 1250 mg for adults and children over 4 years of age

Table 12.3 Recommended dietary allowances (RDAs) for phosphorus [3]

Age	Male (mg)	Female (mg)	Pregnancy(mg)	Lactation (mg)
Birth to 6 months[a]	100	100		
7–12 months[a]	275	275		
1–3 years	460	460		
4–8 years	500	500		
9–13 years	1250	1250		
14–18 years	1250	1250	1250	1250
19+ years	700	700	700	700

[a]Adequate Intake

Table 12.4 Receptors involved in active transport of phosphorus in the gut

Area of absorption	Receptor	Gene
Duodenum and jejunum	NaPi2b, PiT1, PiT2	SLC34A2, SLC20A1, SLC20A2

Intestinal Absorption

- It is mainly absorbed in the small intestine—duodenum and jejunum through paracellular diffusion in between tight junctions.
- This is the main mode of absorption during normal or high availability of dietary phosphate.
- Active intracellular transport in intestines is mediated by transporters (as noted in Table 12.4) in the apical surfaces and is stimulated by calcitriol, estrogen, and acidosis.
- Glucocorticoids decrease phosphate absorption.
- Active transport is important during periods of low dietary availability of phosphate [4].

Table 12.5 Receptors involved in renal reabsorption of phosphorus

Area of absorption	Receptor	Gene
PCT—80% of absorption	NaPi2a, NaPi2c, PiT2	SLC34A1, SLC34A3, SLC20A2

Renal Excretion

- Most people consume more than average recommended daily allowance (RDA) of phosphorus through diet.
- Therefore, levels are mainly controlled via excretion through kidneys.
- Nearly 60–70% of filtered phosphate is absorbed back in the proximal tubules. Further absorption (10–15%) occurs in the distal tubules as well.
- Reabsorption in renal tubules is mainly regulated by NaPi2a and NaPi2c receptors as noted in Table 12.5. PiT receptors also play a minor role [5, 6].

Hormonal Control of Serum Phosphorus Levels

- Various hormones and factors control serum phosphorus levels such as parathyroid hormone (PTH), 1, 25-dihydroxy vitamin D, Fibroblast growth factor 23 (FGF23), α-klotho, growth hormone and insulin-like growth factor, thyroid hormone, etc. (Tables 12.6 and 12.7).
- Of these, PTH and FGF23 are primary regulators of serum phosphorus levels.
- Hypo- and hyperkalemia and acidosis and alkalosis also influence serum levels [7].

Table 12.6 Effect of different hormones on serum phosphorus levels and their action on various tissues

	Bone	Kidney	Intestine	Net effect
PTH	↑ Through bone resorption	↓↓ Through phosphaturia	↑ Indirect effect through increasing 1, 25 $(OH)_2D$	↓↓ (Phosphaturic effect predominates)
1, 25 $(OH)_2D$			↑↑	↑ Through increased intestinal absorption
FGF 23 (secreted from osteocytes and osteoblasts)		↓↓↓		↓↓↓

Table 12.7 Interaction between the various hormones

	PTH	1, 25 $(OH)_2D$	FGF23
PTH		↑	↑
1, 25 $(OH)_2D$	↓		↑
FGF23	↓	↓	

Sensing of Phosphorus

- The main receptor for sensing seems to be the CasR (calcium sensing receptor) present in the parathyroid glands.
- If serum phosphorus levels rise, then there is enhanced PTH release, which lead to phosphaturia [8].

Effect of Primary Hyperphosphatemia

- Elevated serum phosphorus level directly increases PTH and FGF 23 levels to increase phosphaturia.

- High phosphorus usually suppresses 1, 25-dihydroxy vitamin D level.
- However, severe acute increase in phosphate level will cause lowering of serum calcium level due to increased calcium phosphate binding, which will then increase PTH and calcitriol.

Causes of Hypophosphatemia [9, 10]

Due to Decreased Intestinal Absorption

- Premature infants fed exclusive breast milk due to low phosphate content of breast milk, starvation, anorexia, malabsorption due to celiac, Crohn's disease, chronic diarrhea or persistent vomiting, vitamin D deficiency or resistance and use of phosphate binders such as calcium, aluminum, or magnesium containing antacids or newer phosphate binders such as sevelamer.

Due to Increased Renal Loss

- Hyperparathyroidism, renal tubular defects such as Fanconi syndrome, osmotic diuresis such as uncontrolled diabetes and diabetic ketoacidosis, drugs such as diuretics, glucocorticoids, cisplatin, ifosamide. Genetic conditions resulting in primary tubular defects in phosphate transporters such as NaPi2a and 2c resulting in some types of autosomal recessive (AR) hypophosphatemic rickets.
- Increased renal loss due to excess FGF 23: fibrous dysplasia, McCune Albright syndrome, oncogenic or tumor-induced osteomalacia, X-linked dominant hypophosphatemic rickets due to PHEX gene mutation, autosomal dominant (AD) hypophosphatemic rickets due to FGF23 activating mutations, AR hypophosphatemic rickets due to DMP1 and ENPP1 mutations [11].

Due to Cellular Shift of Phosphate into Cells

- Refeeding, insulin therapy in uncontrolled diabetes and diabetic ketoacidosis, hungry bone syndrome, respiratory alkalosis, hyperventilation, sepsis, salicylate intoxication.

Clinical Features

- Mild hypophosphatemia may be clinically asymptomatic.
- Severe acute hypophosphatemia (serum Phos levels <1 mg/dL): symptoms are mainly due to energy depletion due to decreased ATP generation—muscle weakness including respiratory muscles leading to respiratory failure, tremors, seizures, neuropathies, bone pain and bone loss, hemolysis, anemia, metabolic acidosis, and insulin resistance.
- Chronic hypophosphatemia results in rickets and osteomalacia.

Causes of Hyperphosphatemia [9, 10]

- *Increased phosphate load*: Phosphate containing laxatives and enemas, vitamin D excess.
- *Decreased excretion*: Hypoparathyroidism, pseudohypoparathyroidism, renal failure, growth hormone excess, hyperthyroidism, tumoral calcinosis, genetic causes such as loss of function mutations in FGF23, GALNT3 mutations, leading to accelerated degradation of FGF23.
- *Cellular shift* of phosphate into the extracellular space: rhabdomyolysis, hemolysis, tumor lysis, crush injuries, respiratory or metabolic acidosis, malignant hyperthermia.

Clinical Features [10]

- Hyperphosphatemia causes hypocalcemia and symptoms related to hypocalcemia including tetany, stridor, respiratory distress, seizures.

- Chronic gradual rise: can cause ectopic calcifications of vessels, increased cardiovascular mortality and morbidity.

Lab Evaluation [10]

- Serum phosphorus, calcium, alkaline phosphatase, magnesium, PTH, 25-hydroxy vitamin D and 1, 25-dihydroxy vitamin D level, FGF 23 levels.
- Spot urine phosphorus and urine creatinine levels, tubular reabsorption of phosphate (TRP).

  TRP can be calculated using the formula as follows:

$$\text{TRP} = 1 - \frac{\text{Urinary phosphorus} \times \text{Serum creatinine}}{\text{Urinary creatinine} \times \text{Serum phosphorus}}$$

Treatment [10]

Hypophosphatemia

- Acute severe: will need IV repletion.
- Chronic mild: oral phosphate supplements.
- If FGF 23 mediated, may need calcitriol as well.
- Recently, FGF 23-mediated conditions are managed via FGF23 antibody—burosumab with good benefits [12]

Hyperphosphatemia

- Reduced intake/dietary restriction.
- Addition of phosphate binders such as sevelamer, calcium carbonate.
- Hydration.

Specific Pediatric Conditions

Osteopenia or Metabolic Bone Disease (MBD) of Prematurity

- Poor mineral accrual due to preterm delivery and reduced movement against the uterus wall decreases bone mineralization in preterm infants.
- Develops within 6–16 weeks after birth.
- Hypophosphatemia and elevated alkaline phosphatase levels are noted.
- Alkaline phosphatase greater than 500 IU/L and serum phosphorus less than 5.6 mg/dL are suggestive of MBD.
- Tubular reabsorption of phosphorus (TRP) >95% is suggestive of depleted phosphorus stores and phosphate supplementation is indicated.
- Total requirement of phosphate may range between 50 and 100 mg/kg/day.
- Additionally, calcium supplementation may also be needed especially if PTH level is elevated. Total calcium requirement can be up to 120–200 mg/kg/day [13, 14].

References

1. Wagner CA. The basics of phosphate metabolism. Nephrol Dial Transplant. 2024;39(2):190–201.
2. Root AW. Disorders of mineral metabolism: normal homeostasis. In: Sperling pediatric endocrinology. Elsevier; 2021. p. 220–78.
3. National Institutes of Health, Office of Dietary Supplements. Phosphorus – Health Professional Fact Sheet. Health Professional Fact Sheet; 2023. p. 1.
4. Peacock M. Phosphate metabolism in health and disease. Calcif Tissue Int. 2021;108(1):3–15.
5. Blaine J, Chonchol M, Levi M. Renal control of calcium, phosphate, and magnesium homeostasis. Clin J Am Soc Nephrol. 2015;10(7):1257–72.
6. Walker V. The intricacies of renal phosphate reabsorption – an overview. Int J Mol Sci. 2024;25(9)

7. Lederer E. Regulation of serum phosphate. J Physiol. 2014;592(18):3985–95.
8. Zechner C, Rhee EP. Phosphate sensing in health and disease. Curr Opin Nephrol Hypertens. 2024;33(4):361–7.
9. Root AW, Levine MA. Disorders of mineral metabolism II. Abnormalities of mineral homeostasis in the newborn, infant, child, and adolescent. In: Sperling pediatric endocrinology. Elsevier; 2021. p. 705–813.
10. Ward LM, et al. Bone fragility disorders in childhood and adolescence. In: Paediatric endocrinology: management of endocrine disorders in children and adolescents. Cham: Springer International Publishing; 2024. p. 1–47.
11. Bitzan M, Goodyer PR. Hypophosphatemic rickets. Pediatr Clin N Am. 2019;66(1):179–207.
12. Baroncelli GI, Grandone A, Aversa A, Sessa MR, Pelosini C, Michelucci A, et al. Safety and efficacy of burosumab in improving phosphate metabolism, bone health, and quality of life in adolescents with X-linked hypophosphatemic rickets. Eur J Med Genet. 2024;70(May):104958.
13. Rayannavar A, Calabria AC. Screening for metabolic bone disease of prematurity. Semin Fetal Neonatal Med. 2020;25(1):101086.
14. Kehinde F, Marinescu A, Turchi R. Catch it before it breaks!: managing metabolic bone disease of prematurity. Curr Opin Pediatr. 2021;33(6):676–83.

Magnesium 13

Andrew R. Lavik

Magnesium: Recommended Dietary Allowance (RDA)

- The recommended dietary allowance (RDA) for magnesium is detailed in Table 13.1.

Table 13.1 Recommended dietary allowance for magnesium

Age	Male and female RDAs	
0–6 months	30 mg[a]	
7–12 months	75 mg[a]	
1–3 years	80 mg	
4–8 years	130 mg	
9–13 years	240 mg	
	Male RDA	**Female RDA**
14–18 years	410 mg	360 mg
19–30 years	400 mg	310 mg

[a]Denotes adequate intake, the level of daily intake assumed to ensure nutritional adequacy in age groups where there is insufficient evidence to determine an RDA

A. R. Lavik (✉)
Section of Pediatric Endocrinology, Cleveland Clinic Children's Hospital, Cleveland, OH, USA
e-mail: lavika2@ccf.org

K. Radhakrishnan (ed.), *Handbook of Clinical and Practical Pediatric Nutrition*, https://doi.org/10.1007/978-3-031-97759-6_13

Recommended Dietary Allowance (RDA) for Magnesium [1]

RDA: The average daily level of magnesium intake that is sufficient to meet the nutrition requirements of 97–98% of healthy individuals in the respective group.

Physiology

Body Distribution

- Magnesium is the fourth most abundant electrolyte in the body after calcium, potassium, and sodium [2].
- Total body magnesium content by age is detailed in Table 13.2.

- Total Body Magnesium.
  - ~99% in bone, muscle, and non-muscle soft tissue [2, 3]
    - Bone comprises ~60% of total body magnesium: complexed with calcium and phosphorus in hydroxyapatite crystals [2, 3]
      - About 30% of bone magnesium exists as an exchangeable pool that functions to stabilize serum magnesium concentrations [2, 3]
    - Within cells, ~95% of magnesium is bound to ligands such as ATP, ADP, nucleic acids, and proteins, while the remainder is free ionized magnesium [4]
  - ~1% is extracellular and exists in three states [4, 5]:

Table 13.2 Total body magnesium content by age

	Total body magnesium
Birth	760 mg
4–5 months	5 g
Adulthood	20–28 g

- Ionized magnesium (60% of the extracellular magnesium): as with calcium, *ionized magnesium is the only physiologically active form of magnesium.*
- Protein bound (30%): primarily bound to albumin and often linked via free fatty acids.
- Complexed to serum anions (10%) such as phosphate, bicarbonate, citrate, or sulfate.

Functions of Magnesium

- In cells:
  - Magnesium is the second most prevalent intracellular cation after potassium [4, 5]
  - Magnesium is an essential cofactor in 600+ enzymatic reactions, including ALL reactions involving ATP and ATPases [2, 4, 5]
  - Magnesium can be considered "nature's calcium blocker" [4]: magnesium plays an important role in regulating all functions dependent on intracellular calcium signaling [5]
  - Magnesium regulates metabolism of glucose, proteins, and lipids [2, 4] and utilization of nutrients such as B vitamins, vitamin D, and glutathione [3]
  - Magnesium complexes with proteins, nucleic acids, and ribosomes and is integral to DNA and RNA production and stability [2, 3]
  - Magnesium is important for intracellular signal transduction, specifically through regulation of various ion channels and tyrosine kinases (including growth factors) [2, 3]. Like calcium, magnesium is also an intracellular second messenger [4]
- In tissues:
  - Magnesium is a key structural component of bone [3]
  - Magnesium regulates muscle contraction and relaxation, including of the cardiovascular system [3] such as contractility of cardiomyocytes and vasodilatory function of endothelial cells [2]

  - Magnesium regulates ion channels involved in cardiac action potentials, thereby modulating cardiomyocyte excitation, cardiac signal transduction, contraction, and risk of arrhythmias [2]
  - Magnesium regulates neurotransmitter release and action potential conduction [3]
- In general:
  - Magnesium is essential for regulating calcium and phosphorus levels in the body as well as vitamin D function.
    - Magnesium is essential for the synthesis and secretion of parathyroid hormone (PTH), which in turn regulates total body calcium and phosphorus; thus, *hypomagnesemia must be corrected before hypocalcemia can be corrected* [2, 4]
    - Magnesium is needed to produce the biologically active form of vitamin D [2]

Magnesium Hemostasis

- Like calcium, total body magnesium is maintained by the following three mechanisms [2]:

  1. Intestinal absorption.
  2. Renal excretion/reabsorption.
  3. Reversible exchange from the body pool of magnesium (primarily bones).

Intestinal Absorption

- Magnesium is primarily absorbed as an ion through the small intestine with a small percentage being absorbed in the colon [2]
- Magnesium absorption is dependent on total body magnesium status, not dietary intake of magnesium [3, 6]

- Magnesium absorption occurs by two mechanisms:
  - Passive paracellular diffusion through tight junctions between intestinal epithelial cells.
    - Accounts for 80–90% of total magnesium absorption [3, 6]
    - Major absorption mechanism used in small intestine with regions of highest absorption in ileum and distal jejunum [3]
  - Active transcellular transport via magnesium transporters and channels.
    - Accounts for 10–20% of total magnesium absorption.
    - Key transporters/channels: TRPM6, TRPM7 (most selective for magnesium), MAGT1, SLC41A1, SLC41A2, SLC41A3, CNNM1-4, MRS2, and paracellin-1 [2, 6]
    - Primarily occurs in the colon via TRPM6 (and to some degree TRPM7) [4, 6]
    - Uptake can be actively enhanced if dietary magnesium intake is poor (from ~25% uptake of all dietary magnesium to ~75%) in order to maintain magnesium homeostasis [5–7]

Nutritional Sources of Magnesium

- About 10% of daily magnesium intake can occur through water ingestion, though magnesium content of water can vary widely depending on water mineral content/hardness [2, 3]
- Unrefined sea salt is an excellent dietary source of magnesium [2]
- Unrefined whole grains, nuts, cocoa, and dark chocolate are also good dietary sources of magnesium [2]
- Legumes, fruit (especially some dried fruits), fish, meat, and milk contain a moderate amount of magnesium [2, 3]
- Most non-milk dairy products are low in magnesium [3]
- Considerable nutritional magnesium is lost as more foods are processed or refined [2]

- Foods high in calcium decrease intestinal magnesium absorption [2]
- Phosphorus in carbonated beverages and phosphate additives in processed meats decrease intestinal magnesium absorption due to the formation of phosphate–magnesium salts [2]
- Green leafy vegetables have historically been considered high in magnesium, but recent reports suggest that actual magnesium absorption from these sources is relatively insignificant [2]

Renal Excretion

- Regulation of magnesium excretion in the kidneys is critical to maintaining serum magnesium homeostasis. This is a highly modifiable process [3]
- Under physiologic conditions, ~95% of plasma magnesium filtered by the glomeruli is reabsorbed (fractional/tubular reabsorption of magnesium = ~95%) and ~ 3–5% is excreted in the urine [3]
- In states of magnesium deficiency, renal reabsorption of magnesium can increase to 99.5%, leading to daily renal magnesium losses as low as 12 mg [2, 5]
- In hypermagnesemia states or in the setting of low glomerular filtration rate, renal magnesium reabsorption can fall to nearly zero [5]
- Magnesium handling in the nephron:
  - *Proximal tubule*: location of ~20% of magnesium reabsorption; primarily by paracellular transport [3, 4]
  - *Loop of Henle*: ~70% of magnesium reabsorption, primarily in the thick ascending limb of the loop of Henle; also by paracellular transport [3]
  - *Distal convoluted tubule*: ~10% of renal magnesium reabsorption; where "fine-tuning" of reabsorption occurs; process occurs via transcellular transport by proteins TRPM6 and TRPM7 [4]

- Magnesium reabsorption and excretion is regulated by:
  - Hormones, like estrogen, parathyroid hormone (PTH), calcitonin, and epidermal growth factor (EGF) [3, 6]
  - Membrane receptors, like the calcium-sensing receptor (CaSR) [6]
  - Other factors that regulate concentration gradients and membrane potentials in the renal collecting system, like acid–base status [3, 6]

Bone Matrix Homeostasis

- About 30% of bone magnesium exists as an exchangeable pool (like calcium) that functions to stabilize serum magnesium concentrations [2, 3]

Evaluation of Magnesium/Magnesium Measurement

- Serum magnesium is **NOT** an accurate estimation of total body magnesium stores, yet (1) it is commonly assessed and (2) is accepted as the standard for laboratory magnesium status evaluation [2, 3]
  - Like calcium, serum magnesium content is affected by serum albumin level and sample preparation (i.e., hemolysis, specimen tube EDTA content) [4]
- Urinary magnesium is a poor indicator of total body magnesium since magnesium excretion is highly dependent on endogenous and exogenous factors [2]
- Ionized magnesium (unlike ionized calcium) is not routinely measured at present but may become more standard in the future [5, 6]
- Assessment of bone and tissue magnesium is impractical [2]
- **A practical approach for determining magnesium status is to evaluate serum magnesium while also considering dietary magnesium intake, bone health, and urinary losses.**

Pathophysiology: Hypomagnesemia

Definition: Hypomagnesemia

- Serum magnesium concentration below 0.70–0.85 mmol/L (<1.7 mg/dL), though as noted before, serum magnesium is not a perfect reflection of total body magnesium [2–4]
- Hypomagnesemia is much more common than hypermagnesemia; present in 3–10% of full-grown individuals, especially those hospitalized and in intensive care units or with type 2 diabetes [4]
- Hypomagnesemia is often a result of chronic low magnesium ingestion and/or excess magnesium losses [4]
- Hypomagnesemia is associated with an overall increased risk of death as well as death specifically from a cardiovascular cause [4]

Causes: Hypomagnesemia

- Extra-renal causes:
  - Chronic low oral magnesium ingestion (rare since magnesium is widely abundant in foods) [2, 5]
  - Individuals dependent on parenteral nutrition [5]
  - Low intestinal magnesium absorption (Crohn's disease, ulcerative colitis, celiac disease, short bowel syndrome, chronic diarrhea, other syndromes resulting in significant bowel inflammation or steatorrhea) [3]
  - Refeeding syndrome [8]
  - Magnesium losses by another non-renal mechanism [3]
    - Endocrine causes:
      - Hyperaldosteronism.
      - Hyperthyroidism.
      - Hyperparathyroidism.
      - "Hungry Bone Syndrome" in which acute changes in parathyroid hormone, vitamin D, and/or other bone constituents cause rapid magnesium sequestration in bone and symptomatic serum hypomagnesemia [5]

    - Excess vomiting (rare but reported) [5]
    - Excess skin losses in burn victims [5]
    - Physical activity [2]
- Renal causes: All caused by excess renal magnesium losses/ renal magnesium wasting:
  - Autoimmune, specifically autoantibodies against claudin-16 [4]
  - Chronic renal failure.
  - Dialysis [3]
  - Genetic syndromes [3]:
    - Autosomal dominant hypomagnesemia (KCNA1).
    - Bartter syndrome.
    - Familial hypomagnesemia with hypercalciuria and nephrocalcinosis (claudin-16 mutation).
    - Familial hypomagnesemia with secondary hypocalcemia (TRPM6 mutation).
    - Gitelman syndrome (Na-Cl-cotransporter mutation).
    - Isolated autosomal recessive hypomagnesemia (EGF/ EGFR mutation).
    - Isolated dominant hypomagnesemia (Na/K-ATPase mutation).
    - Maturity-onset diabetes of the young 5 (MODY5; HNF1B mutation).
    - SeSAME syndrome (KCNJ10 mutation).
- Medications (**mechanism may be renal or extra-renal depending on implicated agent**) [2–4]:
  - Antibiotics (aminoglycosides).
  - Antifungals (amphotericin B).
  - Antimicrobials (pentamidine).
  - Antivirals (foscarnet).
  - Beta adrenergic agonists (fenoterol, salbutamol, theophylline).
  - Biologics.
  - Bisphosphonates (pamidronate).
  - Cardiac medications (digitalis).
  - Chemotherapeutics.
  - Diuretics (loop diuretics, thiazide diuretics, amiloride).
  - Immunosuppressants (i.e., tacrolimus, cyclosporine).

  - Insulin.
  - Monoclonal antibodies (cetuximab, panitumumab).
  - Proton pump inhibitors.
- Renal tubular damage:
  - Acute tubular necrosis.
  - Urinary tract obstruction.
  - Delayed renal allograft function.

Clinical Manifestations: Hypomagnesemia

- Often associated with other electrolyte abnormalities (hypocalcemia, hypokalemia, hyponatremia, metabolic alkalosis) [4, 5]
- Often nonspecific signs/symptoms.
- Chronic hypomagnesemia has been implicated in multiple disorders including insulin resistance, type 2 diabetes, attention-deficit hyperactivity disorder, psychiatric disorders, fractures, and low bone mineral density [2, 3]
- Mild (serum magnesium 1.2–1.7 mg/dL or 0.5 mmol/L–0.7 mmol/L): fatigue, weakness, nausea, vomiting, loss of appetite, insulin resistance, suppression of PTH release, and end-organ PTH resistance [2, 5]
  - **Remember, hypomagnesemia may present with signs and symptoms of hypocalcemia that are persistent until hypomagnesemia is corrected.**
- Moderate-to-severe (serum magnesium <1.2 mg/dL or ≤ 0.5 mmol/L): neuromuscular irritability (including positive Trousseau's and Chvostek's signs despite normal serum calcium), muscle cramping, muscle spasms, paresthesia, tremors, personality changes, carpopedal and coronary spasms, tetany, nystagmus, arrhythmias including torsades de pointes, vasodilation/vasoconstriction abnormalities, or seizure, severe hypocalcemia, hypokalemia, or death [2, 4]

Evaluation: Hypomagnesemia

- Perform a comprehensive assessment to determine the underlying cause of hypomagnesemia; see causes above.

- Determine exposure to medications that can cause hypomagnesemia.
- Assess current and prior dietary magnesium content.

- Obtain:
  - Serum magnesium and other electrolytes.
  - Assess kidney function (creatinine, blood urea nitrogen).
  - Assess acid–base status.
  - Consider PTH, thyroid function, urine studies (urine magnesium, urine creatinine, urine specific gravity).
  - Consider electrocardiogram (ECG) +/− telemetry monitoring.
- Determine renal magnesium handling: Are the kidneys appropriately maximally reabsorbing magnesium, or are they wasting magnesium in the urine? [5]
  - Option 1: Fractional Excretion of Magnesium (FE-Magnesium) [5]

$$FE - Mg2+ = \frac{\left(\text{Magnesium}\left[\text{urine}\right] \times \text{Creatinine}\left[\text{serum}\right]\right)}{\left(0.7 \times \text{Magnesium}\left[\text{serum}\right] \times \text{Creatinine}\left[\text{urine}\right]\right)} \times 100$$

    - FE-Magnesium >2% indicates inappropriate renal wasting.
    - FE-Magnesium <2% indicates appropriate renal reabsorption.
  - Option 2: Total Magnesium in 24-h Urine Collection.
    - 24-h urine magnesium of 12 mg or less in a full-grown adult: suggests an intact renal response to low serum magnesium [5]
    - 24-h urine magnesium of 24 mg greater in a full-grown adult: suggests inappropriate renal magnesium wasting [5]

Management: Hypomagnesemia

- Discontinue the offending agent, if identified.
- If symptomatic hypomagnesemia, treat with IV magnesium (typically magnesium sulfate).
  - Guidelines for full-size adults recommend administering 8–12 g of magnesium sulfate in the first 24 h followed by 4–6 g daily for 3–4 days thereafter to replete body magnesium stores [5]
  - Dosing in pediatric patients should be adjusted accordingly.
  - Use IV magnesium replacement cautiously in individuals with renal impairment: use dose reductions of 50–75%. Monitor serum magnesium levels and deep tendon reflexes closely for signs of serum hypermagnesemia (a decrease in deep tendon reflexes suggest hypermagnesemia) [5]
- Once acute symptoms of hypomagnesemia resolve and IV magnesium is no longer necessary, transition to oral magnesium supplementation, if possible:
  - Inorganic magnesium salts (magnesium chloride, oxide, sulfate).
    - less bioavailable than organic magnesium compounds [2]
  - Organic magnesium compounds (magnesium citrate, malate, pidolate, taurate).
    - more bioavailable than inorganic magnesium salts [2]
  - Target daily magnesium intake of 4–6 mg/kg/day or higher for long-term repletion of magnesium stores; may take 20–40 weeks of supplementation for magnesium stores to reach steady state [2, 3]
  - Since intestinal absorption of different formulations of enteral magnesium varies widely, some patients with poor response to one formulation of magnesium may respond well to another [5]
  - *Note of caution*: unabsorbed magnesium salts cause diarrhea and laxative effects (due to osmotic activity and stimulation of gut motility) [2]

- Potassium-sparing diuretics (or other medications noted earlier that promote renal magnesium retention) may be useful in mitigating chronic renal magnesium wasting by facilitating magnesium reabsorption [5]

Pathophysiology: Hypermagnesemia

Definition

- Serum magnesium >2.55 mg/dL (>1.05 mmol/L):
- Hypermagnesemia is very rare; typically occurs:
  - in individuals with chronic kidney disease who receive magnesium-retaining medications [3, 4] and,
  - in individuals who receive high dose magnesium for other medical reasons [4]
- The renal system typically responds to hypermagnesemia by increasing baseline urinary magnesium excretion from 3–5% to nearly 100% [5]; hence, hypermagnesemia is only seen:
  - in patients with chronic kidney disease and,
  - when magnesium loads are so high that magnesium content rises despite maximal urinary magnesium excretion,

Causes: Hypermagnesemia

- If **renal function is normal, suspect iatrogenic cause:**
- Renal dysfunction:
  - Acute kidney injury [6]
  - Chronic kidney disease [6]
  - Other conditions that reduce renal excretion of magnesium: hyperparathyroidism, adrenal insufficiency, hypothyroidism [6]
- Increased intestinal absorption:
  - Bowel pathology (constipation managed with magnesium containing laxatives, inflammatory bowel disease, GI

bleeding, gastritis, colitis) may lead to breakdown of intestinal epithelium and/or slowed transit time, both of which can lead to increased intestinal magnesium absorption [5, 6]

- Medications:
  - Parenteral magnesium infusions, such as for tocolysis for women in labor, acute headache management, acute asthma exacerbation therapy (1 report) [4–6, 9]
  - Excess oral magnesium supplementation.
  - Magnesium-containing enemas [5]
  - Angiotensin-converting enzyme inhibitors [6]
  - Antacids [5]
  - Anticholinergics [6]
  - Accidental ingestion of Epsom salts [5]
  - Laxative abuse [5]
  - Milk alkali syndrome [6]
  - Nonsteroidal anti-inflammatory drugs (NSAIDs) [6]
- Magnesium leak into extracellular fluid:
  - Hemolysis, such as in tumor lysis syndrome [6]
  - Rhabdomyolysis [6]
  - Metabolic acidosis (movement of magnesium from intracellular to extracellular space) [6]
- Genetic:
  - Familial hypocalciuric hypercalcemia: autosomal dominant disorder in which calcium sensing receptor has altered function, leading to increased renal calcium and magnesium reabsorption [5, 6]

Clinical Manifestations: Hypermagnesemia [6]

- Symptoms based on levels of magnesium are detailed in Table 13.3.

Table 13.3 Symptoms of hypermagnesemia based at various magnesium levels

Serum magnesium 2.55–5.35 mg/dL (1.05–2.2 mmol/L):
Well-tolerated, no symptoms or nonspecific symptoms.
Serum magnesium 5.35–8.5 mg/dL (2.2–3.5 mmol/L):
Nausea/vomiting
Dizziness
Weakness
Slight confusion
Serum magnesium 8.5–15.8 mg/dL (3.5–6.5 mmol/L):
Worsening confusion, drowsiness
Headaches, blurred vision
Flushing
GI problems
Urinary problems (bladder paralysis)
Depressed reflexes
Mild decrease in blood pressure
Serum magnesium 15.8–21.1 mg/dL (6.5–8.7 mmol/L):
Respiratory depression
Muscle paralysis
Paralytic ileus
Hypotension
Cardiac changes: Sinus bradycardia, prolonged PR and QRS intervals, A-V block, possible ST elevation and prominent T waves
Serum magnesium >21.1 mg/dL (>8.7 mmol/L):
Seizure, coma
Asystole, cardiac arrest

Evaluation: Hypermagnesemia [6]

- Perform a comprehensive assessment to determine the underlying cause of hypermagnesemia (see causes above).
  - Determine exposure to therapies containing magnesium.
- Obtain:
  - Serum magnesium and other electrolytes.
  - Assess kidney function (creatinine, blood urea nitrogen).
  - Assess acid–base status.

  - Consider PTH, thyroid function, urine studies (urine magnesium, urine creatinine, urine specific gravity).
  - Consider ECG +/− telemetry monitoring.

Management: Hypermagnesemia

- Discontinue the offending agent, if identified [5]
- Consider normal saline infusion at 1.5–2 times maintenance fluid rate to facilitate renal magnesium excretion [6]
- If severe symptomatic hypermagnesemia, consider acute management with parenteral elemental calcium infusion (as calcium gluconate or calcium chloride).
  - In a full-grown individual, a loading dose of 1 g calcium given over 2–5 min followed by 100–200 mg over 5–10 min can improve hypotension and respiratory depression [5]
    - Mechanism: counteract effects of excess magnesium in neuromuscular junction and heart [5]
- Consider increasing magnesium excretion:
  - If renal function intact, consider loop diuretic (i.e., furosemide at 1 mg/kg) in combination with intravenous saline infusion (to prevent electrolyte imbalance) [5]
  - If renal impairment/failure, use hemodialysis or peritoneal dialysis: often can remove 50% serum magnesium in 3–4 h of treatment [5, 6]
    - Note: monitor calcium levels during dialysis as hypocalcemia can occur, which worsens signs and symptoms of hypermagnesemia [6]

Future Directions: Magnesium

- Magnesium is a common micronutrient implicated in a wide variety of physiologic processes, yet accurate methods to measure total body magnesium are lacking, limiting our understanding of this nutrient.

- It is likely that, in the near future, additional methods of magnesium measurement (i.e., determination of ionized magnesium content) will move beyond the research field and achieve wider acceptance among clinical laboratories. In addition, new techniques for evaluating total body magnesium content may be developed.
- Together, these new tools will help to broaden our understanding of magnesium as an essential micronutrient in human health, increase the number of diseases in which magnesium abnormalities are known to occur, and may lead to new treatment strategies for common conditions.

References

1. Health NIo. Magnesium: Fact Sheet for Health Professionals2022 8/30/2024. Available from: https://ods.od.nih.gov/factsheets/Magnesium-HealthProfessional/
2. Fiorentini D, Cappadone C, Farruggia G, Prata C. Magnesium: biochemistry, nutrition, detection, and social impact of diseases linked to its deficiency. Nutrients. 2021;13(4)
3. Gröber U, Schmidt J, Kisters K. Magnesium in prevention and therapy. Nutrients. 2015;7(9):8199–226.
4. Touyz RM, de Baaij JHF, Hoenderop JGJ. Magnesium disorders. N Engl J Med. 2024;390(21):1998–2009.
5. Topf JM, Murray PT. Hypomagnesemia and hypermagnesemia. Rev Endocr Metab Disord. 2003;4(2):195–206.
6. Aal-Hamad AH, Al-Alawi AM, Kashoub MS, Falhammar H. Hypermagnesemia in clinical practice. Medicina. 2023;59(7):1190.
7. Reddy ST, Soman SS, Yee J. Magnesium balance and measurement. Adv Chronic Kidney Dis. 2018;25(3):224–9.
8. da Silva JSV, Seres DS, Sabino K, Adams SC, Berdahl GJ, Citty SW, et al. ASPEN consensus recommendations for refeeding syndrome. Nutr Clin Pract. 2020;35(2):178–95.
9. Ambrożej D, Adamiec A, Forno E, Orzołek I, Feleszko W, Castro-Rodriguez JA. Intravenous magnesium sulfate for asthma exacerbations in children: systematic review with meta-analysis. Paediatr Respir Rev. 2024;52:23.

Copper

14

Anthony Anani

Introduction

The transition metal copper is an essential micronutrient involved in many enzymatic processes that require redox-chemistry. The redox-activity of copper is potentially harmful. Therefore, intracellular Cu concentration is kept at a relatively low range, and moderate increases can cause cytotoxicity and even lead to cell death; thus, the uptake, distribution, and elimination of Cu are tightly regulated.

Copper is acquired from the diet by intestinal absorption and is subsequently distributed throughout the body. About 0.6–1.6 mg of dietary copper is absorbed from the gut per day, with 50% of dietary copper absorbed. A high copper content will reduce absorption. About 4.5 mg is excreted into the gastrointestinal (GI) system in bile and pancreatic juice and about 0.5–2.5 mg is lost in stool [1].

A. Anani (✉)
Department of Pediatric Gastroenterology, Cook Children's Medical Center Prosper, Prosper, TX, USA
e-mail: Anthony.Anani@cookchildrens.org

K. Radhakrishnan (ed.), *Handbook of Clinical and Practical Pediatric Nutrition*, https://doi.org/10.1007/978-3-031-97759-6_14

Copper (Cu) is an essential micronutrient that acts as a catalytic cofactor in a wide range of biological processes:

- mitochondrial respiration,
- antioxidant defense,
- bio-compound synthesis, neurotransmitter synthesis,
- iron metabolism.

In the following sections of this chapter, we will highlight its metabolism, functions, deficiency states, and an excess of copper, as well as genetic disorders of copper metabolism.

Dietary Sources of Copper

- The richest dietary copper sources include shellfish, seeds and nuts, organ meats, wheat-bran cereals, whole-grain products, and chocolate.
- The absorption of copper is strongly influenced by the amount of copper in the diet; bioavailability ranges from 75% of dietary copper when the diet contains only 400 mcg/day to 12% when the diet contains 7.5 mg/day.
- Tap water and other beverages can also be sources of copper, although the amount of copper in these liquids varies by source (ranging from 0.0005 mg/L to 1 mg/L).

Several food sources of copper are listed in Table 14.1.

Table 14.1 Dietary sources of copper

Food	Micrograms (mcg) per serving	Percent DV[a]
Beef, liver, pan fried (3 ounces)	12,400	1378
Oysters, eastern, wild, cooked, 3 ounces	4850	539
Baking chocolate, unsweetened, 1 ounce	938	104
Potatoes, cooked, flesh and skin, 1 medium potato	675	75
Mushrooms, shiitake, cooked, cut pieces, ½ cup	650	72
Cashew nuts, dry roasted, 1 ounce	629	70
Crab, Dungeness, cooked, 3 ounces	624	69
Sunflower seed kernels, toasted, ¼ cup	615	68
Turkey, giblets, simmered, 3 ounces	588	65
Chocolate, dark, 70–85% cacao solids, 1 ounce	501	56
Tofu, raw, firm, ½ cup	476	53
Chickpeas, mature sees, ½ cup	289	32
Millet, cooked, 1 cup	280	31
Salmon, Atlantic, wild, cooked, 3 ounces	273	30
Pasta, whole wheat, cooked, 1 cup (not packed)	263	29
Avocado, raw, ½ cup	219	24
Figs, dried, ½ cup	214	24
Spinach, boiled, drained, ½ cup	157	17
Asparagus, cooked, drained, ½ cup	149	17
Sesame seeds, ¼ cup	147	16
Turkey, ground, cooked, 3 ounces	128	14
Cereal, cream of wheat, cooked with water, stove top, 1 cup	104	12
Tomatoes, raw, chopped, ½ cup	53	6
Yogurt, Greek, plain, low fat, 7-ounce container	42	5
Milk, nonfat, 1 cup	27	3
Apples, raw, with skin, ½ cup slices	17	2

[a]*DV* daily value

- The U.S. Food and Drug Administration (FDA) developed DVs to help consumers compare the nutrient contents of foods and dietary supplements within the context of a total diet.
- The DV for copper is 0.9 mg (900 mcg) for adults and children age 4 years and older. FDA does not require food labels to list copper content unless copper has been added to the food.
- Foods providing 20% or more of the DV are considered to be high sources of a nutrient, but foods providing lower percentages of the DV also contribute to a healthful diet.
- The U.S. Department of Agriculture's (USDA's) FoodData Central lists the nutrient content of many foods.

Copper Metabolism

Copper absorption and metabolism follows the path below:

Duodenum — > portal circulation — > liver — > blood stream — > target tissues/organs

Duodenum

- Copper transport protein (CTR1) located on the apical side of enterocyte takes the monovalent copper reduced from divalent copper by the action of metalloreductase (six-transmembrane epithelial antigen of the prostrate (STEAP) and duodenal cytochrome b reductase (DCYTB)). Transported out of the enterocytes by Cu-ATPase7A (ATP7A) is found in most cells except the liver [2].

Portal Circulation

- Cu is secreted into the bloodstream and bound to soluble proteins (albumin, transcuprein, histidines, macroglobulins).

Liver

- As the blood flows through the liver, the hepatocytes mediate the uptake of Cu via CTR1. As it moves through the cytoplasm of the hepatocyte, enzymatic activities occur. Cu is either chelated by metallothionen for storage or delivered by Cu chaperones to specific proteins. [2]
- The principal Cu chaperones include COX17 (which delivers Cu to cytochrome *c* oxygenase), CCS (Cu chaperone for superoxide dismutase, which delivers Cu to superoxide dismutase 1), and ATOX1 (which delivers Cu to ATP7A and ATP7B). [2]
- The Cu-ATPases (ATP7B in the case of hepatocytes) pump Cu ions from the liver back into the blood, where it again binds to soluble chaperones and is transported to specific tissues and organs [2].

Target Tissues/Organs

- Copper catalyzes reactions in a wide range of physiological processes, including mitochondrial energy production, tyrosine and neurotransmitter metabolism, redox homeostasis, and extracellular matrix remodeling.
- In the body, Cu is stored primarily in the liver, and excess of Cu is eliminated in the feces, either through biliary excretion or as unabsorbed metal ions. Other pathways for Cu elimination such as urine, sweat, and menses play a relatively minor role in Cu loss. Taken together, the systemic Cu status is regulated by duodenal absorption and/or biliary excretion [1].
- The Cu-ATPases ATP7A and ATP7B act as the major transporter for exporting cellular Cu.

ATP7A and ATP7B: copper transporters that play a vital role in copper homeostasis and the normal functioning.

- ATP7A is expressed in most tissues/organs, with the exception of the liver, where ATP7B is found to be predominantly expressed [2].
- In other tissues such as the placenta and the blood–brain barrier (BBB), ATP7A mediates the transport of Cu across polarized cells to ensure adequate Cu is delivered for the development of the fetus and brain.
- In the liver, ATP7B mobilizes Cu in secretory vesicles to the bile in order to prevent the accumulation of Cu.
- Severe imbalance of copper homeostasis can occur with some hereditary disorders of copper metabolism due to mutations in ATP7A and ATP7B, which have been recognized as Menkes disease (MD) and Wilson's disease (WD), respectively [2].

Functions/Uses of Copper in the Body [1, 2, 5, 6]

1. Collagen synthesis:
    - Cofactor for lysine oxidase.
    - Important for collagen crosslinking.
    - In severe deficiency, tissue ends up losing tensile strength.
2. Cathecolamines:
    - Copper has an active role in norepinephrine and epinephrine synthesis.
    - Cofactor for dopamine β hydroxylase.
3. Energy metabolism:
    - Copper is important component of cytochrome oxidase.
    - Copper is also important for myelin synthesis—through cytochrome oxidase.
4. Pigment metabolism:
    - Tyrosinase requires copper as a cofactor in the synthesis of melanin in the melanocyte.
5. Iron metabolism: via ceruloplasmin.

- Ceruloplasmin has ferroxidase activity that converts ferrous to ferric ions.
- Four proteins with ferroxidase activity:

(a) Ceruloplasmin,
(b) Membrane bound ceruloplasmin,
(c) Haephastin (basal layer on enterocytes), and.
(d) Zyklopen (placenta).

6. Indirect anti-oxidant properties:
   - Through superoxide dismutase.
   - Ceruloplasmin: By binding copper (being a transitional element) and by reducing iron from ferrous to ferric state and thereby reducing free iron.

Copper Deficiency

Copper deficiency was first described in 1930. The median time from symptoms to diagnosis is about 12 months. Latent copper deficiency occurs 3 months after starting enteral nutrition and manifestations can be hematological or neurological or both [8].

Causes

- Nutritional causes and malnutrition alone in general may be seen but uncommon.
- Zinc toxicity by inducing metallothionein.
- Prematurity with GI complications with less than optimal supplementation.
- After gastric bypass surgery.
- High enterostomy—jejunostomy with excess loss.
- Parenteral/enteral nutrition with inadequate copper supplementation.

Manifestations

- *Hematologic*: decreased oxidation of ferrous to ferric that leads to decreased hemoglobin synthesis: [3]
  - (a) Anemia usually microcytic.
  - (b) Leucopenia–neutropenia.
  - (c) Occasional pancytopenia.
  - (d) Bone marrow changes that could be similar to myelodysplasia.
- *Neurologic*: it can cause myelopathy—copper deficiency myelopathy with motor findings. [7]

Copper Excess

If we are unable to excrete or metabolize copper appropriately, it can cause cell injury from free radical release. Excess copper in the body may be due to our ability to excrete or transport copper.

- High copper content in diet or water source.
- Excess intake when on long-term parenteral nutrition.
- Long-standing cholestatic liver disease when copper intake is not reduced—Wilson's disease (see below).
- Accidental ingestion/suicide attempt can also lead to excess and toxicity to cells.

Genetic Disorders of Copper Metabolism

1. Wilson's disease.
2. Menke disease.
3. Occipital horn syndrome (Milder Alleic variant of Menkes).
4. Distal hereditary motor neuropathy.
5. Aceruloplasminemia.
6. Mednik Syndrome.
7. Huppke–Brendal syndrome.

Wilson's Disease

- A classic example of a Cu-overload condition is Wilson's disease (WD), an autosomal recessive disorder characterized by a variety of mutations in the ATP7B gene.
- The resulting impaired ATP7B function impairs Cu excretion and leads to persistent Cu accumulation in the brain, liver, and other tissues.
- In healthy individuals, hepatic Cu content is generally <55 μg/g dry weight; in patients with WD, hepatic Cu can exceed 250 μg/g dry weight.
- We advise readers to familiarize with the diagnostic aspects of Wilson's disease, which is beyond the scope of this chapter.

Symptoms

Hepatic symptoms

- Fulminant hepatic failure (also known as acute liver failure).
- Persistently elevated levels of serum aminotransferases.
- Jaundice.
- Chronic hepatitis.

Neurological symptoms

- Tremors.
- akinetic-rigid syndrome (Parkinsonism),
- Ataxia.
- Dystonia.
- Other common neurological findings can include dysarthria, spasticity, and a lack of motor coordination. Structural brain MRI scans in patients with MD have shown widespread lesions in the midbrain, putamen, pons, globus pallidus, thalamus, and cerebellum, as well as cortical atrophy. Loss of neurons and the occurrence of abnormal astrocytes are typical neuropathological features in patients with WD.

- Hepatic Cu accumulation will likely lead to the development of hepatic cirrhosis or even fulminant liver failure. In most cases of WD, Cu deposition can be observed in the cornea known as Kayser–Fleischer rings, representing as an ophthalmic manifestation of the disease.
- Non-hepatic and non-neuronal complications associated with WD include osteomalacia, osteoarthritis, hemolysis, cardiac arrhythmia, and renal abnormalities—tubular dysfunction.

Treatment

- Oral zinc to decrease Cu absorption.
- Chelating agents such as D-penicillamine and trientine.
- The choice of treatment generally depends on the disease stage, with Cu chelators recommended for patients with advanced symptomatology.
- Evidence is limited regarding the strategy of restricting dietary Cu for treating WD.

Menkes Disease (MD) [9]

- MD is an X-linked recessive disease that affects Cu metabolism and is caused by mutations in the ATP7A gene.
- The resulting loss of functional ATP7A in the intestine leads to reduced Cu efflux into the blood, an accumulation of Cu in enterocytes, and generalized severe systemic Cu deficiency.
- Almost always manifests in the first 2–3 months of life.
- The disorder was first described in 1962.
- MD is a fatal disorder, and affected patients usually die in early childhood.

Symptoms

- Mental retardation.
- Hypothermia.

- Neuronal degeneration and seizures (from catecholamine deficiency).
- Dysautonomia.
- Bone fractures.
- Hair abnormalities—short, sparse, and twisted.
  - Microscopy—pili torti.
  - Trichoclasis—transverse fracture of shaft.
  - Trichoptilosis—longitudinal fracture of hair.
- Skin abnormalities.
  - Pale skin + loose folds of skin, particularly around neck, axillae, and trunk.
  - Pale skin from decreased melanin synthesis.
  - Sagging cheeks and relatively larger ears.
- Widespread vascular abnormalities.

Diagnosis

- Primarily through genetic screen.
- Plasma copper, ceruloplasmin, and plasma catecholamine are reduced.

Treatment

- Cu salts such as Cu-histidine complexes, subcutaneously injected bypassing the malfunctioning intestinal absorption.
- Notably, treatment has been shown to be effective in patients in which the mutated ATP7A protein that retains the ability to transport Cu across the BBB.
- Early diagnosis and treatment can exhibit gross improvements (fine neuronal development and motor movement) vs. late diagnosis and treatment with a poor prognosis.
- Better general neurological outcome in asymptomatic patients compared to symptomatic patients.

Occipital Horn Syndrome (Milder Allelic Variant of Menkes) [4, 9]

- Similar hair and connective tissue abnormalities as in Menkes.
- Occipital exostosis—at the insertion of trapezius and sterno-cleidomastoid.
- Plasma copper, ceruloplasmin, and plasma catecholamine reduced.
- Though plasma copper may be low to low, normal copper therapy is recommended, if possible early before neurological defects manifest.
- Questionable role of levo-dihydrophenylserine to bolster epinephrine levels by bypassing dopamine-β-hydroxylase.

Distal Hereditary Motor Neuropathy [9]

- Mutation in ATP7A—affects intracellular trafficking.
- Distal muscle weakness—curly fingers and pes cavus.
- Absent reflexes.
- No other biochemical findings like Menke.

Aceruloplasminemia [10]

- Gene on chromosome 3. First detected in 1987.
- Most patients have hardly any detectable cerruloplasmin.
- Most patients are homozygous. Occasional patient may have some ceruloplasmin level (apoceruloplasmin).
- Rarely, heterozygotes may become symptomatic.
- Most patients become symptomatic in fourth and fifth decade.

Symptoms

- Neurological—start after 40 s.
  - Ataxia.
  - Abnormal movement—dystonia/chorea/tremors.
  - Parkinsonism like symptoms.

- Diabetes or abnormal glucose control—as early as 30 s.
- Retinal degeneration.
- Anemia.
  - Elevated ferritin.
  - Low iron and iron refractory anemia.
- Low copper and normal 24 h urine copper.

Treatment

- Desferrioxamine chelation.
  - May induce anemia, so short therapies advised.
  - Deferiprone—no clear role.
  - Deferasirox (oral agent)—may help if others do work well.
  - Best response if started early.
- Role of plasma therapy (to provide ceruloplasmin) + chelation—some patients may benefit.
- Zinc chelation?

MEDNIK Syndrome [11, 12]

- **M**ental Retardation, **E**nteropathy, **D**eafness, Peripheral **N**europathy, **I**cthyosis, **K**eratoderma.
- Mutation in α1A component of Adaptor Protein 1 (AP1).
- Important in Clathrin coat assembly and transvesicular Golgi transport.
- Recently, mutation in β subunit of AP-1 protein also causes the same disorder.
- Basically impairs intracellular trafficking of ATP7A (possibly ATP7B).
- Patients have low copper and normal ceruloplasmin.

Huppke–Brendal Syndrome [13]

- Characterized by.
  - Deafness—sensorineural.
  - Bilateral cataract and ocular lenz dislocation.
  - Severe developmental delay.
- Low copper and ceruloplasmin.
- Mutation involving SLC33A1—involved in acetylation and secretion of ceruloplasmin.

Referees

1. van den Berghe PVE, Klomp LWJ. New developments in the regulation of intestinal copper absorption. Nutr Rev. 2009;67(11):658–72. https://doi.org/10.1111/j.1753-4887.2009.00250.x.
2. Chen L, Min J, Wang F. Copper homeostasis and cuproptosis in health and disease. Signal Transduct Target Ther. 2022;7:378. https://doi.org/10.1038/s41392-022-01229-y.
3. Myint ZW, Oo TH, Thein KZ, Tun AM, Saeed H. Copper deficiency anemia: review article. Ann Hematol. 2018;97(9):1527–34. https://doi.org/10.1007/s00277-018-3407-5.
4. Chen J, Jiang Y, Shi H, et al. The molecular mechanisms of copper metabolism and its roles in human diseases. Pflugers Arch Eur J Physiol. 2020;472:1415–29. https://doi.org/10.1007/s00424-020-02412-2.
5. Tapiero H, Townsend DM, Tew KD. Trace elements in human physiology and pathology: zinc and metallothioneins. Biomed Pharmacother. 2003;57(9):386–98. https://doi.org/10.1016/S0753-3322(03)00012-X.
6. Ali SA, Naaz I. Biochemical aspects of mammalian melanocytes and the emerging role of melanocyte stem cells in dermatological therapies. Int J Health Sci (Qassim). 2018;12(1):69–76.
7. Jaiser SR, Winston GP. Subacute combined degeneration due to copper deficiency. J Neuroimaging. 2008;18:345. https://doi.org/10.1111/j.1552-6569.2007.00235.x.
8. Ito Y, Ando T, Nabeshima T. Recovery and maintenance of copper levels in geriatric patients on enteral feeding for a prolonged period. J Nutr Sci Vitaminol. 2006;52(3):200–4.
9. Kaler SG. Inborn errors of copper metabolism. In: Handbook of clinical neurology, vol. 113; 2013. p. 1745. https://doi.org/10.1016/B978-0-444-59565-2.00045-9.

10. Miyajima H, Hosoi Y. Aceruloplasminemia. In: Rosenberg's molecular and genetic basis of neurological and psychiatric disease; 2025. p. 801–13.
11. Alsaif HS, Al-Owain M, Barrios-Llerena ME, Gosadi G, Binamer Y, Devadason D, et al. Homozygous loss-of-function mutations in AP1B1, encoding beta-1 subunit of adaptor-related protein complex 1, cause MEDNIK-like syndrome. Am J Hum Genet. 2019;105(5):1016–22.
12. Martinelli D, Travaglini L, Drouin CA, Ceballos-Picot I, Rizza T, Bertini E, et al. MEDNIK syndrome: a novel defect of copper metabolism treatable by zinc acetate therapy. Brain. 2013;136(3):872–81.
13. Bindu PS, Chiplunkar S, Vandana VP, et al. Huppke-Brendel syndrome. In: Adam MP, Feldman J, Mirzaa GM, et al., editors. GeneReviews®. Seattle: University of Washington; 2024.

Zinc

15

Aditi Mittal

Introduction

Zinc is the second most prevalent trace element in the body, following iron [1]. In the United States, incidence of zinc deficiency is around 5% in early childhood and doubles itself in young adulthood, mostly involving nonpregnant women of reproductive age [2]. However, more than 50% of children less than 5 years of age and close to 70% of young adults are affected by zinc deficiency worldwide, with three-fourths of the population from southeast Asia and sub-Saharan Africa, mostly due to diet rich in phytates or inadequate caloric intake [3]. Zinc is part of many structural proteins, enzymes, transcription factors, which makes it significant at physiological level in human body.

Roles and Function of Zinc

Please refer to Table 15.1

A. Mittal (✉)
Presbyterian Healthcare Services, Department of Pediatric Gastroenterology, Albuquerque, NM, USA
e-mail: amittal@phs.org

K. Radhakrishnan (ed.), *Handbook of Clinical and Practical Pediatric Nutrition*, https://doi.org/10.1007/978-3-031-97759-6_15

Table 15.1 Physiological role of zinc

Physiological process	Some roles [3, 4]
Cognitive function	Zinc inhibits GABA-A receptor, which reduces inhibitory signaling in brain, thus exhibiting antidepressant-like activity
Growth and development	Zinc is part of DNA and RNA polymerase enzymes that are vital for neural tube formation, stem cell proliferation, and differentiation, and zinc also regulates function of IGF-1 (insulin growth factor-1)
Reproduction	Zinc binds to zinc-sensing receptor in sperm tail and assists with sperm motility, zinc stimulates production of LH (luteinizing hormone) and FSH (follicular stimulating hormone) from pituitary gland, and zinc regulates testosterone levels by inhibiting aromatase enzyme that converts testosterone to estrogen
Bone	Zinc is a cofactor of alkaline phosphatase (ALP) and helps in collagen matrix synthesis, mineralization, and bone turnover
Wound healing	Zinc-dependent metalloproteinases enhance debridement and the movement of keratinocytes
Immunity	Zinc regulates adaptive and innate immunity (NK cells and cytotoxic T-cells), and zinc is also vital in T-helper type 1 cell response with production of cytokines such as IFN, IL-2, TNF-alpha but does not affect T- helper type 2 cytokines
Metabolism	Zinc regulates the synthesis of TSH (thyroid stimulating hormone) and TRH (thyroid releasing hormone), and zinc mediates insulin signaling pathway, thereby stimulating lipogenesis and glucose uptake in adipocytes
Oxidative stress	Zinc inhibits NADPH oxidase decreasing production of superoxide, and zinc stabilizes superoxide dismutase that helps with superoxide removal
Vision	Zinc content is high in retina and due to its antioxidant property, zinc prevents AMD (age-related macular degeneration)

Sources

1. *Animal-based*: Richest sources of zinc include seafood (oysters, fish) and meat (beef, poultry). Other sources are eggs and dairy [2, 3].
2. *Plant-based*: Major sources of zinc include beans, nuts, and whole grains. Bioavailability is lower from plant-based foods as they contain phytates, which binds zinc and forms an insoluble complex, preventing zinc absorption in intestine [2, 3].

Digestion and Metabolism

1. Zinc is absorbed primarily in duodenum and jejunum. Free Zn^{2+} ions released from food are absorbed via ZIP 4 (zinc/iron regulated transporter) into the enterocyte and transported to portal vein via ZnT (zinc transporters).
2. Metallothioneins (MTs) are proteins present in the enterocyte, which have the affinity to metals such as zinc and copper and help in homeostasis of zinc. MTs bind to zinc ions and decrease intracytoplasmic concentration and release them when the cell needs it.
3. Zinc is mostly bound to albumin in the systemic circulation before getting absorbed in peripheral tissues. Other protein carriers include α2-macroglobulin.
4. About 50% of the zinc is excreted via feces and the rest via urine, sweat, menstrual flow, semen, loss of skin, nails, and hair.
5. In the state of zinc deficiency, there is upregulation of ZIP transporters, decreasing fecal and urinary excretion and increasing endogenous zinc secretion via pancreas/liver, bone marrow, and testes. Skin, skeletal muscle, and heart conserve their zinc levels [5, 6].
6. Bioavailability of zinc ranges from 5% to 60% depending upon the amount of phytate in the diet [3]:

(a) *Factors that increase bioavailability*: amino acids (in animal protein) and citrate (in human milk) increase solubility of zinc, fermentation and germination of grains/seeds leads to increased phytase production that hydrolyzes phytates [7], and supplements such as zinc citrate and zinc gluconate have highest bioavailability.

(b) *Factors that decrease bioavailability*: calcium, casein in cow's milk, phytates in legumes, beans and grains, medications such as diuretic (chlortalidone), angiotensin-converting enzyme inhibitors (ACEIs), or angiotensin-receptor blockers (ARBs). Supplements with elemental iron of 25 mg or more can reduce zinc absorption; however, iron fortified foods do not interfere with zinc absorption.

Assessment of Zinc Status

1. Recommended daily allowance of zinc ranges from 2 to 5 mg in less than 8 years of age and 8 to 11 mg in above 9 years of age [8].
2. Zinc intake of more than 200 mg/day leads to acute toxicity, whereas chronic toxicity occurs with intake of 50–150 mg/day for a longer period of time [3].
3. Normal serum zinc is 80–120 mcg/dL in a healthy adult (variations in level could occur diurnally and due to other factors such as illness, weight loss, and chronic liver disease) [2].
4. Serum zinc less than 70 mcg/dL in women and 74 mcg/dL in men indicates inadequate zinc status. In pediatrics, zinc status is assessed based on risk factors and signs of zinc deficiency (e.g., impaired growth) in addition to lab values [2].

Zinc Deficiency

1. Causes and risk factors:
   (a) *Inadequate intake*: food insecurity in low- and middle-income countries; other high-risk groups include preterm infants, pregnant females, vegetarians (particularly vegan) [2, 3].
   (b) *Inadequate absorption*: acrodermatitis enteropathica, inflammatory gastrointestinal (GI) disorders (celiac disease, IBD), short bowel syndrome, chronic alcohol use [2, 3].
   (c) *Excess loss*: burns, hemodialysis, diarrhea, urinary loss due to diuretics [2].
2. Acrodermatitis enteropathica [5]:
   (a) An autosomal recessive condition.
      - Affecting 1 in 500,000 children with equal incidence in males and females.
      - Mutation in SLC39A4 on chromosome 8 that encodes ZIP 4 protein, thus zinc absorption is affected leading to zinc deficiency.
   (b) Presents in infancy, typically 4–6 weeks after weaning from breastfeeding.
3. Signs and symptoms of zinc deficiency [3, 5]:
   (a) *CNS*: emotional lability, depression, impaired taste and smell, photophobia.
   (b) *GI*: diarrhea, anorexia, low ALP.
   (c) *Immunology*: thymic atrophy, frequent infections, delay in wound healing.
   (d) *Skin and hair*: hair loss, acrodermatitis (psoriasiform lesions affecting perioral, perianal, perineal, and acral areas).
   (e) *Reproductive system*: hypogonadism, oligospermia, impaired fetal development, reduced birth weight.
   (f) *Bone*: decreased bone mineral density, growth retardation.

4. Management of zinc deficiency:
   (a) In May 2004, the WHO/UNICEF jointly recommended oral zinc supplementation for acute diarrheal illness in children to decrease severity and duration of illness (10 mg/day in <6 months, 20 mg/day from ages 6 months to 5 years for 10–14 days) [9].
   (b) In *acrodermatitis* enteropathica, treatment with oral zinc 1–3 mg/kg/day for lifetime is the standard therapy. The zinc levels and ALP are monitored every 3–6 months to assess therapy response [10].
   (c) Zinc *requirement* is 2–4 mg/kg/day in malnourished children and could be higher than 50 mg/day in severe deficiency due to malabsorption disorders such as Crohn's disease or short bowel syndrome [5].

Zinc Toxicity

1. Causes include excessive intake of over-the-counter zinc supplements, exposure to pesticides, exposure to compounds in paints, rubber, dyes, and dental fixtures [3].
2. GI symptoms such as nausea, diarrhea, and abdominal pain are prominent with intake of zinc doses more than 50 mg/day.
3. Chronic zinc toxicity can decrease copper absorption by increasing MTs in enterocyte, which have high affinity for copper. This condition is called zinc-induced copper deficiency. Consequently, copper deficiency can affect iron absorption. It can lead to anemia, neutropenia, leukopenia, and reduced immune function. Long-term copper deficiency can lead to irreversible neurological complications such as gait imbalance and paresthesia.
4. Tests to evaluate zinc poisoning include serum zinc, copper, ceruloplasmin, and liver function tests. Treatment includes using oral copper gluconate, IV copper sulfate or chelating agents such as DTPA (diethylenetriamine pentaacetate).

Future Directions

More research is needed to know the proportion of zinc bound to albumin in systemic circulation and if albumin supplementation along with zinc supplementation is beneficial in scenarios with albumin deficiency. More studies are needed to determine benefit of using zinc in shortening the course of infections other than acute diarrheal illness, e.g., viral infections such as COVID-19.

References

1. Saper RB, Rash R. Zinc: an essential micronutrient. Am Fam Physician. 2009;79(9):768–72.
2. National Institutes of Health (NIH) Office of Dietary Supplements (ODS). Zinc [Fact Sheet for Health Professionals]; 2022. https://ods.od.nih.gov/factsheets/Zinc-HealthProfessional/#disc
3. Stiles LI, Ferrao K, Mehta KJ. Role of zinc in health and disease. Clin Exp Med. 2024;24(1):38. https://doi.org/10.1007/s10238-024-01302-6.
4. Devi CB, Nandakishore T, et al. Zinc in human health. IOSR J Dent Med Sci. 2014;13:18–23.
5. Sangeetha VJ, Dutta S, Moses JA, Anandharamakrishnan C. Zinc nutrition and human health: overview and implications. eFood. 2022;3(5):e17. https://doi.org/10.1002/efd2.17.
6. Maares M, Haase H. A guide to human zinc absorption: general overview and recent advances of in vitro intestinal models. Nutrients. 2020;12(3) https://doi.org/10.3390/nu12030762.
7. Agnoli C, Baroni L, Bertini I, et al. Position paper on vegetarian diets from the working group of the Italian Society of Human Nutrition. Nutr Metab Cardiovasc Dis. 2017;27(12):1037–52. https://doi.org/10.1016/j.numecd.2017.10.020.
8. Institute of Medicine. Food and Nutrition Board. Dietary reference intakes for Vitamin A, Vitamin K, Arsenic, Boron, Chromium, Copper, Iodine, Iron, Manganese, Molybdenum, Nickel, Silicon, Vanadium, and Zinc. Washington: National Academy Press; 2001.
9. Larson CP, Roy SK, Khan AI, Rahman AS, Qadri F. Zinc treatment to under-five children: applications to improve child survival and reduce burden of disease. J Health Popul Nutr. 2008;26(3):356–65. https://doi.org/10.3329/jhpn.v26i3.1901.
10. Ciampo IRLD, Sawamura R, Ciampo LAD, Fernandes MIM. Acrodermatitis enteropathica: clinical manifestations and pediatric diagnosis. Rev Paul Pediatr orgao Of da Soc Pediatr Sao Paulo. 2018;36(2):238–41. https://doi.org/10.1590/1984-0462/;2018;36;2;00010.

Manganese

16

Michael James Schmalz

Introduction

Manganese (Mn) is an abundant and easily oxidized metal naturally found in air, water, and soil [1]. It is essential for many cellular functions such as antioxidant defense, blood sugar regulation, coagulation, immune function, neurotransmitter synthesis, growth, and bone formation. Deficiency is rare but can be iatrogenic or related to transport deficiencies. Toxicity is almost completely limited to environmental/occupational or iatrogenic exposures, but inherited disorders exist. This chapter serves as a brief review of the biochemical function of manganese, highlights our metabolic needs, and how to identify disease states associated with abnormal manganese levels.

M. J. Schmalz (✉)
GI Associates, LLC, Pediatric Gastroenterology, Milwaukee, WI, USA
e-mail: Mike.schmalz@giassociates.com

K. Radhakrishnan (ed.), *Handbook of Clinical and Practical Pediatric Nutrition*, https://doi.org/10.1007/978-3-031-97759-6_16

Manganese Function in the Body

Mn Superoxide Dismutase (MnSOD)

Cellular death and aerobic respiration create superoxide species, which are toxic to iron–sulfur-containing proteins. Detoxifying metalloproteases called superoxide dismutases evolved to process these normal by-products of metabolism by converting them into hydrogen peroxide [2].

- MnSOD resides in the mitochondria and is responsible for superoxides produced through aerobic respiration.
- Deficiency in this enzyme increases cell death and has been associated with the development of chronic disease such as insulin-dependent diabetes mellitus and metabolic syndrome.
- Furthermore, MnSOD alleviates the oxidative stress produced during bacterial infections and supports immune function [3].

Growth, Bones, and Collagen

Mn partially regulates IGF-1 activity that facilitates bone turnover, collagen formation, and growth in children.

- Mn deficiency along with vitamin D, phosphate, and calcium increases the risk of osteopenia.
- Mn acts as a cofactor for glycosyltransferase enzymes necessary for collagen production. Deficiency can result in poor wound healing and increase the risk of developing osteoporosis [2, 4].

Blood Glucose

Studies of Korean diabetic patients found them to have significantly lower Mn serum levels, suggesting a role in serum glucose homeostasis [2].

- Mn is also a vital cofactor for pyruvate carboxylase synthesis and is involved in the first step of gluconeogenesis [1, 2].
- More research is needed to understand this relationship and the development of diabetes mellitus.

Ceruloplasmin

Ceruloplasmin is a copper-containing metalloprotein that oxidizes Fe and Mn for loading onto transferrin.

- Low levels of ceruloplasmin may cause abnormal distribution into the brain, leading to toxicity and *manganism* [5, 6].

Cholesterol

Mn is a cofactor for mevalonate kinase, geranyl pyrophosphate synthetase, and farnesyl pyrophosphate synthase. All of these enzymes are important for cholesterol synthesis. It is thought that cholesterol deficiencies lead to downstream deficiencies in sex hormones hindering male and female fertility, but more research is needed [2].

Manganese Exposure, Storage, and Excretion

Manganese primarily enters the body through ingestion via drinking water, foods, or supplements with a 3–5% absorption rate (M > F).

- Foods high in manganese include whole grains, rice, nuts, shellfish, spinach, pumpkins, sunflower, pine nuts, chili powder, cloves, and saffron [1].
- The adult Western diet provides between 2.3 and 8.8 mg/day [1]. See Table 16.1 for RDA information and Table 16.2 for total body volume and excretion rates.

Table 16.1 RDA table [2]

Recommended daily allowance of manganese (mg/day)	
Adult male	2.3
Adult female	1.8
Pregnant and lactating women	2.0–2.6
14–18 years old	2.2
0–6 months	0.003

Table 16.2 Manganese storage and excretion [2]

Excretion from liver	3.6 mg/day
Excretion from kidney	0.03 mg/day
Total body magnesium weight	10–20 mg
Whole blood Mn reference range	4–17 mcg/L

- Mn is absorbed in the intestines primarily through divalent metal transporter 1 (DMT1). DMT1 also transports other metals including copper, zinc, iron (Fe), and calcium, which compete with Mn and affect absorption rates [1].
- Individuals with Fe-deficient diets are at an increased risk of Mn toxicity and studies have found upregulated Fe/Mn transporter levels in the brains of rats and pigs. DMT1, along with transferrin receptors, are also found on red blood cells, which transport Mn throughout the body and help distribute it to other organs [1].

Once absorbed, Mn is primarily stored in descending concentrations in the liver, pancreas, bone, kidneys, and brain [1, 2].

- Like many other metabolites, the liver facilitates Mn storage, redistribution, and excretion.
- Conditions causing end-stage liver disease leading to impaired hepatobiliary excretion are associated with hepatocerebral degeneration due in part to Mn overload.

- The solute carrier family 30 member 10 gene (SLC30A10) expressed in the liver is responsible for hepatobilliary excretion of Mn and serum Mn induces its expression.

Disorders of Manganese Absorption, Metabolism, and Excretion

Mn deficiency is rare but can be seen in intentionally depleted diets or patients on total parenteral nutrition deficient in trace elements. Acute findings of Mn deficiency include lightening of body hair, dermatitis (Miliaria Crystallina), decreased growth of hair and nails, nausea and vomiting, and mild weight loss. Symptoms can reverse when the diet is replenished [7]. Long-term Mn deficiency can cause developmental delays, short stature, osteoporosis, low fertility, impaired glucose tolerance, and impaired wound healing [2].

Inhalation is the most reported cause of Mn toxicity, primarily affecting smelters, miners, and welders. Mn is rapidly absorbed through the lungs or olfactory bulb and transported to the brain by zinc transporters ZIP8 and ZIP14. Transdermal absorption is associated with exposure to methylcyclopentadienyl manganese tricarbonyl, a gasoline additive [1, 2].

Lastly, intravenous administration bypasses the gastrointestinal (GI) tract and most relevant when trace elements are added to total parenteral nutrition (TPN) (Table 16.3). Infants on TPN are at highest risk of toxicity by this route.

- In patients receiving long-term TPN, monitoring Mn in whole blood is considered the standard of care.
- Normal whole blood values range from 4 to 17 mcg/L in North America with motor deficits more likely in levels >7.5 mcg/L [7] (Table 16.2).

Table 16.3 Parenteral dosing [7]

Adult	0.06–0.1 mg/day
Children	1–50 mcg/day

Genetic Disorders of Manganese Metabolism

Hypermanganesemia with Dystonia 1 (HMNDYT1)

- Is secondary to SLC30A10 mutations, causes impairment of manganese excretion, and is an autosomal recessive (AR) disorder.
- It presents with developmental/gross motor delays such as high stepping gait and dystonia along with polycythemia, toxic accumulation in the liver, and low iron [2, 8].

HMNDYT2

- Is an AR mutation involving SLC39A14 that also causes neurodegenerative effects but does not involve the liver or cause polycythemia. SLC39A14 codes for ZIP14 and it is thought that deficiency of this protein inhibits Mn reuptake back into the liver, leading to the accumulation in the brain and lack of hepatotoxic effects.
- These patients often present with delayed milestones by 1 year old, relatively earlier than that seen in HMNDYT1.
- T1 weighed MRI studies of patients with Mn toxicity show accumulation in the basal ganglia, subthalamic regions, midbrain, and cerebellum.
- Mn deposition in these tissues causes a constellation of neurologic symptoms known as *manganism* [1, 2].
- These extrapyramidal symptoms gradually become "Parkinson's-like" and include cognitive delays, dystonia, rigidity, and high stepping gait [2] (Table 16.4).

Table 16.4 Symptoms of manganism [2]

Early	Late "Parkinson's-like"
Weakness	Hallucinations
Headache	Mania
Anorexia	Dysonia/gait disturbances
Sleep disturbance	Tremors
Muscle excitability	Rigidity

- Mn chelation with EDTA-CaNa2 and iron supplementation to compete with Mn absorption are the mainstays of treatment for both HMNDYT1 and 2 [8].

Congenital Disorder of Glycosylation Type IIn (CDG2N)

- This is due to SLC39A8 deficiency (AR), and was the first described inherited disorder of Mn deficiency.
- SLC39A8 is involved in the Mn reabsorption from the biliary tract and back into the hepatocyte.
- SLC39A8 deficiency leads to excess excretion and downstream deficiencies in Mn-containing enzymes.
- Patients with CDG2N present with profound developmental delay, dwarfism, short stature, deafness, and liver disease. Patients are reported to have low ceruloplasmin.
- Treatment involves supplementation with Mn sulfate [8].

References

1. Chen P, Bornhorst J, Aschner M. Manganese metabolism in humans. Front Biosci. 2018;23(9):1655–79.
2. Baj J, Flieger W, Barbachowska A, Kowalska B, Flieger M, Forma A, et al. Consequences of disturbing manganese homeostasis. Int J Mol Sci. 2023;24(19) https://doi.org/10.3390/ijms241914959.
3. Robinson BH. The role of manganese superoxide dismutase in health and disease. J Inherit Metab Dis. 1998;21(5):598–603.
4. Rondanelli M, Faliva MA, Peroni G, Infantino V, Gasparri C, Iannello G, et al. Essentiality of manganese for bone health: an overview and update. Nat Prod Commun. 2021;16(5)
5. Jursa T, Smith DR. Ceruloplasmin alters the tissue disposition and neurotoxicity of manganese, but not its loading onto transferrin. Toxicol Sci. 2009;107(1):182–93.
6. Tarnacka B, Jopowicz A, Maślińska M. Copper, iron, and manganese toxicity in neuropsychiatric conditions. Int J Mol Sci. 2021;22(15) https://doi.org/10.3390/ijms22157820.

7. Santos D, Batoreu C, Mateus L, Marreilha Dos Santos AP, Aschner M. Manganese in human parenteral nutrition: considerations for toxicity and biomonitoring. Neurotoxicology. 2014;43:36–45.
8. Anagianni S, Tuschl K. Genetic disorders of manganese metabolism. Curr Neurol Neurosci Rep. 2019;19(6):33.

Selenium

17

Praveen Kumar Conjeevaram Selvakumar

Introduction

Selenium is a naturally occurring trace element with variable biologic functions in children. However, the margin between dietary needs and toxic levels is narrow, indicating a need for strict regulation of intake and selenium stores in the body.

Physiological Role of Selenium

The physiologic functions of selenium are achieved through selenoproteins.

- Majority of the selenoproteins are redox enzymes incorporated into.
  - Glutathione peroxidase.
  - Iodothyronine deiodinase.

P. K. C. Selvakumar (✉)
Bon Secours Pediatric Gastroenterology Associates,
Richmond, VA, USA
e-mail: Praveen_selvakumar@bshsi.org

K. Radhakrishnan (ed.), *Handbook of Clinical and Practical Pediatric Nutrition*, https://doi.org/10.1007/978-3-031-97759-6_17

– Thioredoxin reductase.
– Selenoprotein P.

The above proteins are involved in antioxidant properties, thyroid metabolism, immune function, anticarcinogenic function, and even fertility [1].

- Selenium is an essential component of both cellular and serum glutathione peroxidase, which neutralizes harmful free radicals protecting oxidative tissue injury.
- Selenoprotein-dependent deiodinase catalyzes the conversion of thyroxine (T4) to its active form triiodothyronine (T3), therefore critical for thyroid function.
- Selenoproteins are important for activated T-cell function, differentiation, and proliferation of B-cells and subsequent production of cytokines, explaining therefore selenium deficiency has been associated with impaired immune response against viral infections [2].
- Limited evidence has indicated potential cardiovascular benefits of selenium by preventing oxidative stress in blood vessels and platelets aggregation but evidence has not been consistent [6].
- Similarly, some epidemiological studies have indicated anticarcinogenic benefits of selenium supplementation but results are not consistent across various studies [7].

Dietary Sources of Selenium

Selenium intake is widely variable based on the concentration of the soil where the plants and animals are grown [2].

- Dietary selenium exists in organic forms such as selenomethionine and selenocysteine, whereas inorganic forms include selenite and selenate.
- Organic forms present in plant and animal products are more bioavailable than inorganic forms.

- Selenite is present in food supplements, whereas selenate could be found in plants and fish. Brazil nuts, cereals, seafoods, and milk are the richest sources of selenium [3].

Selenium RDA [12]:

- **Infants**: 20 μg/day.
- **Children (1–3 years)**: 20 μg/day.
- **Children (4–8 years)**: 30 μg/day.
- **Children (9–13 years)**: 40 μg/day.
- **Adolescents (14–18 years)**: 55 μg/day.

Absorption and Metabolism of Selenium

- Absorption of dietary selenium occurs mainly in duodenum where various forms of selenium are converted into hydrogen selenide.
- Hydrogen selenide is then transported in the blood bound to low density and very low density lipoproteins to liver, which plays an integral role in selenium regulation including extrahepatic distribution and producing excretory metabolites.
- In liver, hydrogen selenide is converted into selenophosphate and then incorporated into selenoproteins in the form of selenocysteine through UGA codon in mRNA.
- Transport of selenium to other organs such as brain and kidney occurs primarily in form of selenoprotein P via receptor mediated endocytosis [4].
- Excretion of selenium is mainly through urine; however, it can also occur through respiratory excretion during excessive consumption, leading to garlic breath odor [5].

Selenium Deficiency

- *Keshan disease*: This is an endemic cardiomyopathy occurring in children from areas of China with poor selenium content in the soil. It is characterized by myocardial necrosis and fibrosis, resulting in heart failure and cardiogenic shock and even death. Complex interplay between selenium deficiency and viral infections, especially Coxsackie virus, has also been implicated in pathogenic role. Keshan disease could be prevented by selenium supplementation in at-risk population. Treatment mainly focuses on selenium supplementation and management of heart failure [8].

- *Kashin–Beck disease (KBD)*: This is an endemic chronic osteoarthropathy, mainly affecting children in selenium deficient regions in remote western China, Tibet, Southeast Siberia, and North Korea. KBD causes cartilage necrosis resulting in joint swelling, stiffness, and even deformities, short stature, and osteoarthrosis. Similar to Keshan disease, selenium supplementation has been associated with prevention of KBD [9].
- Selenium deficiency has been associated with hypothyroidism, increased the risk of autoimmune thyroid diseases and goiter [10].
- Growth retardation, cognitive impairment, pseudoalbinism, and erythrocyte macrocytosis.
- *Special patient populations*: Selenium deficiency can be seen in children on long-term total parenteral nutrition (TPN) not supplemented with selenium. Selenium is not included in currently available pediatric TPN solutions in the United States, so selenium supplementation at 2–3 mcg/kg/day is recommended with a maximum of 40–60 mcg/day. Requirements might be as high as 5–7 mcg/kg/day in preterm infants [11]. Selenium levels are also shown to be lower in children with phenylketonuria (due to selenium-limiting low-protein diet) and also in cystic fibrosis [10].

Diagnosis and Treatment

- Diagnosis of selenium deficiency is multifaceted, including a combination of clinical features and assessment, dietary questionnaire, and laboratory evaluation.
- Labs include assessment of serum selenium levels (normal range: 70–150 mcg/L based on age) and functional assessment

by measuring selenoprotein activity such as plasma glutathione peroxidase.
- Treatment involves dietary changes, selenium supplementation (selenomethionine or sodium selenite), and management of any related diseases.

Selenium Toxicity

Selenium toxicity can occur in children mostly from accidental overdose of supplementation (acute toxicity), excessive supplementation over a period of time (chronic toxicity or selenosis), and toxic environmental exposure rather than dietary sources.

- Acute toxicity causes gastrointestinal symptoms, respiratory symptoms, neurologic symptoms, and even renal failure.
- Chronic toxicity (selenosis) can result in hair loss, nail loss and brittleness, mood changes, irritability, garlic odor, and metallic taste [4].

Future Research

Antioxidant properties with various physiologic functions have led to numerous research possibilities and new findings, indicating future therapeutic and preventive possibilities.

- With potential anticancer properties, future studies could explore physiology of selenium in cancer prevention, use of selenium as synergistic therapy with current conventional cancer therapy, and even personalized therapy based on genetic profiles.
- Future studies on role of selenium in reducing oxidant stress and inflammation in atherosclerosis progression can lead to finding adjunct therapy in cardiovascular diseases.
- Investigation into role of selenium in glucose metabolism and insulin sensitivity could lead to new therapeutic possibilities in the management of type 2 diabetes and metabolic syndrome [13].

- Function of selenium in immune cell responses (especially T-cells and macrophages) to various infections and autoimmune diseases need to be studied further.
- Selenium is vital for maternal health during pregnancy, so exploring selenium supplementation in preventing maternal complications, preventing birth defects, and overall fetal neurodevelopmental outcome is of growing interest [14].

References

1. Fairweather-Tait SJ, Bao Y, Broadley MR, Collings R, Ford D, Hesketh JE, Hurst R. Selenium in human health and disease. Antioxid Redox Signal. 2011;14:1337–83.
2. Rayman MP. Selenium and human health. Lancet Lond Engl. 2012;379:1256–68.
3. Navarro-Alarcon M, Cabrera-Vique C. Selenium in food and the human body: a review. Sci Total Environ. 2008;400:115–41.
4. Ferreira RLU, Sena-Evangelista KCM, De Azevedo EP, Pinheiro FI, Cobucci RN, Pedrosa LFC. Selenium in human health and gut microflora: bioavailability of Selenocompounds and relationship with diseases. Front Nutr. 2021;8:685317.
5. Hadrup N, Ravn-Haren G. Absorption, distribution, metabolism and excretion (ADME) of oral selenium from organic and inorganic sources: a review. J Trace Elem Med Biol. 2021;67:126801.
6. Shimada BK, Alfulaij N, Seale LA. The impact of selenium deficiency on cardiovascular function. Int J Mol Sci. 2021;22:10713.
7. Kuršvietienė L, Mongirdienė A, Bernatonienė J, Šulinskienė J, Stanevičienė I. Selenium anticancer properties and impact on cellular redox status. Antioxid Basel Switz. 2020;9:80.
8. Ge K, Xue A, Bai J, Wang S. Keshan disease-an endemic cardiomyopathy in China. Virchows Arch A. 1983;401:1–15.
9. Schepman K, Engelbert RHH, Visser MM, Yu C, de Vos R. Kashin Beck disease: more than just osteoarthrosis. Int Orthop. 2011;35:767–76.
10. Dobrzyńska M, Kaczmarek K, Przysławski J, Drzymała-Czyż S. Selenium in infants and preschool children nutrition: a literature review. Nutrients. 2023;15:4668.
11. Zemrani B, McCallum Z, Bines JE. Trace element provision in parenteral nutrition in children: one size does not fit all. Nutrients. 2018;10:1819.

12. Compounds I of M (US) P on DA and R (2000) Selenium. Diet. Ref. Intakes Vitam. C Vitam. E Selenium Carotenoids.
13. Ozturk A, Cakir M. The role of selenium in the development of type 2 diabetes mellitus. Crit Rev Food Sci Nutr. 2018;58(14):2252–63.
14. Biswas K, McLay J, Campbell FM. Selenium supplementation in pregnancy-maternal and newborn outcomes. J Nutr Metab. 2022;4:4715965.

Iodine, Cobalt, Molybdenum, and Chromium

18

Rasha Abi Radi Abou Jaoudeh
and Kadakkal Radhakrishnan

Introduction

This chapter delves into the roles, metabolism, deficiencies, and potential toxicities of iodine, cobalt, molybdenum, and chromium in human health.

Iodine, a vital trace element, is primarily stored in the thyroid gland and is crucial for thyroid hormone synthesis. Iodine deficiency disorder (IDD) is a global public health concern, leading to intellectual disabilities and other health issues. Cobalt serves as the central metal ion in vitamin B12, impacting various physiological functions such as red blood cell synthesis and neurotransmitter regulation. Deficiency in cobalt can lead to megaloblastic anemia and neurological complications. Molybdenum, found in enzymes, plays a crucial role in detoxification pathways and

R. A. R. A. Jaoudeh
Department of Pediatrics, Cleveland Clinic Children's Hospital, Cleveland, OH, USA

K. Radhakrishnan (✉)
Division of Pediatric Gastroenterology, Hepatology and Nutrition, Cleveland Clinic Children's Hospital, Cleveland, OH, USA
e-mail: radhakk@ccf.org

K. Radhakrishnan (ed.), *Handbook of Clinical and Practical Pediatric Nutrition*, https://doi.org/10.1007/978-3-031-97759-6_18

catalytic activities. Molybdenum deficiency, while rare, presents diagnostic challenges and can lead to severe neurological complications. Chromium, particularly the trivalent form, is essential for metabolism and insulin function. Chromium deficiency is common in certain populations and can result in glucose intolerance and neuropathy.

Understanding the roles and potential imbalances of these trace elements is essential for maintaining human health.

Iodine

Iodine, a vital trace element, plays a critical role in human health despite being needed in minute quantities (only 5 g required throughout a 70-year lifespan) [1].

- The thyroid gland acts as its primary storehouse [2], containing around 70–80% of the body's total iodine (15–20 mg in a healthy adult).
- Daily iodine intake varies depending on life stage: adults typically need 150 micrograms (mcg), while pregnant and lactating women require slightly more (200 mcg), and newborns have even lower needs (40 mcg/day) [3].
- The thyroid actively captures iodine from the bloodstream at a rate of approximately 120 mcg daily for the crucial synthesis of thyroid hormones, triiodothyronine (T3), and thyroxine (T4) [3]. These hormones act as master regulators, influencing various physiological processes such as metabolism, growth, and development.

Iodine Metabolism

While the bulk of iodine comes from dietary sources, particularly vegetables grown in iodine-rich soil, drinking water can contribute to meeting the body's remaining iodine needs [4].

The thyroid gland occupies a central role in iodine homeostasis. Structurally, the gland is comprised of numerous follicles lined by a basement membrane and follicular epithelial cells. These follicles are filled with a viscous, glycoprotein known as thyroglobulin. This serves as the substrate for subsequent iodine metabolism within the thyroid gland [3].

Within the thyroid gland, a meticulously orchestrated cascade governs iodine metabolism.

- The initial step, iodide trapping [2], defies concentration gradients through the action of the sodium/iodide symporter (NIS) on the basolateral membrane of follicular cells, actively transporting iodide from the bloodstream into the follicular lumen.
- The second step is thyroglobulin synthesis by follicular cells. Thyroglobulin is a protein rich in tyrosine residues, which serves as the scaffold for thyroid hormone synthesis [3, 4]. Packaged within vesicles, thyroglobulin is then released into the follicular lumen.
- A separate transporter, pendrin, facilitates the movement of iodide into the follicular lumen. Here, iodide oxidation and organification [3, 4] take place.
- The enzyme thyroid peroxidase (TPO) catalyzes the oxidation of iodide, enabling its subsequent attachment to tyrosine residues on thyroglobulin. This iodination follows a specific sequence, first forming monoiodotyrosine (MIT) and then diiodotyrosine (DIT).
- The final step involves thyroid hormone formation and storage. DIT molecules couple to form thyroxine (T4), the primary storage hormone. Alternatively, MIT and DIT can combine to create the more potent triiodothyronine (T3) [3, 4].
- These hormones are stockpiled within the follicular lumen, embedded in a viscous material called colloid, for controlled release into the bloodstream as needed by the body. This stored reservoir can last for several months [3, 4].

Following intrathyroidal storage within the follicular lumen as thyroglobulin-bound iodine, a series of meticulous retrieval steps ensure optimal hormone production and efficient iodine utilization.

- Endocytosis by follicular epithelial cells reclaims the iodinated thyroglobulin from the colloid. Within the cytoplasm, lysosomal fusion facilitates proteolytic degradation of the thyroglobulin complex, liberating not only the active hormones triiodothyronine (T3) and thyroxine (T4), but also residual monoiodotyrosine (MIT) and diiodotyrosine (DIT) molecules.
- T3 and T4 readily diffuse across the basolateral membrane for delivery into the bloodstream, while deiodinase enzymes rapidly process DIT and MIT to recover the valuable iodide component.

This intricate recycling mechanism guarantees the efficient use of intrathyroidal iodine for ongoing hormone synthesis [3, 4].

Iodine Deficiency

Iodine deficiency disorder (IDD) represents a significant global public health concern, ranking as the most common preventable cause of intellectual disability [5].

- Insufficient iodine intake is the primary culprit behind IDD, often linked to low iodine content in staple foods grown on iodine-depleted soil.
- Additionally, limited access to seafood, a rich natural source of iodine, and the presence of goitrogenic substances in certain dietary components can further exacerbate iodine deficiency.
- IDD disrupts the synthesis of thyroid hormones, triiodothyronine (T3) and thyroxine (T4), essential for proper growth and development across all organ systems hormones [6].
- Initially, the thyroid gland may attempt to compensate by releasing stored hormones.
- However, prolonged iodine deficiency triggers a series of compensatory mechanisms [3, 4].
- The pituitary gland increases production of thyroid-stimulating hormone (TSH) in a futile attempt to stimulate the thyroid gland and bolster T4 synthesis.

- Thus, the thyroid gland undergoes cellular hyperplasia and hypertrophy in a desperate effort to increase iodine uptake and hormone production.

The most concerning consequences of IDD manifest during critical developmental periods, particularly fetal development and infancy.

- The brain is highly susceptible to the detrimental effects of thyroid hormone deficiency during these stages.
- Severe iodine deficiency during pregnancy and early childhood can lead to permanent intellectual disability.
- Therefore, ensuring adequate iodine intake for pregnant women, infants, and children remains a crucial public health strategy for preventing this devastating condition.

Patients with intestinal failure (IF) are at an increased risk of nutrient deficiency due to their impaired digestion and absorption, necessitating reliance on parenteral nutrition (PN) for survival and growth.

- Historically, iodine deficiency (ID) in children on long-term PN was rare because of iodine absorption through topical antiseptics.
- However, with the replacement of iodinated antiseptics by chlorhexidine-based compounds, recent studies indicate a high prevalence of insufficient iodine levels in these children despite iodine-rich PN.
- Thus, current PN guideline of 1 μg/kg/day of iodine for children may be inadequate, and iodine intake from oral or enteral formulas is important as it has shown to decrease the frequency of ID in this population [7].

To manage iodine deficiency in the general population, it is important to ensure adequate intake through iodized salt, iodine-rich foods, and supplementation according to recommended dietary allowance (Table 18.1). Tailored interventions, public

Table 18.1 Iodine recommended dietary allowances (RDAs) by age [8]

Age	RDA in males and females (mcg)	RDA during pregnancy (mcg)	RDA during lactation (mcg)
0–6 mo	110		
7–12 mo	130		
1–3 yrs	90		
4–8 yrs	90		
9–13 yrs	120		
14–18 yrs	150	220	290
19 yrs+	150	220	290

Abbreviations: *mcg* microgram, *mo* months, *yrs* years

health measures, and awareness programs are essential to address the specific needs of at-risk populations.

Cobalt

Cobalt, a trace element, exerts a profound influence on human health through its role as the central metal ion within cobalamin (vitamin B12), which is the only naturally occurring organometallic compound harboring a cobalt–carbon bond [9]. Vitamin B12 itself has a remarkably intricate molecular structure, featuring a corrin ring that coordinates the cobalt center with four equatorial nitrogen atoms in a square–planar arrangement. Additional axial ligands further diversify the various forms of vitamin B12, each with distinct functional roles within the body.

For details on B12, its role, absorption and function, please refer to the chapter on "Vitamin B12."

Cobalt Deficiency and Overload

Consequences of cobalt deficiency are directly related to a disturbed synthesis of vitamin B12, which can lead to:

- megaloblastic anemia,

- various neurological complications, myelopathy caused by spinal compression, optic neuropathy, and dementia.

A third of patients with vitamin B12 deficiency have normal levels of cobalamin and thus levels of methylmalonic acid and homocysteine should be checked.

In contrast, cobalt toxicity leads to an abnormal functioning of the thyroid gland and increased erythropoiesis due to bone marrow stimulation [10].

Molybdenum

Molybdenum, a trace element found in highest concentrations within the liver, kidneys, and small intestine, is essential for various biological processes. Organisms can only assimilate molybdenum in the form of the oxyanion molybdate $[Mo(VI)O_4]^{2-}$ [11]. The cellular import mechanism for molybdate differs between prokaryotes and eukaryotes. Prokaryotic uptake is well-characterized, involving ATP-binding cassette (ABC) transporters [12]. In contrast, the finer details of molybdate transport in eukaryotes remain under investigation.

- Molybdate transporter1 (MOT1) and molybdate transporter 2 (MOT2) have been identified as potential molybdate transporters in eukaryotes, with MOT1 being specific to plant-type eukaryotes [13].

Both prokaryotic and eukaryotic organisms possess a repertoire of molybdenum-containing enzymes, with estimates suggesting around 50 such enzymes present in bacteria alone [12].

- These molybdenum enzymes play a vital role in detoxification pathways within their respective organisms.
- Following import into the cell, molybdate undergoes enzymatic conversion for incorporation into a specialized metal cofactor known as molybdenum cofactor (Moco) [13].

- The functional versatility of Moco stems from molybdenum's ability to exist in multiple oxidation states (+4, +5, +6). This property allows molybdenum-coordinated Moco to catalyze diverse reactions involving the transfer of one or two electrons.
- Three distinct enzyme families, namely xanthine oxidase, sulfite oxidase, and DMSO (dimethyl sulfoxide) reductase, all rely on Moco for their catalytic activity [13].

Molybdenum Deficiency and Overload

Molybdenum deficiency, while uncommon, presents significant diagnostic challenges due to its heterogeneous symptomatology and often-nonspecific disease course, leading to potential misdiagnoses.

- Molybdenum cofactor deficiency (MoCD) can manifest across the lifespan, impacting neonates to adults [14]. In recent years, researchers have employed more systematic cohort studies to elucidate the underlying pathways associated with Molybdenum enzyme dysfunction.
- Three distinct subtypes of MoCD have been identified, each resulting from mutations in specific genes: MOCS1 for Type A, MOCS2 for Type B, and MOCS3 for Type C [15].
  - Neonatal presentation of MoCD is characterized by feeding difficulties, inconsolable crying, and neurological impairments that can progress to intellectual disability and social anxiety disorders. Neurological complications are the most severe consequence of MoCD, with disease progression, leading to cerebral atrophy as evidenced by MRI-confirmed psychomotor impairment. Unfortunately, the prognosis for infants with MoCD who survive the neonatal period remains guarded, with limited neurological improvement observed and most succumbing to the disease within a few years [15].

Intriguingly, molybdenum exhibits an antagonistic relationship with copper [16]. Excessive molybdenum intake can disrupt copper homeostasis, leading to potentially fatal copper-dependent disorders.

Chromium

Chromium (Cr) is a transition element with various valence states. Cr IV, V, and VI are carcinogenic, while the biologically active trivalent chromium is an essential trace element and is a component of metalloenzymes [17].

Chromium affects metabolism by [17]:

- increasing the number of insulin receptors,
- altering insulin-receptor binding dynamics,
- promoting internalization of insulin,
- facilitating the translocation of glucose transporters such as Glut1 and Glut4.

The recommended oral intake of chromium, expressed as the adequate intake (AI), is 25–35 μg/day [18].

- Its absorption in the small intestine typically ranges from 0.4% to 2.5%, with the actual rate depending on the individual's total body chromium concentration [17].
- Once absorbed, chromium is transported in the bloodstream, primarily bound to proteins such as transferrin and albumin [17].
- Most of the absorbed chromium is rapidly excreted through urine; hence, dose adjustment is necessary in renal failure.

Chromium is stored in various tissues including liver, spleen, soft tissue, and bone [17].

Chromium Deficiency and Overload

Insufficient chromium intake most commonly occurs in older adults, and patients at risk include those with [19]:

- acute illnesses such as burns, trauma, or infection,
- reduced absorption or intake due to short bowel syndrome or parenteral nutrition (PN) without chromium supplementation.

Clinical symptoms of deficiency include [17]:

- glucose intolerance,
- weight loss,
- elevated plasma free fatty acids,
- neuropathy, which can be reversed with daily chromium supplementation in PN solutions,
- Due to some degree of chromium present, particularly in amino acids mix, chromium deficiency is rare these days.

Ingestion of chromium rarely leads to toxicity given its poor absorption. Parenteral chromium has a higher potential to cause toxicity, specifically in pediatric patients, and those with impaired renal function [20].

References

1. Dhaar G, Robbani I. Foundations of community medicine. Elsevier; 2006.
2. Khurana I, Khurana A, Kowlgi NG. Textbook of medical physiology. Elsevier Health Sciences; 2019.
3. Pal G. Textbook of medical physiology. 4th ed. Elsevier Health Sciences; 2021.
4. Ahad F, Ganie SA. Iodine, iodine metabolism and iodine deficiency disorders revisited. Indian J Endocrinol Metab. 2010;14(1):13–7.
5. Patrick L. Iodine: deficiency and therapeutic considerations. Altern Med Rev. 2008;13(2):116–27.
6. Hetzel BS. Iodine deficiency disorders (IDD) and their eradication. Lancet. 1983;2(8359):1126–9.
7. Leite HP, Hatanaka EF, Sabio GSG, Evangelista NMA, de Camargo MFC. Iodine status in children with intestinal failure. J Pediatr Gastroenterol Nutr. 2024;78(3):691–8.
8. Trumbo P, Yates AA, Schlicker S, Poos M. Dietary reference intakes: vitamin A, vitamin K, arsenic, boron, chromium, copper, iodine, iron,

manganese, molybdenum, nickel, silicon, vanadium, and zinc. J Am Diet Assoc. 2001;101(3):294–301.

9. Hapke M, Hilt G. Introduction to cobalt chemistry and catalysis. In: Cobalt catalysis in organic synthesis; 2020. p. 1–23.
10. Depuis Z, Gatineau-Sailliant S, Ketelslegers O, Minon J-M, Seghaye M-C, Vasbien M, Dresse M-F. Pancytopenia due to vitamin B12 and folic acid deficiency – a case report. Pediatric Reports. 2022;14(1):106–14.
11. Tejada-Jiménez M, Galván A, Fernández E. Algae and humans share a molybdate transporter. Proc Natl Acad Sci. 2011;108(16):6420–5.
12. Hille R, Hall J, Basu P. The mononuclear molybdenum enzymes. Chem Rev. 2014;114(7):3963–4038.
13. Leimkühler S, Wuebbens MM, Rajagopalan KV. The history of the discovery of the molybdenum cofactor and novel aspects of its biosynthesis in bacteria. Coord Chem Rev. 2011;255(9):1129–44.
14. Tian Q, Cao Y, Shu L, Chen Y, Peng Y, Wang Y, et al. Case report: compound heterozygous variants in MOCS3 identified in a Chinese infant with molybdenum cofactor deficiency. Front Genet. 2021;12
15. Spiegel R, Schwahn BC, Squires L, Confer N. Molybdenum cofactor deficiency: a natural history. J Inherit Metab Dis. 2022;45(3):456–69.
16. Thorndyke MP, Guimaraes O, Kistner MJ, Wagner JJ, Engle TE. Influence of molybdenum in drinking water or feed on copper metabolism in cattle – a review. Animals. 2021;11(7):2083.
17. Hua Y, Clark S, Ren J, Sreejayan N. Molecular mechanisms of chromium in alleviating insulin resistance. J Nutr Biochem. 2012;23(4):313–9.
18. Berger MM, Shenkin A, Schweinlin A, Amrein K, Augsburger M, Biesalski HK, et al. ESPEN micronutrient guideline. Clin Nutr. 2022;41(6):1357–424.
19. Roussel AM, Andriollo-Sanchez M, Ferry M, Bryden NA, Anderson RA. Food chromium content, dietary chromium intake and related biological variables in French free-living elderly. Br J Nutr. 2007;98(2):326–31.
20. Balali-Mood M, Naseri K, Tahergorabi Z, Khazdair MR, Sadeghi M. Toxic mechanisms of five heavy metals: mercury, Lead, chromium, cadmium, and arsenic. Front Pharmacol. 2021;12:643972.

Part IV

Water Soluble Vitamins

Vitamin B1: Thiamine

19

Noy Lapidot Alon
and Kadakkal Radhakrishnan

History

Thiamine is a water soluble vitamin of the B group (vitamin B1). Thiamine deficiency, historically referred to as "beriberi" in English, has been recognized for over four millennia in Chinese and Japanese medical manuscripts. It emerged as a significant public health issue in Eastern and Southern Asia and Europe due to the widespread consumption of polished rice, which lacks the thiamine-rich aleurone layer. Until just over a century ago, the prevailing view was that thiamine deficiency was caused by an infection or a toxin. The first person to conclusively show that thiamine deficiency is a nutritional disease, and to combat it with nutritional measures, was Japanese naval surgeon Admiral Takaki.

N. L. Alon
Division of Pediatric Gastroenterology, Hepatology, and Nutrition, Cleveland Clinic Children's Hospital, Cleveland, OH, USA

Department of Gastroenterology Nutrition and Liver Diseases, Schneider Children's Medical Center of Israel, Petach Tikva, Israel

Sackler Faculty of Medicine, Tel Aviv University, Tel Aviv, Israel

K. Radhakrishnan (✉)
Department of Pediatric Gastroenterology, Hepatology, and Nutrition, Cleveland Clinic Foundation, Cleveland, OH, USA
e-mail: RADHAKK@ccf.org

K. Radhakrishnan (ed.), *Handbook of Clinical and Practical Pediatric Nutrition*, https://doi.org/10.1007/978-3-031-97759-6_19

In 1878, Takaki demonstrated that the prevalence of beriberi could be reduced in the Japanese navy by substituting the sailors' usual diet of polished rice and dried fish with meat, wheat, and milk. Further progress was made in 1890 when Dutch medical officers Eijkman and Grijns showed that a paralytic condition, known as polyneuritis, resembling beriberi, could be induced in chickens by feeding them a diet consisting solely of polished rice. This line of inquiry eventually led to significant developments. In 1926, Jansen and Donath isolated rice polishing extracts that cured beriberi in humans, enhancing the understanding of the disease's dietary causes. In 1936, Robert Williams finally published the chemical structure of thiamine [1, 2].

Structure, Dietary Sources, Absorption and Metabolism of Thiamine

The chemical structure of thiamine consists of a pyrimidine nucleus and a thiazole ring linked by a methylene bridge.

- While bacteria, fungi, and plants can synthesize thiamine, humans cannot and therefore primarily depend on dietary sources.
- Intestinal microbiota can also generate thiamine, therefore providing a secondary source of the vitamin [3].

There are several dietary sources of thiamine including

- meat, yeast, grains, cereals, legumes, peas, lentils, and potatoes.
- Thiamine absorption can be significantly interfered with, as thiamine denatures at high pH and high temperatures. Food processing methods such as cooking, baking, and canning may have an impact on the final thiamine content.
- Consumption of thiaminases, anti-thiamine factors in the diet (e.g., tea leaves, herring, shellfish, raw carp, fermented fish, betel nuts), protein and folate nutrition levels, and the ingestion

of beverages such as coffee, tea, and especially alcohol can all contribute to or even directly cause, in different mechanisms, thiamine deficiency [4].
- Diets based on polished rice are a risk factor for thiamine deficiency because they are poor sources of the vitamin.
- Ingestion of juices from citrus fruits increases the bioavailability of thiamine because of their citric acid and ascorbic acid content [4].
- In many high-income countries, wheat flour, cereals, and infant formulae are fortified with thiamine; thiamine-fortified foods contribute about half of the total amount of the vitamin consumed in these settings [5].

Since the body cannot store thiamine and the vitamin has a high turnover rate, a continuous supply is necessary.

- The limited stores may be depleted within 2 weeks or less on a thiamine-free diet, with clinical signs appearing shortly thereafter.

Thiamine absorption and transport:

- Thiamine phosphate esters, derived from dietary sources, initially hydrolyzed into thiamine or thiamine monophosphate (ThMP) by intestinal alkaline phosphatase [6].
- After hydrolysis, free thiamine is transported across the enterocytes brush border membrane, predominantly within the jejunum and ileum.
- At lower concentrations, thiamine absorption occurs via an active, carrier-mediated, pH-dependent, and rate-limited mechanism involving two transporter proteins: the human thiamine transporter-1 (hTHTR-1), which is the product of SLC19 A2 gene, and hTHTR-2, the product of SLC19 A3.
- At higher concentrations, however, absorption proceeds through passive diffusion [6].
- Once in the portal system, thiamine is transported and phosphorylated into its principal active form, thiamine diphosphate

(ThDP), primarily in the liver and, to a lesser extent, in the erythrocytes, which contain ~80% of the total thiamine in whole blood.
- Excess thiamine and its metabolites are eliminated via urinary excretion, which is notably reduced during periods of fasting.

Thiamine Biologic Activity

ThDP is the cofactor of several enzymes involved in key metabolic pathways of carbohydrates and branched-chain amino acids metabolism (Table 19.1). One of thiamin's primary functions is acting as a cofactor for the mitochondrial enzymes: pyruvate

Table 19.1 Thiamin-dependent enzyme

Enzyme	Biological activity	Relevance
Pyruvate dehydrogenase complex	Oxidative decarboxylation of pyruvic acid, converting pyruvate to acetyl CoA in mitochondria	Essential for mitochondrial oxidative metabolism, crucial for cell survival, especially in neurons
α-Ketoglutarate dehydrogenase complex	Oxidative decarboxylation of α-ketoglutaric acid into succinyl CoA, a rate-limiting step in the Krebs cycle	Vital for energy production in cellular metabolism, accumulation of α-KG may also be a diagnostic indicator of thiamine deficiency
Branched-chain 2-oxo acid dehydrogenase	Degradation of branched-chain amino acids leucine, isoleucine, and valine	Central in amino acid metabolism; deficiency leads to maple syrup urine disease due to toxic accumulations
Transketolase	Part of the cytosolic pentose phosphate pathway, non-oxidative carbohydrate metabolism, generation of NADPH, and nucleic acid	Crucial for nervous system integrity and myelin sheath repair
2-Hydroxyacyl-CoA lyase	Functions in the α-oxidation of 3-methyl-branched fatty acids	Produces long-chain aldehydes, involved in fatty acid metabolism

dehydrogenase complex, oxoglutarate dehydrogenase complex, and branched-chain 2-oxo acid dehydrogenase [7].

As described above, thiamine deficiency impairs numerous enzymes and cellular processes; as a result, lactate accumulate in the brain and blood leads to lactic acidosis.

In addition, thiamine deficiency leads to a decrease in the synthesis of neurotransmitters, such as acetylcholine and γ-aminobutyric acid (GABA), which may further contribute to the neurological manifestations.

Risk Factors for Thiamine Deficiency

Thiamine deficiency can arise from several etiological factors, commonly due to insufficient dietary intake (e.g., exclusively breastfed infants of thiamine-deficient mothers, low-income countries, refugee camps) [8], inadequate supplementation in enteral or parenteral nutrition, enhanced metabolic demands (refeeding syndrome), or by increased losses via gastrointestinal (short bowel syndrome, IBD), or renal pathways (renal failure and hemodialysis) [9, 10], or uncommonly due to genetic inborn errors of thiamine metabolism (e.g., mutations in SLC19A2, SLC19A3, SLC25A19). Other significant risk factors in the pediatric population include diabetes mellitus with DKA, etc. are detailed in Table 19.2. Primarily in adults, significant risk factors for thiamine deficiency notably include histories of alcoholism, AIDS, pregnancy, lactation, and advanced age.

All these conditions demand rigorous monitoring due to their increased prevalence and potential for severe deficiency. Often, thiamine deficiency coexists with other micronutrient deficiencies, which may exacerbate the clinical symptoms [10]. The awareness of the multifactorial nature of thiamine deficiency and the wide range of risk factors involved can guide more effective prevention and intervention strategies in clinical practice [3, 9].

Table 19.2 Causes of thiamine deficiency

Alcoholism
Malnutrition
Refeeding syndrome
Malabsorption states
Bariatric surgery
Critical illness
Diabetes mellitus
Chronic kidney disease and hemodialysis
Malignancy
HIV infection
Polished rice-based die
Chronic vomiting
Drugs (e.g., proton-pump inhibitors, metformin, high-dose diuretics)
High dietary intake of thiaminases (e.g., betel nuts and raw fish)

Clinical Manifestations

Thiamine deficiency impacts multiple enzymatic metabolic pathways, as detailed above, thereby presenting with a diverse clinical spectrum.

Infantile Beriberi

Infantile beriberi arises from thiamine deficiency and mainly affects breastfed infants around 3 months old. Symptoms include

- hoarse crying, vomiting, lack of appetite, swelling, reduced urine output, seizures, and heart failure signs (e.g., tachypnoea, tachycardia, pulmonary edema, and hepatomegaly).
- The condition can quickly become fatal without immediate thiamine supplementation.
- This deficiency is often linked to inadequate thiamine in the diets of breastfeeding mothers, leading to thiamine-deficient

breast milk. The high growth rate of the fetus amplifies his thiamine needs, increasing the risk of beriberi if the mother is deficient [11].

- Maternal thiamine deficiency also was reported as a risk factor for intrauterine growth retardation [12].
- Three primary forms of infantile thiamine deficiency have been identified: the pure cardiologic form, aphonic form, and pseudo-meningitic form.
- The pure cardiologic form typically presents in infants aged 1–3 months with symptoms of heart failure such as edema, cyanosis, and breathlessness, or even cardiogenic shock.
- The aphonic form, seen in older infants aged 4–6 months, involves a loss of voice resulting from neuritis, leading to paresis or paralysis of the vocal cords.
- In infants 7–9 months old, the pseudo-meningitic form can mimic bacterial meningitis, presenting with symptoms such as a bulging fontanelle, agitation, vomiting, and seizures [3, 13].

Infantile beriberi has been recognized in several regions of sub-Saharan Africa, central and Southeast Asia, especially in Myanmar, Laos, and Cambodia [14].

The long-term consequences of infantile beriberi were highlighted in a 2003 case series, where several hundred infants fed a thiamine-deficient, soy-based formula suffered severe outcomes. Those who survived, experienced significant long-term sequelae, including motor and cognitive impairments, severe epilepsy, and skeletal deformities such as kyphoscoliosis [15, 16].

Adult Beriberi

Historically, this disorder is classified into two primary forms based on the affected organ systems

- "Wet" beriberi primarily impacts the cardiovascular system, leading to symptoms such as tachycardia, congestive heart failure, and cardiomegaly with pulmonary congestion.

Hemodynamic changes include high cardiac output and low peripheral resistance.
- Rarely, patients have fulminant or "shoshin" beriberi, presenting with acute circulatory collapse.
- Conversely, "dry" beriberi mainly affects the peripheral nervous system, characterized by symmetric polyneuropathy impairment of sensory, motor, and reflex functions that affects distal more than proximal limb segments, as well as progressive muscle weakness [17].

Wernicke–Korsakoff Syndrome

This syndrome manifests in two phases:

- Wernicke encephalopathy (WE) occurs early and may presents with the classic full triad of encephalopathy, ophthalmoparesis, and ataxia in only 17% of the pediatric case. Polyneuropathy and gait abnormalities may be present as well.
- If left untreated, it can eventually evolve into Korsakoff psychosis with signs of severe short-term amnesia, disorientation, confabulation, and hallucinations.
- The reported prevalence of WE in autopsy studies ranges from 0.4% to 2.8% [18].
- Usually associated with alcoholism in adults (excessive alcohol consumption is linked to low thiamine intake and impaired absorption and storage) [18].
- WE can also occur in children with other etiologies such as after bariatric surgeries [19], IBD, or prolonged parenteral nutrition [20, 21].
- As a medical emergency, once suspected, high doses of thiamine treatment should be started to decrease comorbidities and improve prognosis.
- Brain MRI is helpful in diagnosis and follow-up, with high specificity and medium sensitivity in WE. Typical findings consist of symmetrical lesions with T2/FLAIR hypersignal in the thalamus, mammillary bodies, periaqueductal area, and tectal plate [20].

Thiamine deficiency has also been linked to increased risk of Alzheimer's disease with ThDP levels that are decreased in post-mortem brains of patients with Alzheimer's disease [22].

Thiamine Metabolism Dysfunction Syndromes

Defects in genes encoding proteins with relevant functions in thiamine transport and metabolism cause inborn errors of metabolism, leading to thiamine metabolism autosomal recessive, dysfunction syndromes. Currently, there are five genetic phenotypes that have been characterized, caused by SLC19A2, SLC19A3, SLC25A19, and TPK1 mutations [23].

- *Thiamine metabolism dysfunction syndrome 1* (thiamine-responsive megaloblastic anemia syndrome) (OMIM 249270)—also known as Rogers syndrome, is caused by mutations in the *SLC19A2* gene, which encodes the thiamine transporter THTR-1, responsible for a syndrome of megaloblastic anemia, diabetes mellitus, and sensorineural deafness. More than 100 cases have been reported, all of them presenting with symptoms in childhood or adolescence. Deafness is usually the last manifestation to develop. Other symptoms also associated with this disorder involving neurological (such as seizures, ataxia, developmental delay, recurrent strokes alternating between right and left MCA), ophthalmological (pigmentary retinopathy, abnormalities of the optic nerve, cone–rod dystrophy), endocrinological (short stature, cryptorchidism), cardiological, and hematological symptoms. Biochemically, low plasma thiamine levels were found. These patients do not usually present elevated lactate levels.
- *Thiamine metabolism dysfunction syndrome 2* (biotin- or thiamine-responsive encephalopathy type) (OMIM 607483)—autosomal recessively inherited disease caused by mutations in the *SLC19A3* gene, which encode the thiamine transporter THTR-2 and have been reported as episodic encephalopathy with two clinical phenotypes. Early infantile Leigh syndrome (progressive subacute necrotizing encephalomyopathy) is the

most severe SLC19A3-related manifestation. It presents a few days or weeks after delivery with feeding difficulties, lethargy, seizures, and respiratory distress. The adult milder subtype is presenting with lethargy, dystonia, and MRI abnormalities characterized by diffuse leukoencephalopathy and sparing of the basal ganglia. *SLC19A3* patients present a profound decrease of free thiamine in cerebrospinal fluid (CSF) and fibroblasts. Some patients showed elevated lactate in blood and CSF. This disease responds to biotin administration, or sometimes to a combination of biotin and thiamine, though biotin is not transported by ThTR2.

- *Thiamine metabolism dysfunction syndrome 3* (microcephaly Amish type) (OMIM 607196)—mutations in *SLC25A19* cause Amish lethal microcephaly, also an autosomal recessive disease characterized by extreme microcephaly, severe 2-oxoglutarate aciduria, and fatal outcome within the first year.
- *Thiamine metabolism dysfunction syndrome 4*—bilateral striatal degeneration and progressive polyneuropathy (OMIM 613710), characterized by episodes of encephalopathy triggered by fever or infections, flaccid weakness, and slowly progressive axonal polyneuropathy in patients with normal psychomotor development.
- *Thiamine metabolism dysfunction syndrome 5* (episodic encephalopathy type) (OMIM 614458)—thiamine pyrophosphokinase deficiency is associated with episodic encephalopathy, also triggered by infections or dehydration.

Laboratory Diagnosis

The identification of thiamine deficiency predominantly relies on clinical judgment, as many of the relevant assays are specialized, not routinely available in hospital laboratories, and may be both costly and time-consuming (Table 19.3).

Table 19.3 Biochemical detection of thiamine deficiency

Test	Description	Comments	Normal range
Thiamine levels	Direct measurement of thiamine in serum or whole blood	Low specificity. Low sensitivity (*only less than 10% from the total body thiamine is contained in the plasma) Fluctuate rapidly with dietary intake	Varies
Transketolase activation test/ transketolase activity assay	Functional indirect measurement of TDP by measuring the activity of transketolase enzyme in erythrocytes before and after the addition of thiamine	Widely used method to detect thiamine deficiency Higher activation suggests deficiency. Expressed by TPPE (thiamine pyrophosphate effect)	Normal values range from 0% to 15%; a value of 15–25% indicates thiamine deficiency, and > 25% indicates severe deficiency

(continued)

Table 19.3 (continued)

Test	Description	Comments	Normal range
High-performance liquid chromatography	Direct measurement. Since 80% of the total thiamine content of whole blood is present as active ThDP in erythrocytes, making this method superior and more reflective of body stores of thiamine	High specificity and sensitivity Preferred assay to detect deficiency	For normal healthy individuals, ThDP in whole blood is 70–180 nmol/L
Urinary excretion of thiamine and its metabolites	Measurement over a 24-h period	Influenced by recent dietary intake, not a very reliable method for assessing tissue stores	Normal range 150–170 μg/g Cr, while 120–150 μg/g Cr suggests deficiency (*age dependent)
Pyruvate and lactate levels		Low specificity and technically difficult test	Normal range: Pyruvate 0.3–1.5 mg/dL Lactate1.0–2.4 mmol/L (*age dependent)

Treatment

The recommended dietary allowance (RDA):

- It is 1.2 mg/day for adult males and 1.1 mg/ day for adult females.
- The RDA is increased to 1.4 mg/day during pregnancy and even 1.5 mg/day for lactating women.
- In children, the RDA increases with age and is 0.5, 0.6, and 0.9 mg/day, respectively, for 1–3, 4–8, and 9–13 years of age [3, 9].

The typical treatment regimen for adult thiamine deficiency:

- Involves administering 500 mg of thiamine, three times daily for 2–3 days. Following this initial phase, the dosage is reduced to 250 mg daily for an additional 3–5 days or until no further improvement is observed. Continuous evaluation is recommended to assess the need for ongoing thiamine supplementation.
- In pediatric cases, treatment protocols can vary significantly based on the associated conditions and may start with an initial dose of 100 mg daily, adjusting to 20 mg/kg/day following genetic confirmation of a thiamine transporter deficiency. It is crucial to administer glucose only after thiamine to prevent exacerbating the deficiency.
- Concurrent severe magnesium deficiency should also be addressed to optimize the response to thiamine treatment. Pediatric patients at risk for thiamine deficiency are recommended to receive a preventive dose of 0.35–0.5 mg/kg/day of thiamine orally [24].

Future direction for thiamine research in pediatric gastroenterology should emphasizes several critical areas. Developing cost-effective screening tools is essential for integrating thiamine status assessments into national health surveys to better monitor and address deficiencies. Additionally, establishing specific deficiency cutoffs for thiamine diphosphate (ThDP) relevant to populations at high risk for endemic thiamine deficiency will improve diagnostic accuracy and intervention strategies. Furthermore, investigating the roles and effects of thiamine supplementation, especially in low-income countries, could provide new insights into preventing and managing these deficiencies effectively in both mothers and infants. Research must also expand into the genetic aspects of thiamine metabolic dysfunction syndromes among various populations, exploring how genetic variability influences the severity of thiamine deficiency impacts. Further use of next-generation sequencing will expand the spectrum of genotypes and phenotypes of this genetic cases. Comprehensive approach will enable more targeted and effective interventions to mitigate the burden of thiamine-related health issues in pediatric populations.

References

1. Duggan C, Watkins JB, Koletzko B, Walker WA, editors. Nutrition in pediatrics: basic science, clinical applications, vol. 1. 5th ed. Shelton: People's Medical Publishing House-USA; 2016.
2. Carpenter KJ. The discovery of thiamin. Ann Nutr Metab. 2012;61(3):219–23.
3. World Health Organization. Thiamine deficiency and its prevention and control in major emergencies; 1999.
4. Polegato BF, Pereira AG, Azevedo PS, Costa NA, Zornoff LAM, Paiva SAR, et al. Role of thiamin in health and disease. Nutr Clin Pract. 2019;34(4):558–64.
5. Berner LA, Keast DR, Bailey RL, Dwyer JT. Fortified foods are major contributors to nutrient intakes in diets of US children and adolescents. J Acad Nutr Diet. 2014;114(7):1009–22.
6. Sriram K, Manzanares W, Joseph K. Thiamine in nutrition therapy. Nutr Clin Pract. 2012;27(1):41–50.
7. Erdman JW, editor. Present knowledge in nutrition. 10th. ed. Ames: Wiley-Blackwell; 2012. p. 1305.
8. Whitfield KC, Smith G, Chamnan C, Karakochuk CD, Sophonneary P, Kuong K, et al. High prevalence of thiamine (vitamin B1) deficiency in early childhood among a nationally representative sample of Cambodian

women of childbearing age and their children. Tickell KD, editor. PLoS Negl Trop Dis. 2017;11(9):e0005814.
9. Frank LL. Thiamin in clinical practice. J Parenter Enter Nutr. 2015;39(5):503–20.
10. Rakotoambinina B, Hiffler L, Gomes F. Pediatric thiamine deficiency disorders in high-income countries between 2000 and 2020: a clinical reappraisal. Ann N Y Acad Sci. 2021;1498(1):57–76.
11. Whitfield KC, Karakochuk CD, Kroeun H, Hampel D, Sokhoing L, Chan BB, et al. Perinatal consumption of thiamine-fortified fish sauce in rural Cambodia: a randomized clinical trial. JAMA Pediatr. 2016;170(10):e162065.
12. Heinze T, Weber W. Determination of thiamine (vitamin B1) in maternal blood during normal pregnancies and pregnancies with intrauterine growth retardation. Z Für Ernährungswissenschaft. 1990;29(1):39–46.
13. Johnson CR, Fischer PR, Thacher TD, Topazian MD, Bourassa MW, Combs GF. Thiamin deficiency in low- and middle-income countries: disorders, prevalences, previous interventions and current recommendations. Nutr Health. 2019;25(2):127–51.
14. Kareem O, Nisar S, Tanvir M, Muzaffer U, Bader GN. Thiamine deficiency in pregnancy and lactation: implications and present perspectives. Front Nutr. 2023;10:1080611.
15. Fattal-Valevski A, Kesler A, Sela BA, Nitzan-Kaluski D, Rotstein M, Mesterman R, et al. Outbreak of life-threatening thiamine deficiency in infants in Israel caused by a defective soy-based formula. Pediatrics. 2005;115(2):e233–8.
16. Mimouni-Bloch A, Goldberg-Stern H, Strausberg R, Brezner A, Heyman E, Inbar D, et al. Thiamine deficiency in infancy: long-term follow-up. Pediatr Neurol. 2014;51(3):311–6.
17. Ross AC, editor. Modern nutrition in health and disease. 11th ed. Philadelphia: Wolters Kluwer Health/Lippincott Williams & Wilkins; 2014. p. 1616.
18. Galvin R, Bråthen G, Ivashynka A, Hillbom M, Tanasescu R, Leone MA. EFNS guidelines for diagnosis, therapy and prevention of Wernicke encephalopathy. Eur J Neurol. 2010;17(12):1408–18.
19. Oudman E, Wijnia JW, Van Dam M, Biter LU, Postma A. Preventing Wernicke encephalopathy after bariatric surgery. Obes Surg. 2018;28(7):2060–8.
20. Forno A, Cunha B, Luís C, Castro A, Moniz M, Escobar C, et al. Wernicke encephalopathy in children. Neurol Clin Pract. 2021;11(5):e777. https://doi.org/10.1212/CPJ.0000000000000973.
21. Oudman E, Wijnia JW, Oey MJ, Van Dam M, Postma A. Wernicke-Korsakoff syndrome despite no alcohol abuse: a summary of systematic reports. J Neurol Sci. 2021;426:117482.

22. Molina JA, Jiménez-Jiménez FJ, Hernánz A, Fernández-Vivancos E, Medina S, De Bustos F, et al. Cerebrospinal fluid levels of thiamine in patients with Alzheimer's disease. J Neural Transm. 2002;109(7–8):1035–44.
23. Marcé-Grau A, Martí-Sánchez L, Baide-Mairena H, Ortigoza-Escobar JD, Pérez-Dueñas B. Genetic defects of thiamine transport and metabolism: a review of clinical phenotypes, genetics, and functional studies. J Inherit Metab Dis. 2019;42(4):581–97.
24. Lallas M, Desai J. Wernicke encephalopathy in children and adolescents. World J Pediatr. 2014;10(4):293–8.

Vitamin B2: Riboflavin

20

Jennifer Donais
and Kadakkal Radhakrishnan

Dietary Sources

- The majority of natural dietary sources of riboflavin come from meat and dairy products [3].
- Notably, organ meats (e.g., liver) contain some of the highest amounts of riboflavin per serving of all natural sources of riboflavin [4].
- Various cuts of beef, lamb, pork, and turkey provide significant amounts of the nutrient as do milk, yogurt, and eggs [4].
- There are many cereals and wheat flour-containing products that are fortified with riboflavin and are readily available in many developed countries [3].
- Recommended daily allowance varies by age, biological sex, and while pregnant or lactating [3]:

J. Donais
Department of Pediatrics, Cleveland Clinic Children's Hospital, Cleveland, OH, USA
e-mail: DONAISJ2@ccf.org

K. Radhakrishnan (✉)
Division of Pediatric Gastroenterology, Hepatology and Nutrition, Cleveland Clinic Children's Hospital, Cleveland, OH, USA
e-mail: radhakk@ccf.org

K. Radhakrishnan (ed.), *Handbook of Clinical and Practical Pediatric Nutrition*, https://doi.org/10.1007/978-3-031-97759-6_20

- 0–6 months: 0.3 mg
- 7–12 months: 0.4 mg
- 1–3 years: 0.5 mg
- 4–8 years: 0.6 mg
- 9–13 years: 0.9 mg
- 14–18 years: females 0.1 mg, males 1.3 mg
- 19–30 years: females 1.1 mg, males 1.3 mg
- Pregnant: 1.4 mg, lactating: 1.6 mg.

Digestion and Metabolism

- Riboflavin exists as one of three forms, the free form, and as one of two coenzymes, flavin mononucleotide (FMN) and flavin adenine dinucleotide (FAD).
- Both FMN and FAD must be hydrolyzed by phosphatases in the small intestine brush border prior to absorption. The free form may be absorbed without further digestion [5].
- Dietary riboflavin exists in all three forms and is primarily absorbed in the small intestine.
- Riboflavin is additionally produced by intestinal microflora, mainly as the free form. It is absorbed in the large intestine [5].
- There are three riboflavin transporters that have thus far been described in humans, all three of which are expressed in enterocytes of the small and large intestines [6, 7].
- In enterocytes, human riboflavin transporter 2 (hRFt-2) is exclusively expressed on the apical surface, the majority of hRFT-1 is expressed along the basolateral membrane, and hRFT-3 is largely found within intracellular vesicles [6].
- While the exact function of each transporter has not yet been elucidated, the specific locations of these transporters on enterocytes and gene knock out studies support hRFT-2 as the main mode of uptake of free RF from the intestinal lumen, hRFT-1 as the main mode of RF transport into the bloodstream, and hRFT-3 being responsible for maintenance of RF homeostasis at the level of the intestines [6].

- hRFT-3 has additionally been identified in the brain, suggesting its importance in maintaining concentrations of free riboflavin, FMN, and FAD in the brain [7].
- Once absorbed into enterocytes, free riboflavin is converted to FMN by the enzyme cytosolic flavokinase. FAD can further be converted to FMN by the enzyme FAD synthetase. If not converted, free riboflavin is rapidly excreted in urine [8].

Function of Riboflavin

- Multiple steps of the electron transport chain require either FMN or FAD to act as cofactors and, as such, riboflavin is crucial in the generation of ATP [2].
- FAD acts as a coenzyme in multiple intermediary metabolism reactions. This includes beta-oxidation of fatty acids, production of acetyl-CoA and succinyl CoA, and cholesterol synthesis [2].
- Conversion of cholesterol to steroid hormones also requires FAD as a coenzyme for multiple steps [2], and normal riboflavin status has been shown to be crucial for normal adrenal function [8].
- FAD plays a key role in the reduction of glutathione by acting as a cofactor for glutathione reductase. Glutathione, in turn, is a crucial cofactor for reactions that protect cells from reactive nitrogen and oxygen species [2]. Additionally, FAD acts as a coenzyme for the antioxidant xanthine oxidase [2].
- FAD is required to convert folate to the active form, which is required to metabolize homocysteine [8].
- Iron may be released from ferritin by unbound riboflavin, in addition to ascorbate and glutathione [2].

Assessment of Vitamin B2 Status

- Vitamin B2 status is not routinely measured clinically.
- Some laboratories may use an erythrocyte glutathione reductase activity assay to assess serum concentrations of vitamin

B2. This assay yields an erythrocyte glutathione reductase activity coefficient (EGRAC), which is inversely proportionate to the concentration of vitamin B2 in serum [9].

Deficiency

- Deficiency of riboflavin, called ariboflavinosis, is often asymptomatic.
- Symptoms of deficiency include cheilitis, glossitis, stomatitis, mucosal membrane edema, sore throat, seborrheic dermatitis, and normocytic normochromic anemia [9].
- Of note, ariboflavinosis often co-occurs with other vitamin deficiencies.
- Stores of riboflavin within the body are limited to tissue-bound riboflavin. As such, deficiency occurs quickly in the setting of poor intake. It can also be quickly repleted via improved intake or supplementation.
- In countries where fortified foods are readily available, riboflavin deficiency is less common. Underdeveloped countries, particularly those with low meat and dairy consumption, have a higher rate of deficiency [9].
- Other populations who are at a higher risk for riboflavin deficiency include the elderly, pregnant or lactating women, young children, those with restricted diets, including those with eating disorders, and those with physiologically limited absorption at the level of the gut (inflammatory bowel disease, celiac disease, short gut, etc.).
- *Enzymatic deficiency states:*
  - Mutations of the FLAD1 gene, leading to decreased of absent production of FAD synthase, have been described. All cases resulted in progressive neuromuscular compromise and the majority of patients died in early infancy or had a shortened lifespan depending upon the type of mutation and even if the patient had received high dose riboflavin supplementation or not [2].

- Brown–Vialetto–Van Laere Syndrome is caused by the reduced expression of membrane riboflavin transporters, thus reducing availability of FMN and FAD in tissues. This results in progressive sensorineural deafness and bulbar palsy. It can be due to deficiency in either hRFT-1 (Brown–Vialetto–Van Laere Syndrome Type 1) or hRFT-2 (Brown–Vialetto–Van Laere Syndrome Type 2) [2]
- Fazio–Londe Syndrome is caused by reduced expression of hRFT-2 and is characterized by progressive bulbar palsy [10].
- Both Brown–Vialetto–Van Laere Syndrome and Fazio–Londe Syndrome lead to respiratory failure if not adequately treated with riboflavin supplementation [2, 10].

- *Mitochondrial deficiency*: Mutations of the SLC25A32 gene resulting in deficiency of the mitochondrial FAD transporter have been described in two case reports. Both patients experienced deficits in motor function and decreased endurance, which improved with riboflavin supplementation [2].

Toxicity

Riboflavin is water-soluble and is not stored within the human body beyond what is enzymatically bound within tissues. As such, riboflavin toxicity has not been described in humans.

Future Research Possibilities

- Riboflavin's potential for reducing risk of cancer via decreasing impact of reactive oxygen and nitrogen species, along with other mechanisms.
- Riboflavin's potential for decreasing an individual's risk of cardiovascular events via its role in metabolism homocysteine.
- Exact mechanism by which riboflavin derivatives release iron from ferritin.

References

1. Aragão MÂ, Pires L, Santos-Buelga C, Barros L, Calhelha RC. Revitalising riboflavin: unveiling its timeless significance in human physiology and health. Foods. 2024;13(14):2255.
2. Aragão MÂ, et al. Revitalising riboflavin: unveiling its timeless significance in human physiology and health. Foods. 2024;13(14):2255.
3. Riboflavin – Fact Sheet for Health Professionals [Internet]. U.S. Department of Health and Human Services; 2022 [cited 2024 Sept 13]. Available from: https://ods.od.nih.gov/factsheets/Riboflavin-HealthProfessional/
4. Fooddata Central Search Results [Internet]. United States Department of Agriculture; [cited 2024 Sept 13]. Available from: https://fdc.nal.usda.gov/fdc-app.html#/food-search?component=1166
5. Said HM. Intestinal absorption of water-soluble vitamins in health and disease. Biochem J. 2011;437(3):357–72.
6. Subramanian VS, et al. Differential expression of human riboflavin transporters −1, −2, and −3 in polarized epithelia: a key role for hRFT-2 in intestinal riboflavin uptake. Biochim Biophys Acta Biomembr. 2011;1808(12):3016–21.
7. Yao Y, et al. Identification and comparative functional characterization of a new human riboflavin transporter hRFT3 expressed in the brain. J Nutr. 2010;140(7):1220–6.
8. Powers HJ. Riboflavin (vitamin B-2) and health. Am J Clin Nutr. 2003;77(6):1352–60.
9. Parkington DA, Koulman A, Jones KS. Protocol for measuring erythrocyte glutathione reductase activity coefficient to assess riboflavin status. STAR Protocols. 2023;4(4):102726.
10. Varadarajan P, Thayanathi V, Pauline L. Fazio Londe syndrome: a treatable disorder. Ann Indian Acad Neurol. 2014;18:87.

Vitamin B3: Niacin

21

Tsering Yangchen Dirkhipa
and Reema Gulati

Introduction

Vitamin B3, also known as niacin, is one of the water-soluble B-complex vitamins and plays an important role in DNA repair, energy production, and numerous metabolic processes. Its discovery as a vitamin was made in the early twentieth century, while efforts were made to understand and find a cure for a widespread condition called Pellagra, which was common among population with poor diet, particularly those reliant on maize [1]. Joseph Golberger is credited for its discovery due to his extensive studies focusing on niacin [1]. Pellagra is a disorder of niacin deficiency and characterized by "4Ds"—diarrhea, dermatitis, dementia, and death, though uncommon now.

T. Y. Dirkhipa
Department of Pediatrics, MetroHealth Medical Center, Case Western Reserve University, Cleveland, OH, USA
e-mail: tdirkhipa@metrohealth.org

R. Gulati (✉)
Pediatric Gastroenterology, Department of Pediatrics, MetroHealth Medical Center, Case School of Medicine, Case Western Reserve University, Cleveland, OH, USA
e-mail: rgulati@metrohealth.org

K. Radhakrishnan (ed.), *Handbook of Clinical and Practical Pediatric Nutrition*, https://doi.org/10.1007/978-3-031-97759-6_21

Sources The main sources of vitamin B3 are whole grain, cereal, soy, nuts, seeds, legumes, yeast, poultry, red meat, and fish [2, 3].

Digestion and Metabolism

- Niacin is a water-soluble vitamin. It is available in different forms in food, mainly as nicotinic acid and nicotinamide. Tryptophan, which is an amino acid, can also be converted into niacin and hence foods rich in tryptophan are considered a dietary source of niacin [4].
- It is mainly absorbed in the small intestine and a small amount in the stomach [4].
- It is converted into active metabolites: nicotinamide adenine dinucleotide (NAD) and nicotinamide adenine dinucleotide phosphate (NADP). Red blood cells take up some of the excess niacin to form a reserve pool while the remaining excess amounts are methylated in the liver and then excreted in the urine [4].
- NAD and NADP serve as important coenzymes in numerous oxidation–reduction reactions in the body, playing an integral role in the metabolism of glycogen, protein, and fatty acids, as well as the synthesis of pentose and high-energy phosphate bonds [2].
- Factors influencing the availability of niacin: Immunomodulators such as azathioprine, 6-mercaptopurine, and isoniazid, an antitubercular drug, decrease tryptophan conversion and production, respectively. Alcohol can decrease niacin absorption [3].

RDA [4]

- Birth to 6 months: 2 mg.
- 7–12 months: 4 mg NE
- 1–3 years: 6 mg NE
- 4–8 years: 8 mg NE
- 9–13 years: 12 mg NE

- 14–18 years: 16 mg NE (male); 14 mg NE (female).

1 NE = 1 mg of niacin or 60 mg of tryptophan.

Upper Limits [4]

- 1–3 years: 10 mg
- 4–8 years: 15 mg
- 9–13 years: 20 mg
- 14–18 years: 30 mg.

Deficiency

Factors increasing risk for deficiency are as follows [4]:

- Undernutrition.
- Low vitamin B2, B6, and iron (since these are required for tryptophan to niacin conversion).
- Hartnup disease—due to mutation in SLC6A19 in enterocytes and renal tubules:
  - Leads to loss of neutral amino acids, particularly tryptophan.
  - Presents with ataxia, features of Pellagra, nystagmus, and failure to thrive.
  - Rare disorder.
- Carcinoid syndrome—due to low tryptophan availability and excess use by tumor cells.

Pellagra

- Niacin deficiency leads to a condition called Pellagra, which is defined by the classic triad of diarrhea, dermatitis, and dementia [3, 4]. Often, death is added to this triad and then termed as "4Ds"—diarrhea, dermatitis, dementia, and death, though uncommon now [2].

- Gastrointestinal manifestations comprise nausea, vomiting, hypersalivation, abdominal/epigastric pain or discomfort, reduced appetite, and diarrhea [2].
- Cutaneous manifestations begin as erythema, which is bilateral at the sites of sunlight exposure and resembling sunburn. Dermatitis over the neck can sometimes give rise to a necklace-like appearance over the C3 and C4 dermatomes (Casal necklace) [2].
- The neurological symptoms can range from headache, fatigue, and depression to loss of memory and behavioral changes (paranoia, suicidal ideations, and hallucinations) [3, 4].
- It can eventually lead to death if not diagnosed and treated on time [2–4].

Toxicity

- Consumption of 30–50 mg or more/day leads to vasodilation of subcutaneous blood vessels causing transient cutaneous flushing, burning, tingling, and pruritis, which can occur acutely or over days to weeks. Sometimes the vasodilation can be severe enough to cause headache and hypotension [2].
- Consumption of 1000–3000 mg/day can lead to falls, nausea/vomiting, heartburn, hyperglycemia, hyperuricemia, hepatotoxicity, blurry vision, and macular edema [3, 4].
- The above side effects are seen more and at lower doses with nicotinic acid than with nicotinamide [4].

Assessment of Vitamin B3 Status

- The two major methylated metabolites of niacin, N1-methyl-nicotinamide and N1-methyl-2-pyridone-5-carboxamide, are the most reliable and sensitive indicators of niacin status [4].
- Other indicators available are the niacin index (ratio of erythrocyte NAD to NADP concentrations) and the niacin number (ratio of NAD to NADP concentrations in whole blood × 100).

These are based on the fact that the level of NAD decreases with a decline in niacin but NADP concentration remains relatively constant [4].

- Blood level of niacin does not offer a reliable assessment of niacin status [4].

Role in Medicine

- *Dyslipidemia*: Niacin may be used as an adjunct to statins and other lipid-lowering agents. According to AHA/ACA, the addition of niacin to statins does not affect ASCVD (atherosclerotic cardiovascular disease) outcomes but may be helpful in hypertriglyceridemia. Due to the risk of adverse effects such as flushing, which is commonly observed in the pediatric population along with incidences of liver failure, myopathy, and glucose intolerance among others, it is not recommended routinely in the treatment of pediatric dyslipidemia [2].
- *Pellagra*: Off-label use. Nicotinamide is preferred in the treatment of Pellagra due to its lack of cutaneous side effects such as flushing, pruritis, and burning sensation [2].

Newer Role/Research in Development

- Role of topical nicotinamide in the management of Discoid lupus erythematosus [2].
- Role of high-dose vitamin B3 in fatal neurodegenerative conditions such as progressive encephalopathy with brain edema and leukoencephalopathy-2 (PEBEL2): defective NADPH oxidoreductase-like protein (NAXD) and progressive encephalopathy with brain edema or leukoencephalopathy-1 (PEBEL1): deficiency of NADPH epoxidase (NAXE) [2] .

References

1. Lanska DJ. The discovery of niacin, biotin, and pantothenic acid. Ann Nutr Metab. 2012;61(3):246–53. https://doi.org/10.1159/000343115. Epub 2012 Nov 26. PMID: 23183297
2. Peechakara BV, Gupta M. Vitamin B3. [Updated 2024 Feb 29]. In: StatPearls [Internet]. Treasure Island: StatPearls; 2024. Available from: https://www.ncbi.nlm.nih.gov/books/NBK526107/
3. Hanna M, Jaqua E, Nguyen V, Clay J. B Vitamins: functions and uses in medicine. Perm J. 2022;26(2):89–97.
4. ods.od.nih.gov [Internet]. Maryland: NIH Office of dietary supplements [updated 2022 Nov, cited 2024 Sep]. Available from: https://ods.od.nih.gov/factsheets/Niacin-HealthProfessional/#disc

22 Vitamin B5: Pantothenic Acid

Mohammad Nasser Kabbany

Introduction

Vitamin B5 or pantothenic acid (PA) is one of the water-soluble vitamins. Being a main component of Coenzyme A (CoA) makes it important for different metabolic functions like release of energy from carbohydrate, synthesis, and degradation of fatty acids [1]. Its name is derived from the Greek word "pantothen," which means "from everywhere," indicating its wide availability in diet [2].

Sources of Pantothenic Acid and RDA

PA is redundant in regular diet [1].

- Dietary sources include meat, fish, poultry, whole grains, and legumes.
- It is also present in breast milk and infant formula. Colonic bacteria produce PA as well.

M. N. Kabbany (✉)
Department of Pediatric Gastroenterology, Hepatology and Nutrition, University of Chicago, Chicago, IL, USA

K. Radhakrishnan (ed.), *Handbook of Clinical and Practical Pediatric Nutrition*, https://doi.org/10.1007/978-3-031-97759-6_22

- Adequate intake (AI) is suggested to be 5 mg/day for adults and children above 11 years of age.
- For infants and younger children, 2 and 4 mg/day is proposed.

Digestion and Metabolism of Pantothenic Acid

- Dietary PA has two forms: CoA and peptide-bound 4′-phosphopantetheine.
- They are then metabolized in the intestinal lumen into PA, which is absorbed by the enterocytes via SLC5A6/SMVT (sodium-dependent multivitamin transporter) carrier.
- PA subsequently circulates in the blood in the free form and in the red blood cells.
- SLC5A6/SMVT is found in the colonocytes and is the same carrier that facilitates passage of PA across the blood–brain barrier.
- CoA is then synthesized from PA through a multistep process.
- Mitochondria has the largest pool of PA in the form of CoA
- PA is released from CoA, and ACP (acyl carrier protein) can be recycled and utilized again. PA is excreted in the urine [4].

Pantothenic Acid Deficiency

Isolated PA deficiency is rare and is usually associated with other vitamin deficiencies. PA deficiency has been associated with wide range of signs and symptoms including [1]

- Depression
- Neuromuscular findings (distal paresthesia, distal weakness, hyperreflexia without Babinskis signs)
- Cardiovascular (labile heart rate, wide pulse pressure, orthostatic hypotension)
- Gastrointestinal (vomiting and slow growth)
- Recurrent respiratory infections, abortion, and infertility

Pantothenate Kinase-Associated Neurodegeneration (PKAN) is an inborn error of CoA synthesis that results from a mutation in pantothenate kinase enzyme 2 and leads to iron accumulation in the brain [4]. Symptoms include limb dystonia and spasticity, toe walking, developmental delay, ADHD, and retinopathy [4].

Assessment of Pantothenic Acid Status

Circulating levels of PA correlate with its status. It can be measured either in whole blood or 24-h urine. Low levels are considered <1 μmol/L in whole blood and urinary excretion <1 mg/day [4].

Pantothenic Acid Toxicity

PA toxicity is rare and large doses of the vitamin are generally tolerated (as high as 2 g/day). Ingesting massive doses of PA (10–20 g) can cause diarrhea, muscle cramps, and water retention [4].

Future Directions

Pantothenic acid deficiency has been linked to dementia in neurodegenerative diseases such as Parkinson's disease [5]. Future studies are needed to determine if supplementation with PA has any preventative or therapeutic effects in these diseases [6].

References

1. Sonneville, Kendrin, and Christopher P. Duggan. Manual of Pediatric Nutrition. 5th ed., People's Medical Publishing House-USA, 2014.
2. Lanska DJ. The discovery of niacin, biotin, and pantothenic acid. Ann Nutr Metab. 2012;61(3):246–53. https://doi.org/10.1159/000343115.
3. Berger MM, Shenkin A, Schweinlin A, et al. ESPEN micronutrient guideline [published correction appears in Clin Nutr. 2024 Apr;43(4):1024.

doi: 10.1016/j.clnu.2024.03.004]. Clin Nutr. 2022;41(6):1357–424. https://doi.org/10.1016/j.clnu.2022.02.015.
4. Freese R, Aarsland TE, Bjørkevoll M. Pantothenic acid – a scoping review for Nordic Nutrition Recommendations 2023. Food Nutr Res. 2023;67 https://doi.org/10.29219/fnr.v67.10255. Published 2023 Dec 13
5. Hogarth P, Kurian MA, Gregory A, et al. Consensus clinical management guideline for pantothenate kinase-associated neurodegeneration (PKAN). Mol Genet Metab. 2017;120(3):278–87. https://doi.org/10.1016/j.ymgme.2016.11.004.
6. Xu J, Patassini S, Begley P, et al. Cerebral deficiency of vitamin B5 (d-pantothenic acid; pantothenate) as a potentially-reversible cause of neurodegeneration and dementia in sporadic Alzheimer's disease. Biochem Biophys Res Commun. 2020;527(3):676–81. https://doi.org/10.1016/j.bbrc.2020.05.015.

Vitamin B_6: Pyridoxine

23

Natalie Bhesania

Introduction

Vitamin B_6 (B_6) is a water-soluble vitamin that is found in a variety of animal and plant products. It is a crucial vitamin involved in a wide array of metabolic and cellular functions (Table 23.1). It encompasses three compounds: pyridoxal (PL), pyridoxine (PN), pyridoxamine (PM) and their corresponding 5′-phosphate esters: pyridoxal 5′-phosphate (PLP), pyridoxamine 5′-phosphate (PMP), and pyridoxine 5′-phosphate (PNP) [1, 2].

N. Bhesania (✉)
Division of Gastroenterology, Hepatology, and Nutrition, Children's Hospital Los Angeles, Los Angeles, CA, USA

K. Radhakrishnan (ed.), *Handbook of Clinical and Practical Pediatric Nutrition*, https://doi.org/10.1007/978-3-031-97759-6_23

Table 23.1 Important enzymes that need pyridoxine as a cofactor and their role [14]

Enzyme	Role
Glycogen phosphorylase	Rate-limiting step in glycogenolysis (glycogen to glucose-1-phosphate)
Aminolevulinic acid synthase	PLP is a coenzyme for aminolevulinic acid synthase, which is important for hemoglobin synthesis. PLP enhances oxygen binding ability of hemoglobin
Sphingosine-1-phosphase lyase	This enzyme is dependent on PLP and is important for lipid metabolism (involved in breakdown of sphingosine-1-phosphate)
Aromatic L-amino acid decarboxylase	Converts 5-HTP into 5-HT (serotonin)

Vitamin B_6 Absorption, Metabolism, and Physiological Role

PLP and PMP are animal-derived foods and PN and PNP are derived from plant-based foods.

- Humans are unable to produce B_6 and require an important enzyme, PDXK, to phosphorylate PL, PN, and PM into their respective 5′-phosphate esters [3].
- B_6 is absorbed in the jejunum via passive diffusion after undergoing dephosphorylation and is excreted as 4-pyridoxic acid in the urine [1, 2].

PLP and PMP are the major active forms of B_6 and are important coenzymes found in muscle bound to phosphorylase.

- These coenzyme forms of B_6 are involved in over 100 different biochemical enzyme reactions [4].
- While this is not an extensive list, they are involved in protein and amino acid metabolism, immune function, neurotransmitter biosynthesis, gluconeogenesis, glycogenolysis, and hemoglobin formation [1, 4].

- Table 23.1 highlights a few important enzymes that require pyridoxine as a cofactor.

Vitamin B_6 Deficiency

In isolation, B_6 deficiency is rare and is typically associated with poor nutritional status and other B-vitamin deficiencies, including vitamin B12 and folic acid [2].

- The majority of Vitamin B_6 is stored in muscle tissue and stores are not affected until there has been several weeks of poor intake of Vitamin B_6.
- Vitamin B_6 deficiency can be seen in certain patient populations including celiac disease, inflammatory bowel disease, other malabsorption conditions, end-stage renal disease, and certain genetic conditions [4].
- In addition, certain medications that interfere with metabolism of PN can lead to B_6 deficiency over an extended period and include, but are not limited to, levodopa/carbidopa, isoniazid, penicillamine, and hydralazine [5, 6].
- Symptomatic presentation can range from irritability, confusion, depression, peripheral neuropathy, weakened immune response, stomatitis, glossitis, cheilosis, microcytic anemia, seborrheic dermatitis, and seizures [1].
- The clinician should have a high index of suspicion in the appropriate clinical setting to consider this deficiency, given the nonspecific clinical presentation and symptomatic overlap with other vitamin deficiencies.

Treatment of Vitamin B_6 Deficiency

- A variety of supplementation options are available (oral and parenteral) for patients with Vitamin B_6 deficiency. Treatment approach should be based on the age of the patient, symptom presentation, and severity.

- 5–25 mg/day (PO, IM, IV) is recommended for 3 weeks duration followed by 2.5–5 mg/day, which can be administered in the form of a daily multivitamin in pediatric patients [7].
- 10–20 mg/day (PO, IM, IV) is recommended for 3 weeks duration followed by 2–5 mg/day, which can be obtained from a daily multivitamin in adolescent patients [7].

Pyridoxine-Dependent Epilepsy (PDE)

- Recurrent, intractable seizures in the neonatal period that are unresponsive to traditional antiepileptic medications in patient without abnormal perinatal history or underlying brain malformation [8].
- Seizure onset typically within the first weeks to months of life.
- PDE is inherited in an autosomal recessive pattern and involves a mutation in *ALDH7A1* (alpha-aminoadipic semialdehyde dehydrogenase or atiquitin) [9].
- This is an enzyme involved in lysine metabolism and the metabolic intermediate that builds up, Δ-piperideine-6-carboxylic acid (P6C), inactivates PLP and causes seizures secondary to effects of pyridoxine deficiency.
- Responsive to large doses of supplemental B_6 (pyridoxine).
- The most recent guidelines recommend treatment of PDE as follows: Newborns: 100 mg/day (IV), infants: 30 mg/kg/day (300 mg/day max dose), age 1 and older: 30 mg/kg/day (500 mg/day max dose) [10].
- Other rare disorders that cause seizures as manifestation secondary to pyridoxine and PLP deficiency include pyridoxamine phosphate oxidase (PNPO) deficiency, alkaline phosphatase deficiency (congenital hypophosphatasia), and hyperprolinemia type II. Seizures may respond to high-dose pyridoxine/PLP supplementation.

Vitamin B_6 Toxicity

Vitamin B_6 toxicity is usually iatrogenic and not related to the isolated ingestion of food sources alone.

- Patients typically ingest significant dosages in the form of supplements, leading to a variety of symptoms that can overlap with symptoms seen with Vitamin B_6 deficiency [11].
- Symptoms usually manifest after long-term ingestion of supratherapeutic doses of Vitamin B_6 and range from nausea, dizziness, photosensitivity, dermatoses to peripheral neuropathy.

Vitamin B_6 Supplementation

- Vitamin B_6 is available on its own and in a variety of supplements and multivitamins. It is most commonly available as pyridoxine. It is available in a variety of formulations including capsules, tablets (chewable, sublingual), and liquid for ease of administration.
- Vitamin B_6 supplements are also absorbed in the jejunum, like its natural animal- and plant-based sources but the majority is excreted in the urine [1, 2].
- In the general population, the tolerable upper intake level (UL) in patients 19 years of age and older is 100 mg daily [12]. It is important to note that this can only be achieved with the intake of supplements and not from dietary sources alone.
- The recommended dietary allowance (RDA) varies by age and requirements are higher in elderly individuals and during pregnancy and lactation.

Vitamin B_6 Dietary Sources

- Most Vitamin B_6 in the United States is consumed from animal sources (poultry and beef products), fortified cereals, whole grains, fish, certain fruits, and starchy vegetables.

Table 23.2 Pyridoxine RDA

Age	Male	Female	Pregnancy	Lactation
Birth to 6 months	0.1 mg	0.1 mg		
7–12 months	0.3 mg	0.3 mg		
1–3 years	0.5 mg	0.5 mg		
4–8 years	0.6 mg	0.6 mg		
9–13 years	1.0 mg	1.0 mg		
14–18 years	1.3 mg	1.2 mg	1.9 mg	2.0 mg
19–50 years	1.3 mg	1.3 mg	1.9 mg	2.0 mg
51+ years	1.7 mg	1.5 mg		

Adapted from NIH vitamin B_6 fact sheet for healthcare professionals

- Particularly high sources of Vitamin B_6 include beef liver, organ meat, fish, chickpeas, milk and other dairy products, eggs, and certain vegetables (spinach and carrots) [13].
- The recommended dietary allowance (RDA) of Vitamin B_6 can vary based on age (Table 23.2).
- We recommend referring to the most recent guidelines as recommendations may change from the time of this publication.
- Special populations to consider that have higher requirements include pregnant (1.9 mg/day) and lactating females (2.0 mg/day).

Future Research Opportunities

Vitamin B_6 plays a vital role in a variety of important biologic and enzymatic reactions. It has been linked with brain performance and metabolism. Future research looking into the role Vitamin B_6 plays in memory and learning abilities could play a valuable role in the pediatric and adult populations in relation to learning difficulties and impaired memory function in our aging population.

References

1. Dietary Reference Intakes for Thiamin, Riboflavin, Niacin, Vitamin B6, Folate, Vitamin B12, Pantothenic Acid, Biotin, and Choline. Dietary Reference Intakes for Thiamin, Riboflavin, Niacin, Vitamin B6, Folate, Vitamin B12, Pantothenic Acid, Biotin, and Choline. National Academies Press; 1998.
2. da Silva VR, Russell KA, Gregory JF. Vitamin B. In: Present knowledge in nutrition. Wiley; 2012. p. 307–20.
3. Stach K, Stach W, Augoff K. Vitamin B6 in health and disease. Nutrients. 2021;13(9)
4. Mackey A, Davis S, Gregory J. Modern nutrition in health and disease. In: Vitamin B6. 10th ed. Baltimore: Lippincott Williams & Wilkins; 2005.
5. Ghavanini AA, Kimpinski K. Revisiting the evidence for neuropathy caused by pyridoxine deficiency and excess [Internet]. J Clin Neuromusc Dis. 16;2014. www.jcnmd.com
6. Lheureux P, Penaloza A, Gris M. 78 Review pyridoxine in clinical toxicology: a review. Eur J Emerg Med. 2005;12
7. Kliegman RM, Behrman RE, Jenson HB. Nelson textbook of pediatrics. 18th ed. Saunders Elsevier; 2007. p. 2955–99.
8. Adam M, Feldman K, Mirzaa G. Pyridoxine-dependent epilepsy – ALDH7A1. Seattle: GeneReviews®; 2022.
9. Bok LA, Struys E, Willemsen MAAP, Been JV, Jakobs C. Pyridoxine-dependent seizures in Dutch patients: diagnosis by elevated urinary alpha-aminoadipic semialdehyde levels. Arch Dis Child. 2007;92(8):687–9.
10. Coughlin CR, Tseng LA, Abdenur JE, Ashmore C, Boemer F, Bok LA, et al. Consensus guidelines for the diagnosis and management of pyridoxine-dependent epilepsy due to α-aminoadipic semialdehyde dehydrogenase deficiency. J Inherit Metab Dis. 2021;44(1):178–92.
11. Plasma pyridoxal 5 phosphate in the US population: the National Health and Nutrition Examination Survey, 2003–2004.
12. Institute of Medicine (US) Standing Committee on the Scientific Evaluation of Dietary Reference Intakes and its Panel on Folate, Other B Vitamins, and Choline. Dietary reference intakes for thiamin, riboflavin, niacin, vitamin B6, folate, Vitamin B12, pantothenic acid, biotin, and choline. Washington, DC: National Academies Press; 1998. Available from: https://www.ncbi.nlm.nih.gov/books/NBK114310/. https://doi.org/10.17226/6015.
13. Cotton PA, Subar AF, Friday JE, Cook A. Dietary sources of nutrients among US adults, 1994 to 1996. J Am Diet Assoc. 2004;104(6):921–30.
14. Combs Jr GF. The vitamins, 3rd ed.

Biotin 24

Christine Seif Pasquarella

Biotin is also known as vitamin B7 or vitamin H.

- Biotin structure consists of two cyclic molecules.
- Initially found in yeast.
- Water-soluble vitamin that acts as an essential cofactor for several carboxylases involved in the cellular metabolism of fatty acids, amino acids, and gluconeogenesis.
- Biotin is a CO_2 carrier on the surface of each enzyme.

Cofactor for four carboxylase enzymes [1]:

1. Acetyl coenzyme A (CoA) carboxylase (ACC).
2. Pyruvate carboxylase (PC).
3. Propionyl CoA carboxylase (PCC).
4. Methylcrotonyl CoA carboxylase (MCC).

Biotinidase is the enzyme responsible for recycling biotin.

It acts as a hydrolase by cleaving biocytin and biotinyl-peptides to allow the availability of biotin from bound dietary sources (Fig. 24.1).

C. S. Pasquarella (✉)
Pediatric Gastroenterology, Hepatology and Nutrition, Akron Children's Hospital, Akron, OH, USA
e-mail: cpasquarella@akronchildrens.org

K. Radhakrishnan (ed.), *Handbook of Clinical and Practical Pediatric Nutrition*, https://doi.org/10.1007/978-3-031-97759-6_24

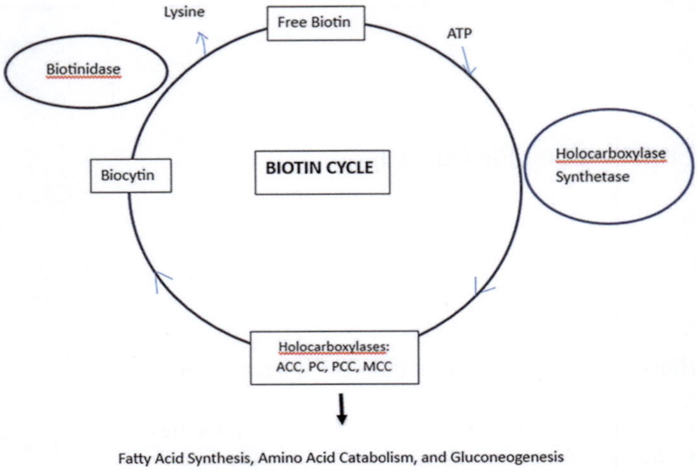

Fig. 24.1 Biotin cycle

Other functions of biotin are as follows: [1].

- Cell proliferation and DNA repair.
- Normal macrophage function.
- Production of antibodies.
- Differentiation of T and B lymphocytes.
- Essential cofactor for mitochondrial carboxylases in hair roots and in keratin production.
  - Although biotin supplementation has been heavily marketed and has gained commercial popularity as useful for hair loss and brittle nails, evidence for this is lacking [2, 3].

Sources of biotin: [1].

1. Dietary source.
   - Found in a variety of plants as most microorganisms and plants are able to synthesize biotin [4].
   - Highest levels are found in egg yolk, soybean products, nuts, yeast, and in organ meat such as liver.

- Biotin is bound to proteins in food and becomes bioavailable after it is released through the action of biotinidase—this occurs in the intestinal lumen.
  - More uptake occurs in proximal compared to distal small intestine.

2. Bacterial source.
   - Biotin is generated in the large intestine by digestive enzymes, bacteria, and by biotinidase.

Excess biotin is excreted in the urine and unabsorbed biotin is excreted in the feces.

Serum concentration of biotin is not sensitive and not routinely tested.

Clinical Manifestations

Biotin Deficiency

Overall, this rarely occurs [5].

Classic manifestations:

- Dermatitis—especially around the eyes, nose, and mouth.
- Conjunctivitis.
- Alopecia.
- Neurologic symptoms.

It was first noted in patients on long-term parenteral nutrition prior to routine biotin supplementation.

Deficiency can occur with consumption of large amounts of raw egg whites as this impairs biotin absorption [1].

- This is due to avidin contained in the egg whites—a substance that binds to biotin and prevents its absorption.
- Cooking the egg whites denatures avidin while biotin remains functional.

Can also occur in patients on long-term anticonvulsant therapy.

Secondary Biotin Deficiency

Multiple carboxylase deficiency: an inherited autosomal recessive disorder of biotin metabolism [6].

- Neonatal form: deficiency of holocarboxylase synthetase (HCLS).
  - Presents in the first week of life.
  - Symptoms: lethargy, hypotonia, seizures, emesis/feeding difficulty.
  - Exhibits metabolic acidosis, organic aciduria, hyperammonemia.
- Later onset: biotinidase deficiency.
  - Slow but progressive loss of biotin in the urine leading to organic aciduria.
  - Symptoms: hypotonia, ataxia, seizures, myoclonus, nystagmus, dermatitis, alopecia, visual and hearing impairments.
  - Exhibits metabolic acidosis, organic aciduria.

Testing for these deficiencies does occur on the newborn screen in most states, as delayed treatment could result in irreversible neurologic symptoms and even death [4, 6].

Both forms can be treated with pharmacologic doses of biotin (5–20 μg/day) [1, 6].

Recommendations for Dosage Intake

The production of biotin from intestinal bacteria is sufficient to meet the body's daily requirements in most healthy individuals (Tables 24.1, 24.2, and 24.3).

No toxicity has been reported.

It is useful to note that pharmacologic doses of biotin supplementation, as low as 10 μg daily, can interfere with laboratory tests for thyroid function. This will result in a pattern that mimics Grave's disease. Biotin supplementation should be held for 48–72 h prior to testing thyroid function [9].

Table 24.1 Recommendations for daily dietary reference intake of biotin [7]

Age	μg/day
0–6 months	5
7–12 months	6
1–3 years	8
4–8 years	12
9–13 years	20
14–18 years	25
>18 years	30

Table 24.2 Recommendations for daily IV intake of biotin [7]

Age	μg/day
Preterm infants	5–8
Term infants and children 1–12 years	20
>12 years	60

Table 24.3 Recommendations for life-long targeted treatment in holocarboxylase and biotinidase deficiency [8]

Enzyme activity	μg/day
<10%	5–10 initially, increasing up to 20 if needed
10–30%	2.5–10 initially, increasing up to 20 if needed

Future Research Possibilities

The role of biotin in the brain has been of increasing interest. High dose (100–300 μg/day) biotin supplementation may represent a therapeutic option to slow progression for patients with multiple sclerosis [10].

Research regarding the implications of biotin nutritional status and deficiency in pregnancy is lacking [5].

References

1. Said HM. Biotin: Biochemical, Physiological and Clinical Aspects. Subcell Biochem. 2011:1–19.
2. Patel DP, Swink SM, Castelo-Soccio L. A review of the use of biotin for hair loss. Skin Appendage Disord [Internet]. 2017;3(3):166–9. Available from: https://www.karger.com/Article/FullText/462981#.
3. Soleymani T, Lo Sicco K, Shapiro J. The infatuation with biotin supplementation: is there truth behind its rising popularity? A comparative analysis of clinical efficacy versus social popularity. J Drugs Dermatol JDD [Internet]. 2017;16(5):496–500. Available from: https://pubmed.ncbi.nlm.nih.gov/28628687/.
4. Ma D, Du G, Fang H, Li R, Zhang D. Advances and prospects in microbial production of biotin. Microb Cell Factories [Internet]. 2024 [cited 2024 Jul 16];23:135. Available from: https://www.ncbi.nlm.nih.gov/pmc/articles/PMC11089781/
5. Said HM. Biotin bioavailability and estimated average requirement: why bother? Am J Clin Nutr. 1999;69(3):352–3.
6. Hymes J, Wolf B. Biotinidase and its roles in biotin metabolism. Clin Chim Acta [Internet]. 1996 [cited 2021 Nov 15];255(1):1–11. Available from: https://www.sciencedirect.com/science/article/abs/pii/0009898196063966
7. Wyllie R, Hyams JS, Kay M. Pediatric gastrointestinal and liver disease. Philadelphia: Elsevier; 2015.
8. Wolf B. Biotinidase deficiency [Internet]. Adam MP, Everman DB, Mirzaa GM, Pagon RA, Wallace SE, Bean LJ, et al., editors. PubMed. Seattle: University of Washington, Seattle; 1993. Available from: https://pubmed.ncbi.nlm.nih.gov/20301497/
9. Ylli D, Soldin SJ, Stolze B, Wei B, Nigussie G, Nguyen H, et al. Biotin interference in assays for thyroid hormones, thyrotropin and thyroglobulin. Thyroid. 2021;
10. Mock DM. Biotin: from nutrition to therapeutics. J Nutr [Internet]. 2017;147(8):1487–92. Available from: https://www.ncbi.nlm.nih.gov/pmc/articles/PMC5525106/pdf/jn238956.pdf.

Vitamin B12

25

Amala Alenchery
and Kadakkal Radhakrishnan

Introduction

Vitamin B12 (cyanocobalamin) is a water-soluble vitamin primarily from animal sources that is an integral cofactor for enzymes involved in fatty acids, myelin, and deoxyribonucleic acid (DNA) synthesis. Its deficiency can result in hematologic and neurologic abnormalities, which may be irreversible if not managed early.

Sources of Vitamin B12 [1, 2]

B12 is predominantly obtained from animal sources such as

A. Alenchery (✉) · K. Radhakrishnan
Division of Pediatric Gastroenterology, Hepatology and Nutrition, Cleveland Clinic Children's Hospital, Cleveland, OH, USA
e-mail: alencherya@upmc.edu; radhakk@ccf.org

K. Radhakrishnan (ed.), *Handbook of Clinical and Practical Pediatric Nutrition*, https://doi.org/10.1007/978-3-031-97759-6_25

- Liver, red meat, dairy, fish, and eggs with minor amounts found in plant sources and foods contaminated or fermented by bacteria such as tempeh and Thai fish sauce (Table 25.1).
- Newborns predominantly depend on maternal B12 stores up to 6 months of age, after which solid food sources are essential.
- About 50% dietary B12 is absorbed with differing age and gender-based recommended dietary allowance (RDA) (Table 25.2) [3].

Table 25.1 Dietary sources of Vitamin B12

Major sources
Liver
Red meat
Oysters
Shellfish/fish
Nutritional yeast (fortified)
Minor sources
Turkey
Chicken
Dairy
Eggs
Breakfast cereal (fortified)
Tempeh

Table 25.2 Age and gender-specific adequate intake (infants) and RDA (older children) for Vitamin B12 [3]

Age	Adequate intake (<1 year of age)	RDA—males	RDA—females
0–6 months	0.4 mcg	–	–
7–12 months	0.5 mcg	–	–
1–3 years	–	0.9 mcg	0.9 mcg
4–8 years	–	1.2 mcg	1.2 mcg
9–13 years	–	1.8 mcg	2.4 mcg
14–18 years	–	1.8 mcg	2.4 mcg

Digestion and Metabolism of Vitamin B12 [1, 2]

- B12 from food binds to salivary R-protein in the mouth until it forms a complex with haptocorrin in the stomach, which is resistant to acid (Fig. 25.1).
- Gastric parietal cells secrete intrinsic factor (IF), which forms the IF-B12 complex in the duodenum responsible for transportation.
- Final site of absorption is the terminal ileum after binding to the receptor protein cubulin, with co-receptors megalin and amnionless.
- In the bloodstream, 80% B12 is inactive, bound to transport protein transcobalamin I (TCI), also known as haptocorrin, with the remaining 20% bound to active transcobalamin II (TC II) to

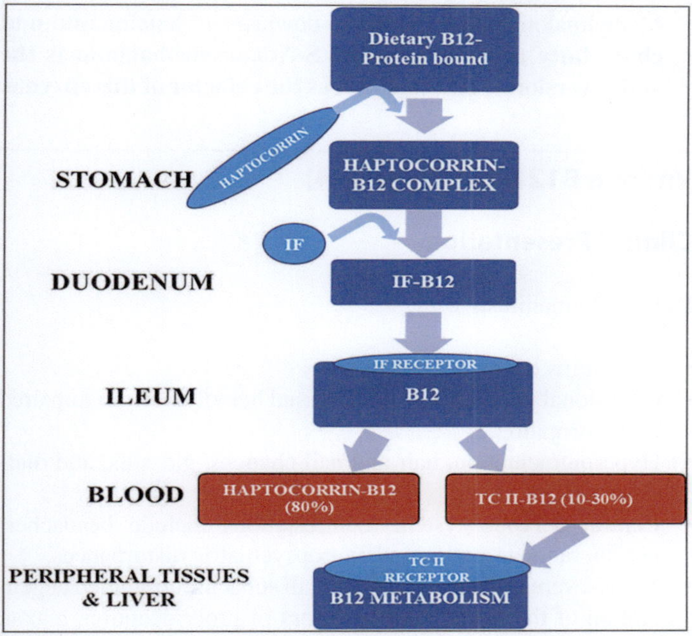

Fig. 25.1 Dietary absorption and transport of Vitamin B12

form holotranscobalamin, which facilitates transport and absorption at peripheral tissues as well as the liver, which serves as the predominant storage site.

- B12 is secreted in bile, reabsorbed via enterohepatic circulation through ileal IF receptors, and excreted in the feces typically with urinary excretion only when levels exceed TC binding capacity.

Role of Vitamin B12

B12 is an important coenzyme for several enzymes such as

- Methionine synthase (essential for methylation of several compounds including DNA, RNA and proteins). **Methylcobalamin, a metabolite of B12 is the cofactor for this enzyme.**
- Methylmalonyl-CoA mutase in downstream **leucine and odd chain fatty acid metabolism. S-Adenosylcobalamin is the active version of B12 that acts as the cofactor of this enzyme.**

Vitamin B12 Deficiency [2–4]

Clinical Presentation

Deficiency manifests with:

- Symptoms of fatigue and pallor.
- Occasional jaundice due to increased hemolysis from impaired RBC formation.
- Hyperpigmentation, hair and nail changes, glossitis, and diarrhea.
- Central nervous system manifestations include headaches, peripheral neuropathy, and neuropsychiatric disturbances.
- More severe deficiency can result in subacute combined degeneration of the spinal cord with loss of proprioception, ataxia, and dementia.
- Infants born to mothers deficient in folate and B12 can develop neural tube defects.

Etiology

There are several causes for deficiency, which may be independent or multifactorial:

- *Dietary insufficiency*: Dietary insufficiency such as strict vegan and some ovo-lacto-vegetarian diets, exclusively breastfed infants of women on vegan diets or with untreated pernicious anemia.
- *Autoimmune*: Pernicious anemia due to antibodies against IF.
- *Malabsorption*:
  - Due to inflammation of small bowel from celiac disease, small bowel bacterial overgrowth, or parasitic infections (due to competition for B12).
  - Decreased IF production from gastric bypass surgery.
  - Impaired absorption due to surgical resection of terminal ileum for any pathology, such as for severe Crohn's disease.
- *Genetic or hereditary defects*:
  - Secondary to intrinsic factor, transcobalamin II deficiency (causing impaired transmembrane B12 transport) or congenital B12 malabsorption (Imerslun–Grasbeck disease).
  - Transcobalamin II deficiency (autosomal recessive): TCII is the plasma protein required for transport of B12 from bloodstream to cells (Fig. 25.1). Deficiency results in a rare disorder presenting in infancy with failure to thrive, pallor, diarrhea, emesis, weakness, developmental delay with lab findings of megaloblastic anemia, and pancytopenia with normal or high plasma B12 levels in the setting of elevated methylmalonic acid (MMA) and homocysteine levels. Treatment involves long-term parenteral B12 supplementation.
  - Disorders of B12 metabolism can be associated with various metabolic disorders (Fig. 25.2): Cbl C, D, and F mutations are associated with combined methylmalonic aciduria and homocystinuria. Cbl A and B mutations are associated

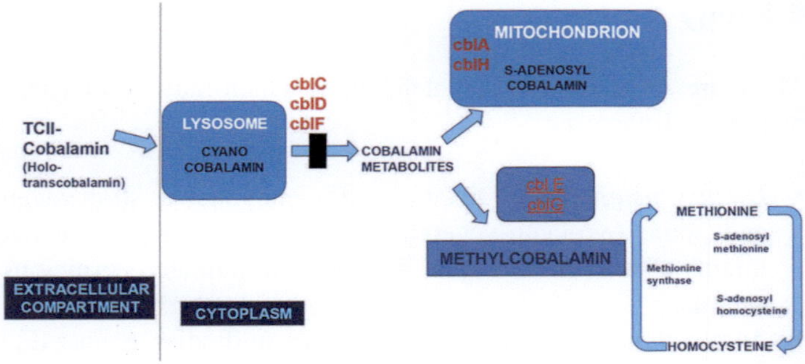

Fig. 25.2 Cellular level metabolism of B12, associated transporters and the role of B12 as a cofactor. THF, tetrahydrofolate; TC-II, transcobalamin II

with methylmalonic aciduria, while Cbl E and G mutations are associated with homocystinuria.

- Certain medication such as metformin, nitrous oxide, (in toxic levels), or acid blockers (PPI or H2 blockers) potentially interact with B12 absorption and can adversely affect serum B12 levels.

Assessment of Vitamin B12 Status

Careful dietary history and physical examination is integral to assess for chronic inflammatory processes such as celiac disease, Crohn's disease, or surgical bowel resection.

- Labs reveal megaloblastic anemia (decreased hemoglobin and elevated MCV >100) on complete blood count (CBC) with macrocytic red cells and hypersegmented neutrophils on peripheral smear.
- Serum folate levels help distinguish it from folate deficiency, which can have a similar presentation or may coexist with B12 deficiency.
- Serum B12 levels are typically <200 pg/mL when deficient.

- Elevated MMA and homocysteine levels aid in the diagnosis, particularly with borderline low B12.
- Schilling test was historically important for diagnosis of pernicious anemia, but is now replaced with IF antibodies and serum gastrin levels in addition to the above testing.
- Megaloblastic anemia in infancy and in toddlers should raise concerns of maternal deficiency or possibility of transcobalamin II deficiency or disorders of B12 metabolism.

Management [4, 5]

Cyanocobalamin is a synthetic form of vitamin B12 available in enteral and parenteral forms, which is approved by the FDA in the United States to treat deficiencies. Hydroxocobalamin is an additional formulation. Limited data is available regarding optimal pediatric dosing regimen with variability in practice. Treatment or supplementation is continued in maintenance phase until symptoms have completely resolved or even longer.

- Enteral formulations (oral, sublingual, intranasal): Absorption through GI tract into bloodstream by binding to IF and other transport proteins. **Enteral option** is safe and effective in children with normal absorptive capability without severe anemia or neurologic symptoms (Table 25.3).
- **Parental formulations** (intramuscular and subcutaneous): peak blood levels in 1 h. Preparation should be stored at room temperature and is light sensitive. In overt deficiency states, parenteral preparation is preferred (Table 25.4).
- Patients require close monitoring for hypokalemia in the setting of myalgias and muscle cramps while correcting the deficient state with parenteral B12 supplementation.

Table 25.3 Enteral/oral dosing of Vitamin B12 supplements in children

Age	Oral formulations	
Sezer et al. [6]	Duration	Dose
6 months to 18 years	1 week	1000 mcg/day daily
	1 week	1000 mcg/day every other day
	2 weeks	1000 mcg/day twice weekly
	3 months	1000 mcg/day weekly
Chandelia et al. [7]		
<1 year	8 weeks	125 mcg/day
1–2 years		250 mcg/day
>2 years		500 mcg/day

Table 25.4 Parenteral dosing of Vitamin B12 supplements in children and adolescents

Parenteral formulation			
Children		Adolescents	
Duration	Dose	Duration	Dose
1 week	100 mcg/day	1 week	1000 mcg/day
1 week	1000 mcg/day every other day	1 month	1000 mcg/week
1 week	1000 mcg/day twice weekly	1 year (maintenance therapy)	1000 mcg/month (cyanocobalamin) or 1000 mcg every 2 months (hydroxycobalamin)
4–8 weeks	1000 mcg/day weekly	–	–

Vitamin B12 Toxicity: Acute and Chronic

Excess nutritional intake does not result in toxicity; however, high-dose oral supplements over a prolonged period can result in some adverse reactions such as erythroderma, acneiform rash, chromaturia, nausea, and headache. There may be rare instances of B12 toxicity from parental administration. Empiric hydroxocobalamin IV therapy is used to curb cyanide toxicity in smoke inhalational injury with the adverse effects of transient hypertension and reflex bradycardia.

Vitamin B12: Future Research Applications

There is ongoing research to identify new cobalamin injectable products for treatment of a range of conditions from IEM to neurological disorders to name a few. There is potential for B12 as an antioxidant and as vectors for xenobiotics, e.g., in drug transport within the body as well as controlled release in malignant cells/ tissues. There is need for further data regarding optimal dosing and other controlled release forms of B12 supplements for therapy, particularly in pediatrics.

References

1. O'Leary F, Samman S. Vitamin B12 in health and disease. Nutrients [Internet]. 2010;2(3):299–316. Available from: https://www.ncbi.nlm.nih.gov/pmc/articles/PMC3257642/.
2. Sobczyńska-Malefora A, Delvin E, McCaddon A, Ahmadi KR, Harrington DJ. Vitamin B12 status in health and disease: a critical review. Diagnosis of deficiency and insufficiency – clinical and laboratory pitfalls. Crit Rev Clin Lab Sci. 2021;58(6):399–429.
3. Folate I of M (US) SC on the SE of DRI and its P on, Vitamins OB, Choline A. Vitamin B12 [Internet]. www.ncbi.nlm.nih.gov. National Academies Press (US); 1998. Available from: https://www.ncbi.nlm.nih.gov/books/NBK114302/.
4. Ankar A, Kumar A. Vitamin b12 deficiency [Internet]. National Library of Medicine. StatPearls; 2022. Available from: https://www.ncbi.nlm.nih.gov/books/NBK441923/.
5. Wang H, Li L, Qin LL, Song Y, Vidal-Alaball J, Liu TH. Oral vitamin B12 versus intramuscular vitamin B12 for vitamin B12 deficiency. Cochrane Database Syst Rev. 2018:3.
6. Sezer RG, Bozaykut A, Akoğlu HA, Özdemir GN. The efficacy of oral vitamin B12 replacement for nutritional vitamin B12 deficiency. J Pediatr Hematol Oncol. 2018;40(2):e69–72.
7. Chandelia S, Chandra J, Narayan S, Aneja S, Chawla HM, Sharma S, et al. Addition of cobalamin to iron and folic acid improves hemoglobin rise in nutritional anemia. Indian J Pediatr. 2012;79(12):1592–6.

Folic Acid

26

Nila Mistry Ambani

Folic acid is a water-soluble vitamin that is an essential nutrient for mammals. Although the terms folic acid and folate are often used interchangeably, folate refers to the naturally occurring form while folic acid refers to the synthetic supplement. It is less commonly called vitamin B9. It was discovered in the 1930s in yeast and liver by Lucy Wills and found to cure macrocytic anemia [1]. In the 1940s, pharmaceutical companies isolated folic acid from spinach, which was then industrially synthesized. Fortification of cereals and grains in the United States became mandatory in 1998.

Physiology of Folic Acid

- Folate is key in one-carbon metabolism [2], which is essential in reactions for:
  - Synthesis of nucleic acids,

N. M. Ambani (✉)
Division of Pediatric Gastroenterology, Hepatology, and Nutrition, Cleveland Clinic Children's Hospital, Cleveland, OH, USA
e-mail: MISTRYN@ccf.org

K. Radhakrishnan (ed.), *Handbook of Clinical and Practical Pediatric Nutrition*, https://doi.org/10.1007/978-3-031-97759-6_26

  - Metabolism of various amino acids such as methionine, serine, glycine, and histidine, and
  - Crucial for formation of hematopoietic cells.

Absorption and Metabolism

- Once ingested, folates need to be hydrolyzed to monoglutamates [2] in the intestinal brush border to be transported into cells.
- There are three transport systems in epithelial cells that assist in this process: the reduced folate carrier (SLC19A1), proton-coupled folate transporter (PCFT, SLC46A1), and the membrane-bound folate receptor [3].
- Folic acid requires reduction to tetrahydrofolate (THF) before it can become active.
- Intracellularly, THF is a key coenzyme that serves as a bridge between the methylation cycle and the DNA biosynthesis cycle [2].

Dietary Sources of Folate

- Food sources of folate include dark green leafy vegetables, fruit and juices, beans, nuts, whole grains, meat, and eggs [4].
- There is variable bioavailability of folate in foods.
- Folic acid is more bioavailable and used to fortify enriched breads and cereals in many countries including the United States (Table 26.1).
- Values are typically based on dietary folate equivalents due to the differences in bioavailability between natural food sources, fortified foods, and folic acid supplements.

Table 26.1 The recommended dietary allowances (RDAs) for folate vary by age [4]

Age	RDA of folate
Birth to 6 months	65 mcg
7–12 months	80 mcg
1–3 years	150 mcg
4–8 years	200 mcg
9–13 years	300 mcg
14–18 years	400 mcg
19+ years	400 mcg
Pregnancy/lactation	500–600 mcg

Causes of Folate Deficiency

Inadequate Intake or Malabsorption

- In pediatrics, poor intake due to highly selective diet such as avoidant/restrictive food intake disorder (ARFID) can lead to nutritional deficiencies including folate deficiency.
- Additionally, malabsorption related to intestinal inflammation (celiac disease or inflammatory bowel disease) or short bowel syndrome can lead to deficiency.

Genetic Causes

- Homozygous mutation of the hPCFT gene associated with the proton-coupled folate transporter in the intestinal mucosa can result in decreased uptake of folate resulting in deficiency.
  - Infants can present with macrocytic anemia and failure to thrive with progression to developmental delays, seizures, and peripheral neuropathy.
- A genetic polymorphism (677C > T) in the methylenetetrahydrofolate reductase (MTHFR) gene resulting in a less active enzyme causes decreased ability to convert folate to an active form [5].
  - This leads to low folate levels and elevated homocysteine levels.

  - Studies have shown that certain genotypes of this polymorphism require higher folate supplementation although its clinical relevance is not fully understood.
  - Mutations of this gene causes homocystinuria.
- Cerebral folate deficiency is a rare condition in which a mutation in the *FOLR1* gene results in decreased ability to transport folate into the cerebrospinal fluid.
  - Symptoms include developmental regression around 2 years of age, seizures, and ataxia.

Medications

- Sulfasalazine is an anti-inflammatory medication used in the treatment of ulcerative colitis and rheumatoid arthritis. It can inhibit intestinal absorption of folate [6].
- Methotrexate, which is used as an antineoplastic agent and for treatment of autoimmune diseases, is a folate antagonist. Folic acid supplementation is recommended to reduce hepatotoxicity and GI side effects of methotrexate [7].

Other Causes of Folate Deficiency

There are also several underlying conditions that require higher folate needs. These include:

- Premature infants.
- Exclusive goat milk diet in an infant.
- Patients with high red blood cell turnover such as chronic hemolytic anemia and sickle cell disease.
- Following gastrointestinal surgery that can impact absorption in the duodenum.

In addition, folate deficiency during pregnancy has been correlated to increased risk of neural tube defects in infants and supplementation before and during pregnancy is universally recommended.

Signs and Symptoms of Folate Deficiency

- Megaloblastic anemia.
- Fatigue.
- Weakness.
- Shortness of breath.
- Difficulty concentrating.
- Hair loss.
- Irregular heartbeat.

Diagnosis of Folate Deficiency

Diagnosis of folate deficiency should include the following tests after a thorough history and exam:

- Complete blood count (CBC) and blood smear.
  - Assess for anemia and macrocytic red blood cells.
- Reticulocyte count.
- Serum folate and Vitamin B12 level.
- Methylmalonic acid (MMA) and homocysteine.
  - Isolated folate deficiency should result in elevated homocysteine and normal MMA.

Management of Folate Deficiency

Folic acid supplementation can be achieved through oral or intravenous routes depending on symptoms. For individuals with neuropsychiatric changes and for neonates and pregnant women for whom development of an infant can be impacted, more urgent repletion with parenteral administration is recommended.

Response can be monitored with assessment of symptoms and laboratory markers of anemia and reticulocytosis in the more immediate setting.

Future Research

Although the role of folic acid supplementation in certain conditions has been well documented, the impact of low levels on the health of individuals including cancer risk and mental health remains to be elucidated [8, 9]. Continued research in epigenetics and polymorphisms in folate metabolism is needed to determine optimal recommendations for additional supplementation.

References

1. Rosenberg IH. A history of the isolation and identification of folic acid (folate). Ann Nutr Metab. 2012;61(3):231–5. https://doi.org/10.1159/000343112.
2. Scaglione F, Panzavolta G. Folate, folic acid and 5-methyltetrahydrofolate are not the same thing. Xenobiotica. 2014;44(5):480–8.
3. Ediger T, Erdman S. Maldigestion and malabsorption. In: Wyllie R, Hyams JS, Kay M, editors. Pediatric gastrointestinal and liver disease. Essay. 6th ed. Elsevier; 2021. p. 328–9.
4. Miller JW. Folic acid. In: Caballero B, editor. Encyclopedia of human nutrition. 3rd ed. Elsevier; 2013. p. 262–9.
5. Schwahn BC, Rozen R. Methylenetetrahydrofolate reductase polymorphisms: pharmacogenetic effects. In: Madame Curie bioscience database [Internet]. Austin: Landes Bioscience; 2000–2013.
6. Halsted CH, Gandhi G, Tamura T. Sulfasalazine inhibits the absorption of folates in ulcerative colitis. N Engl J Med. 1981;305:1513–7.
7. Shea B, Swinden MV, Tanjong Ghogomu E, Ortiz Z, Katchamart W, Rader T, Bombardier C, Wells GA, Tugwell P. Folic acid and folinic acid for reducing side effects in patients receiving methotrexate for rheumatoid arthritis. Cochrane Database Syst Rev. 2013;2013(5)
8. Bender A, Hagan KE, Kingston N. The association of folate and depression: a meta-analysis. J Psychiatr Res. 2017;95:9–18.
9. Pieroth R, Paver S, Day S, Lammersfeld C. Folate and its impact on cancer risk. Curr Nutr Rep. 2018;7(3):70–84.

Vitamin C

27

Suruchi Ramanujan
and Kadakkal Radhakrishnan

Introduction

- Vitamin C is crucial to several processes in the human body; it is important that people maintain stable vitamin C levels.
- It is especially important to monitor vitamin C levels in individuals with chronic conditions and children with critical illnesses, heart and lung disease, and intestinal failure.

Vitamin C's Role in the Body

- Vitamin C primarily acts as an electron donor for several enzymes [1] (Table 27.1).

S. Ramanujan
Department of Medicine, University of California San Diego, San Diego, CA, USA
e-mail: Sramanujan@health.ucsd.edu

K. Radhakrishnan (✉)
Division of Pediatric Gastroenterology, Hepatology & Nutrition, Cleveland Clinic Children's Hospital, Cleveland, OH, USA
e-mail: radhakk@ccf.org

K. Radhakrishnan (ed.), *Handbook of Clinical and Practical Pediatric Nutrition*, https://doi.org/10.1007/978-3-031-97759-6_27

- It is essential to dopamine beta-hydroxylase activity, which is needed for norepinephrine synthesis.
- It is needed for several hypothalamic and gastrointestinal hormones to function (e.g., calcitonin, oxytocin, cholecystokinin, gastrin-releasing peptide, etc.).
- It is required for structurally normal collagen to be produced; not having the structural strength that mature collagen provides can lead to bleeding and poor wound healing [2, 3].
- It is crucial to proper oxygen sensing in multicellular animals; particularly, it plays a role in proline hydroxylation of hypoxia inducible factor-1 (HIF-1a) [4, 5].
- Some vitamin C-dependent enzymes are described in Table 27.1.

Table 27.1 Physiologic functions of vitamin C

Enzyme name ➔ function
Collagen prolyl 4-hydroxylase, Collagen prolyl 3-hydroxylase, Procollagen lysine 2-oxoglutarate-5-dioxygenase ➔ Collagen generation
Prolyl hydroxylase domain-containing proteins Factor inhibiting HIF ➔ HIF-1a hydroxylation and regulation
Dopamine B-hydroxylase ➔ Norepinephrine synthesis
Peptidyl-glycine α-amidating monooxygenase ➔ Peptide hormone amidation
Ten–eleven translocases ➔ Cytosine demethylation
4-Hydroxyphenylpyruvate dioxygenase ➔ Tyrosine metabolism
Jumonji-C domain histone demethylase Lysine demethylases ➔Histone demethylation

Body Stores and Absorption of Vitamin C

- Vitamin C absorption mainly happens in the last section of the small intestine (the distal ileum).
- Absorption happens primarily through ascorbate transporters (SVCT1 and SVCT2) [6–8].
- Since vitamin C is water-soluble, there are low stores in the body; because of this, people must consume adequate amounts of vitamin C through their diets. Stores generally lasts 2 weeks.

Manifestations of Vitamin C Deficiency

- Skin manifestations of vitamin C deficiency include petechiae, bruising, and hemorrhaging around hair follicles [9].
- Infants may present with pseudoparalysis secondary to periostitis.
- Individuals with vitamin C deficiency are also prone to bone and muscle pain and fragile bones [10].
- Some individuals also present with neuropsychiatric presentations such as depression, cognitive changes, and pseudoparalysis [11, 12].
- Skeletal manifestations of vitamin C deficiency include poor bone growth, fractures, and increased fragility. Additionally, low vitamin C intake has been associated with osteoporosis.
- Recommended dietary intake of vitamin C, supplementation options, and foods with high levels of vitamin C are demonstrated in Tables 27.2, 27.3, and 27.4.

Table 27.2 Recommended dietary intake of vitamin C

Category	Recommended daily intake (mg)
Adult women	75
Pregnant women	85
Breastfeeding women	120
Adult men	90
Female teens	65
Male teens	75
Children (age 9–13)	45
Children (age 4–8)	25
Children (age 1–3)	15
Infants (7–12 months)	50
Infants (<6 months)	40

Table 27.3 Dosing suggestions for vitamin C deficiency in high-risk patients

Category	Level of supplementation
Neonates (birth to 28 days)	50 mg orally or IV daily
Premature infants	25 mg orally or IV daily
Less than 10 kg (non-infant)	125 mg orally or 75 mg IV daily
10–39.9 kg	250 mg twice a day orally or 250 mg IV daily
Over 40 kg	500 mg twice a day orally or 500 mg IV daily

Vitamin C levels should be rechecked 2–4 weeks after starting supplementation and dose adjusted accordingly

Table 27.4 Common dietary sources of vitamin C

Guava
Sauerkraut
Red Pepper
Kale
Chives
Coriander
Broccoli
Kiwi
Parsley
Strawberry
Orange
Lemon
Potato

Vitamin C Monitoring in Children

- High-risk groups of children, such as those who are critically ill, have severe asthma, have intestinal failure or short bowel syndrome, receive repeat transfusions (i.e., children with thalassemia) or have developmental delays or severe restrictive food choices, and should be monitored for vitamin C deficiency [13–15].

Areas of Research

- There are no clinical recommendations regarding vitamin C supplementation for healthy individuals in order to decrease risk of respiratory infections although there is active discussion of vitamin C's role in controlling inflammation.
- Another active area of research involves vitamin C's role in modulating cardiovascular disease by preventing endothelial dysfunction.
- In individuals with bone marrow transplants who develop graft versus host disease, studies are being conducted regarding vitamin C supplementation's ability to improve inflammation of the mucosa and improve patients' ability to eat [16].

References

1. Schlueter AK, Johnston CS. Vitamin C: overview and update. https://doi.org/10.1177/1533210110392951.
2. Prockop DJ, Kivirikko KI. Collagens: molecular biology, diseases, and potentials for therapy. Annu Rev Biochem. 1995;64:403–34. https://doi.org/10.1146/annurev.bi.64.070195.002155.
3. Peterkofsky B. Ascorbate requirement for hydroxylation and secretion of procollagen: relationship to inhibition of collagen synthesis in scurvy. Am J Clin Nutr. 1991;54(6 Suppl):1135S–40S. https://doi.org/10.1093/ajcn/54.6.1135s.
4. Yang M, Chowdhury R, Ge W, et al. Factor-inhibiting hypoxia-inducible factor (FIH) catalyses the post-translational hydroxylation of histidinyl

residues within ankyrin repeat domains. FEBS J. 2011;278(7):1086–97. https://doi.org/10.1111/j.1742-4658.2011.08022.x.
5. Padayatty SJ, Levine M. Invited medical review Vitamin C: the known and the unknown and Goldilocks. Oral Dis. 2016;22:463–93. https://doi.org/10.1111/odi.12446.
6. Naidu KA. Vitamin C in human health and disease is still a mystery? An overview. Nutr J. 2003;2:7. https://doi.org/10.1186/1475-2891-2-7.
7. Hellman L, Burns JJ. Metabolism of L-ascorbic acid-1-C14 in man. J Biol Chem. 1958;230(2):923–30.
8. Doseděl M, Jirkovský E, Macáková K, et al. Vitamin C-sources, physiological role, kinetics, deficiency, use, toxicity, and determination. Nutrients. 2021;13(2) https://doi.org/10.3390/nu13020615.
9. Trapani S, Rubino C, Indolfi G, Lionetti P. A narrative review on pediatric scurvy: the last twenty years. Nutrients. 2022;14(3) https://doi.org/10.3390/nu14030684.
10. Thaler R, Khani F, Sturmlechner I, et al. Vitamin C epigenetically controls osteogenesis and bone mineralization. Nat Commun. 2022;13(1):5883. https://doi.org/10.1038/s41467-022-32915-8.
11. Plevin D, Galletly C. The neuropsychiatric effects of vitamin C deficiency: a systematic review. BMC Psychiatry. 2020;20(1):315. https://doi.org/10.1186/s12888-020-02730-w.
12. Paul AJ. Pseudoparalysis secondary to Vitamin C deficiency: a rare presentation in a toddler. JBJS Case Connect. 2023;13(4) https://doi.org/10.2106/JBJS.CC.23.00313.
13. Golriz F, Donnelly LF, Devaraj S, Krishnamurthy R. Modern American scurvy – experience with vitamin C deficiency at a large children's hospital. Pediatr Radiol. 2017;47(2):214–20. https://doi.org/10.1007/s00247-016-3726-4.
14. Al-Subu AM, Long MT, Nelson KL, et al. Risk of hypovitaminosis and vitamin C deficiency in pediatric patients undergoing cardiopulmonary bypass. Pediatr Cardiol. 2023;44(7):1487–94. https://doi.org/10.1007/s00246-023-03243-5.
15. Siripornpanich S, Chongviriyaphan N, Manuyakorn W, Matangkasombut P. Zinc and vitamin C deficiencies associate with poor pulmonary function in children with persistent asthma. Asian Pac J Allergy Immunol. 2022;40(2):103–10. https://doi.org/10.12932/AP-100620-0878.
16. Kletzel M, Powers K, Hayes M. Scurvy: a new problem for patients with chronic GVHD involving mucous membranes; an easy problem to resolve. Pediatr Transplant. 2014;18(5):524–6. https://doi.org/10.1111/petr.12285.

Carnitine in Pediatric Nutrition

28

Elizabeth Hilow

Introduction

Carnitine is a crucial molecule in fatty acid metabolism. It is produced endogenously through the synthesis of amino acids such as lysine and methionine. There are also exogenous dietary sources of carnitine including red meat (lamb and beef), dairy, poultry, and fish. Carnitine's primary role is to facilitate the transport of long-chain fatty acids [1].

Carnitine was first isolated from muscle extracts by Russian researchers Gulewitsch and Krimberg in 1905. It was first used in a therapeutic capacity in 1958 to treat nutritional deficiencies in infants and children, leading the way to its current use in treating infants and children with several inborn errors of metabolism [2].

E. Hilow (✉)
Department of Pediatric Gastroenterology, Phoenix Children's Hospital, Phoenix, AZ, USA
e-mail: ehilow@phoenixchildrens.com

K. Radhakrishnan (ed.), *Handbook of Clinical and Practical Pediatric Nutrition*, https://doi.org/10.1007/978-3-031-97759-6_28

Role of Carnitine

- Carnitine plays a primary role in transport of long-chain fatty acids from the cytosol into the mitochondrial matrix for β-oxidation and generating ATP. This is facilitated through specialized acyltransferases. This process is essential for energy production in several types of tissue including skeletal and cardiac [3].
- Carnitine has been shown to act as a scavenger of reactive oxygen and nitrogen species protecting cells from oxidative damage. This function of carnitine has potential implications for treating conditions resulting from increased oxidative stress including cardiovascular disease, neurodegenerative disease, and aging [11].
- Other roles of carnitine include:
  - Buffering the acyl coenzyme A (CoA)-CoA ratio.
  - Acting in branched-chain amino acid metabolism.
  - Removal of excess acyl groups.
  - Peroxisomal fatty acid oxidation.

Synthesis of Carnitine

- Synthesis of carnitine occurs through a series of enzymatic steps with lysine and methionine serving as precursors. We maintain a balance of carnitine in the body through endogenous synthesis, exogenous dietary intake of carnitine, and renal reabsorption of carnitine.
- In a person with a nonvegetarian diet, a majority of carnitine is dietary (approximately 75%) with endogenous synthesis accounting for approximately 25% of total carnitine [4, 5].
- Defects in any of these enzymes in the carnitine synthesis process can lead to inborn errors of metabolism. These are primary causes of carnitine deficiency that may present with symptoms including hypoketotic hypoglycemia, cardiomyopathy, and liver disease (Fig. 28.1).

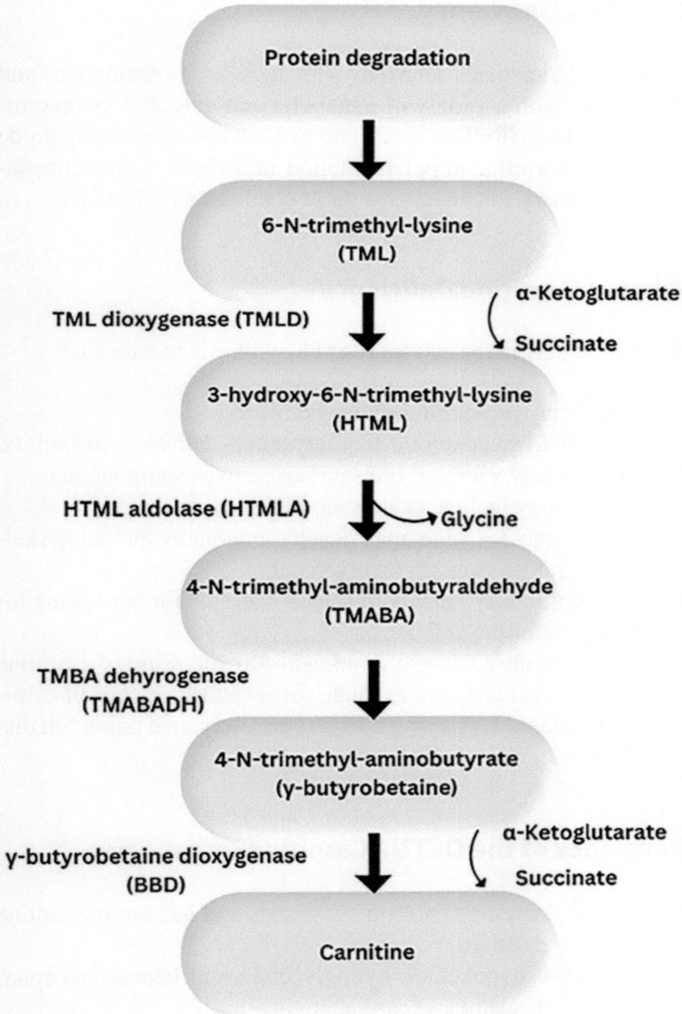

Fig. 28.1 Endogenous synthesis of carnitine: enzymatic pathways [6]

Carnitine Deficiency

Carnitine deficiencies interfere with fatty acid metabolism and can present with a variety of metabolic and muscular symptoms. Labs including carnitine levels and genetic testing can help guide diagnosis. Carnitine supplementation and dietary supplementation are primary treatments for these conditions [7, 8, 15].

Primary Carnitine Deficiency

Genetic defects in the transport or biosynthesis of carnitine:

- Several may present in infancy before age 2.
- Can lead to hypoketotic hypoglycemia, lethargy, irritability, hepatomegaly, elevated transaminases, hyperammonemia.
- Triggers may include acute viral illness.
- Children age 2–4 years may develop myopathy including skeletal and cardiac muscle involvement.
- Low carnitine on a newborn screen warrants further testing for primary carnitine deficiency.
- Urine organic acids are nondiagnostic for primary carnitine deficiency but can help evaluate for secondary causes of carnitine deficiency (organic acidemias and fatty acid oxidation disorders).

Deficiency of the OCTN2 Carnitine Transporter

- Leads to decreased carnitine in tissues and increased carnitine loss through urine.
- Symptoms: hypoketotic hypoglycemia and hepatic encephalopathy or skeletal and cardiac myopathy.
- Treatment: carnitine supplementation.

Defects in CPT1

- Present with recurrent episodes of fasting hypoketotic hypoglycemia or acute liver injury.
- Usually heart and muscle are NOT affected.
- Patients can have elevated carnitine levels.

CACT Deficiency

- Presents most often in neonatal period.
- Symptoms: hypoglycemia, hyperammonemia.
- Additional symptoms: cardiomyopathy with arrythmia—can lead to cardiac arrect.
- Very low plasma carnitine levels.

CPT2 Deficiency

- More frequently presents in adults.
- Rhabdomyolysis triggered by prolonged exercise.
- More severe variants present in neonatal period—may be associated with congenital anomalies.

Treatment for CPT1, CPT2, CACT

- Low-fat diet.
- Medium-chain triglycerides—metabolized by the mitochondria without carnitine.
- Carnitine supplement.
- Avoiding fasting and sustained exercise.

Secondary Carnitine Deficiency

Treated with carnitine supplementation and treatment of underlying cause when possible [9, 10].

Inborn errors of metabolism—accumulate toxic metabolites that deplete carnitine stores:

- Organic acidemias.
- Fatty acid oxidation defects (very long-chain acyl-CoA dehydrogenase-VLCAD deficiency).
- Medium-chain acyl-CoA dehydrogenase (MCAD) deficiency.
- Propionic acidemia.

Chronic Disease

- Cirrhosis.
- Chronic renal failure.
- Diabetes mellitus.
- Heart failure.
- Preterm neonates (due to immature renal function and decreased biosynthesis).
- Malnutrition.
- Catabolic state (i.e., epidermolysis bullosa).

Medications

- Valproate.
- Zidovudine.
- Antibiotics (Pivampicillin).

Carnitine Supplementation

While there is not a particular recommended daily allowance of carnitine, supplementation should be targeted to the individual and their disease process and diet. Pediatric dosing for L-carnitine:

- For treatment of metabolic disorders and enzyme defects: 50–100 mg/kg in divided doses: maximum of 3 g/day.
- For nutritional carnitine deficits: 10–30 mg/kg per day.

In people with omivore diet and in the absence of disease process causing carnitine deficiency, additional supplementation should not be required.

Role of Carnitine in Cardiovascular Disease

- L-carnitine has been shown to have protective effects in the setting of ischemic and reperfusion injury.
- This protective mechanism is thought to be due to reducing oxidative stress and preventing accumulation of toxic metabolites.
- Some clinical studies have demonstrated improved left ventricular dilation and reduction in remodeling with carnitine supplementation after myocardial infarction [12, 13].
- Carnitine supplementation has been shown to improve left ventricular ejection fraction and reduce myocardial stress in pediatric patients with left ventricular dysfunction [14].
- For patients with primary carnitine deficiency, appropriate supplementation is needed to prevent cardiovascular complications, including myopathy, sudden cardiac death, and myocardial scarring [16].
- For some patients with secondary carnitine deficiency, including those with epidermolysis bullosa, carnitine deficiency may lead to dilated cardiomyopathy [17].

Future Directions Research Potential

While carnitine has been shown to have cardioprotective effects, it may also play a role in atherosclerosis [18, 19].

- Carnitine is metabolized by gut microbiota into trimethylamine (TMA). Trimethylamine dehydrogenase is the enzymatic catalyst for conversion of TMA to TMAO.
- TMAO elevation has been associated with increased incidence of atherosclerosis through several mechanisms including:

– Enhancing cholesterol deposition in arterial walls.
– Impairing reverse cholesterol transport.

Several additional clinical applications for carnitine supplementation are being investigated including:

- Nonalcoholic fatty liver disease.
- Oxidative stress and aging.
- Neuroprotection.
- Obesity and CNS damage.
- Metabolic disorders.
- Sepsis management.
- Cancer treatment.

References

1. Borum PR. Carnitine. Annu Rev Nutr. 1983;3:233–59. https://doi.org/10.1146/annurev.nu.03.070183.001313. PMID: 6357236
2. Buist NR. Historical perspective on clinical trials of carnitine in children and adults. Ann Nutr Metab. 2016;68(Suppl 3):1–4. https://doi.org/10.1159/000448320. Epub 2016 Dec 9. PMID: 27931034
3. Hoppel C. The role of carnitine in normal and altered fatty acid metabolism. Am J Kidney Dis. 2003;41(4 Suppl 4):S4–12. https://doi.org/10.1016/s0272-6386(03)00112-4. PMID: 12751049
4. Almannai M, Alfadhel M, El-Hattab AW. Carnitine Inborn errors of metabolism. Molecules. 2019;24(18):3251. https://doi.org/10.3390/molecules24183251. PMID: 31500110; PMCID: PMC6766900
5. Strijbis K, Vaz FM, Distel B. Enzymology of the carnitine biosynthesis pathway. IUBMB Life. 2010;62(5):357–62. https://doi.org/10.1002/iub.323. PMID: 20306513
6. Li N, Zhao H. Role of carnitine in non-alcoholic fatty liver disease and other related diseases: an update. Front Med. 2021;8 https://doi.org/10.3389/fmed.2021.689042.
7. Longo N, di San A, Filippo C, Pasquali M. Disorders of carnitine transport and the carnitine cycle. Am J Med Genet C Semin Med Genet. 2006;142C(2):77–85. https://doi.org/10.1002/ajmg.c.30087. PMID: 16602102. PMCID: PMC2557099
8. Pons R, De Vivo DC. Primary and secondary carnitine deficiency syndromes. J Child Neurol. 1995;10(Suppl 2):S8–24. PMID: 8576570
9. Evangeliou A, Vlassopoulos D. Carnitine metabolism and deficit–when supplementation is necessary? Curr Pharm Biotechnol. 2003;4(3):211–9. https://doi.org/10.2174/1389201033489829. PMID: 12769764

10. El-Hattab AW, Almannai M. Primary carnitine deficiency. 2012 [updated 2024 Dec 5]. In: Adam MP, Feldman J, Mirzaa GM, Pagon RA, Wallace SE, Amemiya A, editors. GeneReviews® [Internet]. Seattle: University of Washington, Seattle; 1993–2024. PMID: 22420015.
11. Gülçin I. Antioxidant and antiradical activities of L-carnitine. Life Sci. 2006;78(8):803–11. https://doi.org/10.1016/j.lfs.2005.05.103. Epub 2005 Oct 25. PMID: 16253281
12. Wang ZY, Liu YY, Liu GH, Lu HB, Mao CY. l-Carnitine and heart disease. Life Sci. 2018;194:88–97. https://doi.org/10.1016/j.lfs.2017.12.015. Epub 2017 Dec 11. PMID: 29241711
13. Ferrari R, Merli E, Cicchitelli G, Mele D, Fucili A, Ceconi C. Therapeutic effects of L-carnitine and propionyl-L-carnitine on cardiovascular diseases: a review. Ann N Y Acad Sci. 2004;1033:79–91. https://doi.org/10.1196/annals.1320.007. PMID: 15591005.
14. Ikeda N, Loomba RS, Patel R, Dorsey V, Yousaf F, Nelson-McMillan K. Effect of carnitine supplementation in pediatric patients with left ventricular dysfunction. Pediatr Cardiol. 2023;44(3):720–6. https://doi.org/10.1007/s00246-022-03003-x. Epub 2022 Sep 15. PMID: 36107209
15. Virmani MA, Cirulli M. The role of l-carnitine in mitochondria, prevention of metabolic inflexibility and disease initiation. Int J Mol Sci. 2022;23(5):2717. https://doi.org/10.3390/ijms23052717. PMID: 35269860; PMCID: PMC8910660
16. Kyhl K, Róin T, Lund A, Vejlstrup N, Madsen PL, Engstrøm T, Rasmussen J. Cardiac function and incidence of unexplained myocardial scarring in patients with primary carnitine deficiency – a cardiac magnetic resonance study. Sci Rep. 2019;9(1):13909. https://doi.org/10.1038/s41598-019-50458-9. PMID: 31558765; PMCID: PMC6763485
17. Lara-Corrales I, Mellerio JE, Martinez AE, Green A, Lucky AW, Azizkhan RG, Murrell DF, Agero AL, Kantor PF, Pope E. Dilated cardiomyopathy in epidermolysis bullosa: a retrospective, multicenter study. Pediatr Dermatol. 2010;27(3):238–43. https://doi.org/10.1111/j.1525-1470.2010.01127.x. PMID: 20609141
18. Koeth RA, Wang Z, Levison BS, Buffa JA, Org E, Sheehy BT, Britt EB, Fu X, Wu Y, Li L, Smith JD, DiDonato JA, Chen J, Li H, Wu GD, Lewis JD, Warrier M, Brown JM, Krauss RM, Tang WH, Bushman FD, Lusis AJ, Hazen SL. Intestinal microbiota metabolism of L-carnitine, a nutrient in red meat, promotes atherosclerosis. Nat Med. 2013;19(5):576–85. https://doi.org/10.1038/nm.3145. Epub 2013 Apr 7. PMID: 23563705. PMCID: PMC3650111
19. Tang WH, Hazen SL. The contributory role of gut microbiota in cardiovascular disease. J Clin Invest. 2014;124(10):4204–11. https://doi.org/10.1172/JCI72331. Epub 2014 Oct 1. PMID: 25271725. PMCID: PMC4215189

Coenzyme Q10 in Pediatric Nutrition

29

Nishaben Patel

History

Frederick Crane and colleagues discovered coenzyme Q in 1957. The name coenzyme Q10 derives from its chemical structure, a benzoquinone ring with a side chain composed of 10 isoprene units. It is commonly referred to as ubiquinone because it is found in almost every cell in all living organisms, making it ubiquitous in nature. [1]

Physiology of CoQ10

- CoQ10 is endogenously synthesized lipid-soluble antioxidant, protecting all types of cellular membranes from free radical-induced oxidative damage.
- CoQ10 is both located in the mitochondria and in extramitochondrial structures with the highest concentration found in the heart, kidneys, muscles, and brain.

N. Patel (✉)
Department of Pediatric Gastroenterology, Hepatology and Nutrition, University of Rochester Medical Center, Golisano Children's Hospital, Rochester, NY, USA
e-mail: Nishaben_Patel@URMC.Rochester.edu

K. Radhakrishnan (ed.), *Handbook of Clinical and Practical Pediatric Nutrition*, https://doi.org/10.1007/978-3-031-97759-6_29

- It can exist in three different oxidation states: the fully oxidized state (ubiquinone), the partially reduced state (ubisemiquinone), and the fully reduced state (ubiquinol) [3].
- Within mitochondria, CoQ10 has a key role in the generation of ATP via oxidative phosphorylation, as an electron carrier from complex I and II to complex III in the mitochondrial electron transport chain.
- CoQ10 can potentially increase the production of vital antioxidants, such as superoxide dismutase, an enzyme that effectively mitigates vascular oxidative stress.
- CoQ10 lowers lipid peroxidation levels by diminishing pro-oxidative compounds.
- CoQ10 also has a role in the metabolism of lysosomes, pyrimidines, sulfides, amino acids, and cholesterol.
- CoQ10 may also mediate the expression of several genes, particularly those involved in inflammation.

CoQ10 Deficiency

Deficiency of CoQ10 is broadly divided into:

1. Primary CoQ10 deficiency.
2. Secondary CoQ10 deficiency.

Primary CoQ10 deficiency results from mutations in genes involved in the CoQ10 biosynthetic pathway.

- In humans, CoQ10 is synthesized from phenylalanine and isoprenyl repeats and at least 10 genes are required for the biosynthesis of functional CoQ10, a mutation in any one of which can result in a deficit in CoQ10 status.
- Primary CoQ10 deficiency is a very rare disorder, the prevalence and incidence of which have been estimated to be less than 1 per 100,000 population, respectively.
- Primary CoQ10 deficiency is associated with a heterogeneous spectrum of clinical phenotypes.

  - the disorder typically has a neonatal, infantile, or childhood age of onset;
  - patients typically present with neurological dysfunction (encephalopathy, psychomotor delay, cerebellar atrophy/ataxia, optic atrophy), nephropathy, cardiomyopathy, or any combination thereof;
  - the outcome for patients is typically either serious disability or fatality. [4]
- The only treatment for primary CoQ10 deficiency is oral supplementation with CoQ10. The reduced form of CoQ10 (ubiquinol) has been approved for the treatment of genetic CoQ10 deficiencies [5].
- However, the condition must be recognized sufficiently early as damage to the kidney or the nervous system can be irreversible. CoQ10 doses used in clinical studies typically range from 10 to 30 mg/kg/day for varying time periods from several months upward. [4]

Secondary Coenzyme Q10 Deficiency results from mutations in genes that are not directly related to the CoQ10 biosynthetic pathway or to nongenetic factors associated with various childhood disorders that result in mitochondrial dysfunction, impaired cellular energy production, and oxidative stress.

Supplementation with CoQ10 has not been universally successful and controversial in most secondary or acquired CoQ10 deficiency disorders in childhood such as:

- Duchenne muscular dystrophy.
- Down's syndrome.
- Attention-deficit hyperactivity disorder (ADHD).
- Autism spectrum disorder.
- Idiopathic cardiomyopathy.
- Friedreich's ataxia.
- Metabolic dysfunction-associated fatty liver disease (MAFLD).
- Prader–Willi syndrome.
- Leigh's syndrome.
- Cyclic vomiting syndrome.

Absorption and Metabolism [7]

- **Absorption:** CoQ10 is a hydrophobic (lipophilic) molecule and absorption of dietary CoQ10 is slow but is improved in the presence of fatty meals.
- **Distribution:** CoQ10 is primarily absorbed from the small intestine, and CoQ10 is incorporated into chylomicrons and is redistributed via the bloodstream, primarily within VLDL, LDL, and HDL. Preclinical studies indicate that CoQ10 in large doses is taken up by all tissues, including heart and brain mitochondria; consequently, a beneficial effect is observed in cardiovascular and neurodegenerative diseases. The highest levels of CoQ10 in human tissues exist in the heart, liver, kidneys, and muscles (high energy requirements) [2].
- **Metabolism:** CoQ10 is reduced to ubiquinol during or after absorption in the small intestine, and the reduced form represents approximately 95% of the circulating CoQ10 in humans.
- **Elimination:** The primary route of elimination is biliary and fecal.

Sources and Available Dosage Forms of CoQ10

What are the Different Forms of CoQ10?

The two main forms of CoQ10 supplements are ubiquinone and ubiquinol.

- Ubiquinone is the oxidized form of CoQ10 and the most widely available and researched form used in supplements. The body has to convert ubiquinone into ubiquinol for it to be useful in cellular energy production.
- Ubiquinol is the reduced, active antioxidant form of CoQ10. It is more bioavailable, meaning it gets absorbed better into the bloodstream and is more readily used by the body's cells. Ubiquinol also acts as an antioxidant, meaning it can neutral-

ize harmful free radicals in the body, while ubiquinone does not have this property to the same extent.

- As we age the body's ability to convert ubiquinone to ubiquinol may decrease, making exogenous ubiquinol a more attractive option for older adults.
- CoQ10 oral supplementation is available in various forms, such as tablets, capsules, soft gels, and liquid formulations and doses range from 30 to 600 mg per unit and are easily accessible over the counter.
- Meat has the highest amount of CoQ10, followed by dairy, eggs, and plant-based food sources (oils and legumes).
- In patients with primary CoQ10 deficiency, early treatment with high-dose supplementation (ranging from 5 to 50 mg/kg/day) can limit disease progression [6].

Safety and Side Effects

- CoQ10 supplements appear to be safe and produce few side effects when taken as directed.
- Mild side effects might include digestive problems such as:
  - Upper abdominal pain.
  - Loss of appetite.
  - Nausea and vomiting.
  - Diarrhea.
- Other possible side effects may include:
  - Headaches and dizziness.
  - Insomnia.
  - Fatigue.
  - Skin itching or rashes.
  - Irritability or agitation.

The safety of use of CoQ10 during pregnancy and breastfeeding has not been established.

Drug Interactions

- **Anticoagulants:** CoQ10 is chemically similar to vitamin K, and there is potential for warfarin and CoQ10 interaction, which could result in warfarin treatment failure and increased risk of blood clots.

Future Research Possibilities

The current gold standard approach for CoQ10 deficiency diagnosis is genetic testing or biochemical detection of CoQ10 deficiency via muscle biopsy. However, minimally invasive measurements of CoQ10 levels in the plasma cannot be used to diagnose deficiency, because it is influenced by dietary or exogenous CoQ10 sources. Studies show that there are clear discrepancies between blood CoQ10 levels and bioavailability at a tissue level. Future studies are needed to find a form of exogenous CoQ10 supplement that yields the highest bioavailability at a tissue level.

References

1. Raizner AE. Coenzyme Q(10). Methodist Debakey Cardiovasc J. 2019;15(3):185–91. https://doi.org/10.14797/mdcj-15-3-185.
2. Bhagavan HN, Chopra RK. Coenzyme Q10: Absorption, tissue uptake, metabolism and pharmacokinetics. Free Radic Res. 2006;40(5):445–53. https://doi.org/10.1080/10715760600617843.
3. Hargreaves I, Heaton RA, Mantle D. Disorders of human coenzyme Q10 metabolism: an overview. Int J Mol Sci. 2020;21(18):6695. https://doi.org/10.3390/ijms21186695.
4. Mantle D, Millichap L, Castro-Marrero J, Hargreaves IP. Primary coenzyme Q10 deficiency: an update. Antioxidants (Basel). 2023;12(8):1652. https://doi.org/10.3390/antiox12081652.
5. Hernández-Camacho JD, Bernier M, López-Lluch G, Navas P. Coenzyme Q(10) supplementation in aging and disease. Front Physiol. 2018;9:44. https://doi.org/10.3389/fphys.2018.00044.

6. Salviati L, Trevisson E, Agosto C, Doimo M, Navas P. Primary coenzyme Q(10) deficiency overview. In: Adam MP, Feldman J, Mirzaa GM, et al., editors. GeneReviews(®). Seattle: University of Washington, Seattle. GeneReviews is a registered trademark of the University of Washington, Seattle. All rights reserved; 1993.
7. Sood B, Patel P, Keenaghan M. Coenzyme Q10. [Updated 2024 Jan 30]. In: StatPearls [Internet]. Treasure Island: StatPearls; 2024. Available from: https://www.ncbi.nlm.nih.gov/books/NBK531491/

Alpha Lipoic Acid

30

Elizabeth Robinson
and Kadakkal Radhakrishnan

Introduction

The place of alpha lipoic acid (LA) as a vitamin is controversial. It is component of key enzymatic reactions in the mitochondria. Importantly, it is a potent antioxidant given its ability to chelate free radicals. LA can chelate heavy metals and also has the ability to enhance intracellular glutathione levels (GSH) by recycling cellular GSH levels.

What Is Alpha Lipoic Acid

- Alpha lipoic acid (LA) is a naturally occurring antioxidant synthesized in the mitochondria [9].
- It is an organosulfur compound produced in nature and has a chiral center with two thiol groups.
- It can therefore occur in two forms: oxidized form (i.e., LA) and reduced form (i.e., dihydrolipoic acid (DHLA)). Both are potent antioxidants.

E. Robinson · K. Radhakrishnan (✉)
Division of Pediatric Gastroenterology Hepatology and Nutrition, Cleveland Clinic Children's Hospital, Cleveland, OH, USA
e-mail: ROBINSE10@ccf.org; RADHAKK@ccf.org

K. Radhakrishnan (ed.), *Handbook of Clinical and Practical Pediatric Nutrition*, https://doi.org/10.1007/978-3-031-97759-6_30

- LA has two enantiomers: R-enantiomer (R LA or + LA) and S-enantiomer (S LA or – LA). The R-enantiomer is the naturally present variant and the S-structure mirrors R; it is, however, not present in nature [3]. Synthetic LA is a racemic mixture of +LA and – LA.

Role of LA: Physiology

- LA is an important component/cofactor of multiple enzymes in the body:
  - Glycine cleavage system.
  - Pyruvate dehydrogenase.
  - Alpha ketoglutarate dehydrogenase.
  - Branched chained alpha ketoacid dehydrogenase.
  - Transketolase enzyme.
- *Antioxidant properties*: Both LA and DHLA are potent antioxidants, can scavenge hydroxyl radicals and hypochlorous acid, and LA can scavenge superoxide.
- *Chelation*: LA and DHLA can chelate transitional elements and this works in line with its antioxidant effect as well. LA can chelate copper, zinc, and lead and DHLA can chelate copper, zinc, mercury, lead, and iron.
- *Inducer of endogenous antioxidants*: DHLA and LA can regenerate other endogenous antioxidants such as vitamin C and E as well as glutathione.
- *Cellular signaling*: [6].
  - LA secondary to its prooxidant activity augments Nrf2 (nuclear factor-erythroid 2-related factor 2) signaling that protects cells from oxidative stress and regulates cellular and tissue homeostasis.
  - LA can also activate PKCδ, ERK 1/2, p38 MAPK, PI3 kinase, and ATK signaling pathway.

Sources of LA

- LA is inherently synthesized in the body from octanoic acid though a series of enzymatic pathways.
- Generally, it is synthesized in the liver and heart, as well as testes in males [8].
- Therefore, muscle meats, heart, liver, and kidney are natural sources of LA, and plant sources include spinach, broccoli, carrots, and potato [4, 8].

Dose Recommendations and Potential Use of LA

- As mentioned, the majority of LA is synthesized in the body, but some studies recommend additional dosing [9]. However, there is no good consensus on optimal dosing recommendations.
- According to guidelines, the recommended dose for adult patients is 200–1800 mg daily, whereas other sources recommend 200–2400 mg daily.
- LA may help improve vision in patients with type 1 and 2 diabetes.
- Intravenous dosing of LA may help patients with neuropathy. There has been research into diabetic neuropathy and metabolic syndromes with high-dose LA for improvement of symptoms [2, 4].
- Due to its antioxidant nature and free radical scavenging, LA has been shown to help with diabetes management and insulin resistance [6].
- Generally, LA is well tolerated without significant toxicity. Very high doses of LA may be associated with abnormal liver enzymes and concerns for hepatic dysfunction.

Cellular Transport of LA

- Cellular uptake of LA is mediated by sodium-dependent multivitamin transporter (SMVT)—SLC5A6 [7].
- This transporter is also involved in transport of biotin and pantothenic acid.
- Mutation of this protein is associated with failure to thrive, acidosis, development delay [1].
- Patients may show benefit to high-dose supplementation with LA, biotin, and pantothenic acid [5].

Future Research

Further research is required into the role of LA in improving visual disturbance and neuropathy in diabetes. Disorders associated with mutations of SMVT and roles of LA, biotin, and pantothenic acid require further investigation.

References

1. Holling T, Nampoothiri S, Tarhan B, Schneeberger PE, Vinayan KP, Yesodharan D, Roy AG, Radhakrishnan P, Alawi M, Rhodes L, Girisha KM, Kang PB, Kutsche K. Novel biallelic variants expand the SLC5A6-related phenotypic spectrum. Eur J Hum Genet. 2022;30(4):439–49. https://doi.org/10.1038/s41431-021-01033-2.
2. Najafi N, Mehri S, Ghasemzadeh Rahbardar M, Hosseinzadeh H. Effects of alpha lipoic acid on metabolic syndrome: a comprehensive review. Phytother Res. 2022;36(6):2300–23. https://doi.org/10.1002/ptr.7406.
3. Packer L, Cadenas E. Lipoic acid: energy metabolism and redox regulation of transcription and cell signaling. J Clin Biochem Nutr. 2010;48(1):26–32. https://doi.org/10.3164/jcbn.11-005FR.
4. Salehi B, Berkay Yılmaz Y, Antika G, Boyunegmez Tumer T, Fawzi Mahomoodally M, Lobine D, Akram M, Riaz M, Capanoglu E, Sharopov F, Martins N, Cho WC, Sharifi-Rad J. Insights on the use of α-lipoic acid for therapeutic purposes. Biomolecules. 2019;9(8):356. https://doi.org/10.3390/biom9080356.

5. Schwantje M, De Sain-van Der Velden M, Jans J, Van Gassen K, Dorrepaal C, Koop K, Visser G. Genetic defect of the sodium-dependent multivitamin transporter: a treatable disease, mimicking biotinidase deficiency. JIMD Rep. 2019;48(1):11–4. https://doi.org/10.1002/jmd2.12040.
6. Shay KP, Moreau RF, Smith EJ, Smith AR, Hagen TM. Alpha-lipoic acid as a dietary supplement: molecular mechanisms and therapeutic potential. Biochim Biophys Acta Gen Subj. 2009;1790(10):1149–60. https://doi.org/10.1016/j.bbagen.2009.07.026.
7. Subramanian VS, Constantinescu AR, Benke PJ, Said HM. Mutations in SLC5A6 associated with brain, immune, bone, and intestinal dysfunction in a young child. Hum Genet. 2017;136(2):253–61. https://doi.org/10.1007/s00439-016-1751-x.
8. Theodosis-Nobelos P, Papagiouvannis G, Tziona P, Rekka EA. Lipoic acid. Kinetics and pluripotent biological properties and derivatives. Mol Biol Rep. 2021;48(9):6539–50. https://doi.org/10.1007/s11033-021-06643-z.
9. Tibullo D, Volti G, Giallongo C, Grasso S, Tomassoni D, Anfuso CD, Lupo G, Amenta F, Avola R, Bramanti V. Biochemical and clinical relevance of alpha lipoic acid: antioxidant and anti-inflammatory activity, molecular pathways and therapeutic potential. Inflamm Res. 2017;66:947–59.

Part V

Fat Soluble Vitamins

Vitamin A

31

Charles B. Chen

Vitamin A is an important micronutrient involved in multiple cellular processes. The presence of vitamin A was described by Frederick Gowland Hopkins in 1912 and for his discovery, he received the Nobel Prize in Physiology or Medicine in 1929. Deficiency of vitamin A is an important preventable cause of blindness in the world, particularly in children.

Role of Vitamin A

Vitamin A is a fat-soluble vitamin which plays critical roles including:

- Immune function and immuno-regulation.
- Epithelial integrity.
- Formation and maintenance of the epithelium.
- Maintenance of vision.

C. B. Chen (✉)
Division of Gastroenterology, Department of Pediatrics, University of Missouri School of Medicine, Columbia, MO, USA

K. Radhakrishnan (ed.), *Handbook of Clinical and Practical Pediatric Nutrition*, https://doi.org/10.1007/978-3-031-97759-6_31

Vitamin A Derivatives [1]

- Retinol
  - Functions in vitamin A transport and storage
  - Produced from beta-carotene
- Retinal
  - Plays important roles in vision
  - Synthesized from oxidation of retinol
- Retinoic acid
  - Functions in embryologic development and immune function
  - Synthesized from oxidation of retinaldehyde

Vitamin A Sources

- Humans are unable to synthesize vitamin A and obtain the micronutrient primarily from dietary sources.
- Vitamin A is obtained from many foods such as fish, eggs, organ meats, and yellow and leafy green vegetables (Table 31.1) [2].
- Two main forms of vitamin A.
  - Retinyl esters
  - Carotenoids
- Retinyl esters are derived from animal products, while carotenoids are obtained from plants.
- One IU retinol is equivalent to 0.3 mcg retinol activity equivalent (RAE).

Table 31.1 Foods high in vitamin A

Dairy
Fish
Eggs
Organ meats
Green vegetables (broccoli, spinach)
Liver

Vitamin A Digestion, Absorption, Transport, and Stores

- Retinyl esters are much more readily absorbed than carotenoids, with absorption rates of greater than 75% for the former compared to generally 20–50% for the latter [3].
- Vitamin A is absorbed in the proximal small intestine and is mediated by both carrier-dependent proteins and passive diffusion [3].
- Digestion of retinyl esters by intestinal and pancreatic enzymes leads to subsequent uptake of retinol by enterocytes.
- Bile acids regulate vitamin A uptake.
- Carotenoids may be absorbed directly by the intestinal mucosa or may be converted to retinol.
- Retinol is converted to retinyl esters, carried by chylomicrons, and transported through the lymphatic system and eventually reaches the liver after additional modifications [4].
- Up to 80% of vitamin A is stored in the liver, and excess retinol is stored in the liver as retinal esters [5].
- Transport to the plasma occurs in a bound form with retinol-binding protein.
- Excretion of vitamin A occurs through urine and feces.

Vitamin A Deficiency

Vitamin A deficiency is seen more frequently in developing nations, where micronutrient deficiencies are more common. The prevalence is higher in pediatric patients, with almost up to 15% of children and adolescents in a review of 165 low- and middle-income countries having vitamin A deficiency [6].

- Clinical manifestations include vision defects, dermatologic findings, and increased susceptibility to infections.
- Ophthalmic effects most notably include night blindness (due to degeneration of retinal rods), conjunctival xerosis, Bitot's

spots (at corneal limbus), corneal xerosis, and xerophthalmia (Table 31.2).
  - Ophthalmic effects are one of the most preventable manifestations.
- Conditions that cause cholestasis or exocrine pancreatic insufficiency often result in vitamin A deficiency.
- Gastrointestinal conditions such as inflammatory bowel disease have also been associated with vitamin A deficiency, with the prevalence reported at 16% in one study [7].
- Infections such as measles are well reported to bring out vitamin A deficiency .
- Early diagnosis is crucial given the potential implications of untreated vitamin A deficiency as well as the impact on quality of life.
- The degree of improvement in clinical symptoms is variable and often may depend on the duration of those symptoms; vitamin A recommended daily allowance and dosing in deficiency states are presented in Tables 31.3 and 31.4.

Table 31.2 Ophthalmic manifestations of vitamin A deficiency

Stage 1	Night-blindness
Stage 2	Bitots spots and other conjunctival changes (xerosis)
Stage 3	Corneal manifestations and scarring

Table 31.3 Vitamin A recommended daily allowance

	RAE (mcg)
Infants 12 months and under	400–500
2–18 years	300–600
Adults	700–900

Table 31.4 Vitamin A dosing in deficiency states

Infants	Up to 600 mcg
Young children	600–900 mcg
Adolescents	1700–2800 mcg
Adults	3000 mcg

- Ophthalmic findings such as night blindness often improve or resolve with vitamin A supplementation, while other manifestations such as corneal ulceration may persist and lead to long-term loss of vision.
- Morbidity and mortality from infections are also increased with vitamin A deficiency, especially in children [8].

Assessment of Vitamin A Status

- Serum plasma retinol concentration is used to monitor vitamin A status, with a level of 20 mcg/dL or higher being generally considered normal [9].
- However, serum retinol levels often do not decrease unless hepatic stores of vitamin A are low.
- Plasma levels are affected by a variety of nutritional and clinical conditions deficiency as well.
- In clinical practice, vitamin A levels are often not routinely checked unless there is a known deficiency or other condition that puts the patient at risk for fat-soluble vitamin deficiency.
- Impression cytology, characterized by removal of the superficial layers of the ocular conjunctival surface epithelium for histologic analysis, may indicate vitamin A deficiency.
- Retinol/RBP ratio (ratio close to 1:1 suggests appropriate vitamin A levels).
- Retinol loading test assesses change in serum retinol after administration of a vitamin A supplement.
- Retinol dose response (RDR) measures the percentage increase in retinol level 5 hours after oral dose of vitamin A and is used more often in research settings.
  - Rise over 20% from baseline is an indication of vitamin A deficiency.
- Retinol isotope dilution test assesses total body vitamin A stores and is used in research settings.

Vitamin A Toxicity

Compared to vitamin A deficiency, vitamin A toxicity is uncommon and generally results from excessive intake through supplementation or diet.

Acute Vitamin A Toxicity

- Generally due to excessive vitamin A supplementation (greater than 100,000 IU over a period of 6 months).
- Symptoms include nausea, vomiting, irritability, and cutaneous changes [4].
- Diagnosis is made by history, clinical symptoms, and serum vitamin A levels.
- Management.
  - Identification and discontinuation of vitamin A intake or supplementation.
  - Supportive therapy and management of complications such as increased intracranial pressure and hepatic injury.
  - Correction of electrolyte abnormalities (hypercalcemia).
- Clinical symptoms often resolve within 4 weeks.

Chronic Vitamin A Toxicity

- Often due to consumption of vitamin A-rich foods or prolonged use of vitamin A supplementation.
- Often presents with cutaneous manifestations (dry, scaly skin) and bone changes (bone pain, calcinosis, bone spurs, bone resorption, osteoporosis, and higher risk of fractures).
- Central nervous system effects may occur and include elevations in intracranial pressure, although vitamin A-induced pseudotumor cerebri is an uncommon manifestation.
- Risk of hepatic fibrosis.
- Fetal malformations may occur in pregnant women with hypervitaminosis A.

- Management.
  - Identification and discontinuation of vitamin A intake or supplementation.
  - Supportive therapy .

Uses of Vitamin A Derivatives

- Vitamin A derivatives are used frequently in medicine.
- All-trans retinoic acid is highly effective in treating acute promyelocytic leukemia by inducing the PML-RARα gene which eventually inhibits proliferation of leukemic cells [10].
- Retinol is used to treat acne and mediates a number of processes including increasing epithelial turnover as well as modulating inflammatory pathways [11].
- Retinoids are also used in other dermatologic conditions such as psoriasis and ichthyosis.
- Vitamin A supplementation also has been used in treating ophthalmic conditions such as retinitis pigmentosa, with studies showing that it can slow down loss of cone function in pediatric patients [12].

Future Research

There are multiple future directions for vitamin A research. There is an ongoing investigation into vitamin A dosing and duration of supplementation and its impact on morbidity and clinical outcomes in the pediatric population. In addition to its uses in the fields of dermatology and oncology, vitamin A derivatives are also being investigated in the treatment of neurological conditions given evidence suggesting a role of vitamin A in cognitive functioning. Finally, as measles is prevalent in certain regions of the world such as Africa and Asia, further clinical and epidemiological studies are needed to analyze the role of vitamin A in affecting disease course and long-term outcomes.

References

1. Zhong M, Kawaguchi R, Kassai M, Sun H. Retina, retinol, retinal and the natural history of vitamin A as a light sensor. Nutrients. 2012;4(12):2069–96.
2. Conaway HH, Henning P, Lerner UH. Vitamin a metabolism, action, and role in skeletal homeostasis. Endocr Rev. 2013;34(6):766–97.
3. Reboul E. Absorption of vitamin A and carotenoids by the enterocyte: focus on transport proteins. Nutrients. 2013;5(9):3563–81.
4. Penniston KL, Tanumihardjo SA. The acute and chronic toxic effects of vitamin A. Am J Clin Nutr. 2006;83(2):191–201.
5. Chen G, Weiskirchen S, Weiskirchen R. Vitamin A: too good to be bad? Front Pharmacol. 2023;14:1186336.
6. Song P, Adeloye D, Li S, Zhao D, Ye X, Pan Q, et al. The prevalence of vitamin A deficiency and its public health significance in children in low- and middle-income countries: a systematic review and modelling analysis. J Glob Health. 2023;13:04084.
7. Alkhouri RH, Hashmi H, Baker RD, Gelfond D, Baker SS. Vitamin and mineral status in patients with inflammatory bowel disease. J Pediatr Gastroenterol Nutr. 2013;56(1):89–92.
8. Imdad A, Mayo-Wilson E, Haykal MR, Regan A, Sidhu J, Smith A, et al. Vitamin A supplementation for preventing morbidity and mortality in children from six months to five years of age. Cochrane Database Syst Rev. 2022;3(3):CD008524.
9. Miller M, Humphrey J, Johnson E, Marinda E, Brookmeyer R, Katz J. Why do children become vitamin A deficient? J Nutr. 2002;132(9 Suppl):2867S-80S.
10. Szymański Ł, Skopek R, Palusińska M, Schenk T, Stengel S, Lewicki S, et al. Retinoic Acid and its derivatives in skin. Cells. 2020;9(12):2660.
11. Motamedi M, Chehade A, Sanghera R, Grewal P. A clinician's guide to topical retinoids. J Cutan Med Surg. 2022;26(1):71–8.
12. Berson EL, Weigel-DiFranco C, Rosner B, Gaudio AR, Sandberg MA. Association of Vitamin A Supplementation with disease course in children with retinitis pigmentosa. JAMA Ophthalmol. 2018;136(5):490–5.

Vitamin D

32

Rishi Gupta

Vitamin D Physiology

- Vitamin D is a fat-soluble vitamin playing an important role in calcium homeostasis.
- Cholecalciferol (vitamin D3) and ergocalciferol (vitamin D2) are derived from animal and plant sources, respectively.
- Vitamin D2 and D3 are converted to storage form Calcidiol (25-hydroxyvitamin D (25OHD)) by 25-hydroxylation in liver.
- The active form Calcitriol (1,25-dihydroxyvitamin-D (1,25 OHD)) is formed by 1-alpha-hydroxylation of 25-OHD mainly in the kidneys. This conversion is regulated by parathyroid hormone (PTH) and hypophosphatemia besides other factors.
- 1,25 OHD binds to intracellular receptor and affects gene expression by interacting with vitamin D response elements—leading to increased calcium and to some extent phosphorus absorption in intestine, suppresses PTH secretion and inhibits its own synthesis in kidneys completing negative feedback loop.

R. Gupta (✉)
Division of Pediatric Gastroenterology, Hepatology and Nutrition, Golisano Children's Hospital at University of Rochester Medical Center, Rochester, NY, USA
e-mail: rishi_gupta@urmc.rochester.edu

K. Radhakrishnan (ed.), *Handbook of Clinical and Practical Pediatric Nutrition*, https://doi.org/10.1007/978-3-031-97759-6_32

- **Fortified foods and dermal synthesis are the major natural sources of vitamin D. Very few foods in natural state have vitamin D except fatty fish.**
- **Unfortified cow's milk has no vitamin D and human milk has 10 IU vitamin D in 8 oz whereas fortified milk has 100–150 IU of vitamin D in 8 oz.**
- Cutaneous synthesis involves conversion of 7-dehydrocholesterol to vitamin D3. Increased skin melanin, less sun exposure, covered skin, sunscreen application, and less ultraviolet B light exposure in winter sun and in northern climates decrease cutaneous synthesis of vitamin D [1].
- 25-OH vitamin D levels no consensus but levels >20 ng/ml are considered sufficient by institute of medicine (IOM) in North America where as other organizations including endocrine society recommends normal levels to be >30 ng/ml targeting lower blood PTH levels [2].
- Daily vitamin D requirement—Infants—400 IU daily and children- 600 IU daily **(see** Table 32.1**).**
- **Children with cholestatic disorders like biliary atresia due to inadequate intestinal absorption and obese children due**

Table 32.1 Recommended vitamin D intake in children and adults [3]

Age group	Daily vitamin D intake RDA	Special considerations
Term infants (<1 year of age)	400 IU	Exclusive breast fed and with intake of infant formula <800 ml/day
Premature infants (<1 year of age)	400–1000 IU	Guidelines differ in terms of exact supplementation
Children 1–18 years of age	600 IU	
Adults (<70 years of age)	600 IU	
Adults (>70 years of age)	800 IU	

to visceral fat sequestration of vitamin D might require higher daily vitamin D intake to maintain normal levels though there are no guidelines on how high that daily intake should be.

- **Low vitamin D levels in general should be rechecked 3–4 months after starting therapy.**

Treatment of Vitamin D Deficiency [4]

Children with Serum Vitamin D < 20 ng/ml without Rickets

1. Vitamin D 2000 IU daily for 3 months followed by daily maintenance dose of 600–1000 IU daily.
2. Vitamin D 50,000 IU weekly for 6 weeks followed by daily maintenance dose of 600–1000 IU daily.

Children with Serum Vitamin D < 20 ng/ml with Rickets

1. Vitamin D 3000–6000 IU daily for 12 weeks followed by daily maintenance dose of 600–1000 IU daily.
2. Vitamin D 50,000 IU weekly for 12 weeks followed by daily maintenance dose of 600–1000 IU daily.
3. Oral elemental calcium at 30–75 mg/kg/day is needed till high dose daily vitamin D is given, usually for initial 6–12 weeks and then after 500 mg daily calcium dose.
4. Stoss therapy is an accepted method to treat vitamin D deficiency rapidly by giving a single dose of 300,000–600,000 IU injection of vitamin D intramuscularly where available or oral vitamin D 50,000 IU daily for total cumulative dose of 300,000–600,000 IU [5].

Vitamin D Deficiency States-

1. Nutritional vitamin D deficiency Rickets.
2. Vitamin D-dependent Rickets, type-1.
3. Vitamin D-dependent Rickets, type-2.
4. Chronic kidney disease (CKD) induced vitamin D deficiency.

Nutritional Vitamin D Deficiency Rickets- Rickets is a disease of growing bones due to under mineralization of matrix at growth plates in children.

- It can manifest clinically from craniotabes, wide anterior fontanel, and delayed dentition to rachitic rosary, widened wrists and ankles, valgus and varus deformities of legs, failure to thrive.
- Deficiency can lead to hypocalcemic seizures in infants and children.
- Underlying cause is vitamin D deficiency leading to low phosphate and calcium levels in blood and bone.
- Diagnosis is made by classic radiographic abnormalities showing widened metaphysis of long bones and supported by low vitamin D and phosphate levels and increased alkaline phosphatase levels.
- Serum calcium levels can be normal due to secondary hyperparathyroidism.
- Treatment consists of daily vitamin D 2000 IU or even higher doses along with appropriate calcium and phosphate supplementation.
- Children with severe hypocalcemia might also need intravenous calcium supplementation initially.
- In certain situations, due to compliance or logistics reasons—Stoss therapy of 300,000 to 600,000 IU of vitamin D oral/intramuscular is also a reasonable option.
- Follow-up is needed with repeat X-ray and serum vitamin D and calcium, phosphate, and alkaline phosphatase levels after 4–8 weeks to make sure those are normalizing.

Vitamin D-Dependent Rickets (VDDR), Type-1 and Type-2-

- Type-1 disorders are due to mutation in genes either encoding 25-hydroxylase (leading to less 25-OHD levels) or 1,25 hydroxylase (leading to low 1,25-OHD levels).
- Type-2 disorders are due to mutation in genes encoding for either vitamin D receptor (type 2A) or in the hormone response element-binding protein interfering with 1,25-OHD action (type 2A) (Please see Table 32.2).
- In both these conditions, serum alkaline phosphatase and parathyroid hormone levels are elevated, and phosphate levels are low. Calcium levels can be low to normal.
- Treatment consists of high-dose vitamin D (25-OHD or 1,25-OHD depending on the mutation) and high-dose calcium while monitoring for development of any nephrocalcinosis (Table 32.3).

Table 32.2 Causes of vitamin D insufficiency in infants and children

1.	Low maternal vitamin D levels.
2.	Premature birth, given less time for transplacental transfer of vitamin D from mother to the fetus.
3.	Exclusive breast feeding without vitamin D supplementation to the infant.
4.	Low consumption of dairy products and vitamin D-fortified foods.
5.	Less sun exposure specially in higher latitudes.
6.	Increased skin pigmentation leading to less vitamin D formation in skin.
7.	Obesity due to sequestration of vitamin D in visceral fat.
8.	Conditions associated with intestinal malabsorption such as exocrine pancreatic insufficiency, inflammatory bowel disease, and cholestatic liver disorders like biliary atresia.
9.	Conditions leading to decreased activation or increased metabolism of vitamin D- liver and kidney diseases and medications like ketoconazole (decreased activation) and medications like certain anticonvulsants (increased metabolism).
10.	Genetic disorders leading to 25-hydroxylase deficiency, 1,25-hydroxylase deficiency, and hereditary resistance to vitamin D.

Table 32.3 Vitamin D deficiency disorders

Disease	Pathophysiology	Serum 25-OHD levels	Treatment supplementation
Vitamin D deficiency	Nutritional vitamin D deficiency	Low	25-OHD (2000 IU daily)
VDDR, type 1A	Mutation in renal 1-α-hydroxylase	Normal	1,25-OHD (0.25–2 mcg daily)
VDDR, type 1B	Mutation in 25-hydroxylase	Low	25-OHD (3000 IU or higher dose daily)
VDDR, type 2A	Mutation in vitamin D receptor	Normal	Very high dose of 25-OHD or 1,25-OHD with high dose calcium
VDDR, type 2B	Overexpression of hormone response element-binding protein interfering with 1,25-OHD action	Normal	Very high dose of 25-OHD (>5000 IU daily) or 1,25-OHD (2 mcg/day) with high dose calcium (1000–3000 mg/day)
CKD-induced vitamin D deficiency	Low activity of renal 1-α-hydroxylase	Normal	1,25-OHD supplementation and phosphate restriction

Extraskeletal Effects of Vitamin D-

- Activated vitamin D receptor (VDR) (after binding to 1,25-OHD) binds in a ligand-dependent fashion to hundreds of genomic loci responsible for cellular differentiation, innate and adaptive immunity, and other functions [6].
- This has been postulated as a mechanism for extra skeletal beneficial effects of vitamin D including prevention of inflammation, autoimmunity, antioxidant, cancer and cardiovascular diseases risk reduction, alleviation of depression, etc.
- Even though epidemiological data exists linking low vitamin D (<20 ng/ml) levels to above mentioned pathological states, but there are no randomized controlled good trials demonstrating

that vitamin D supplementation reduces risk or improves prognosis for above mentioned conditions.

- Therefore, there are no guidelines or recommendations for vitamin D supplementation to prevent or treat these conditions.

Future Directions for Research for Vitamin D Role in Disease Prevention-

- The knowledge gained so far about vitamin D receptor binding-induced molecular signaling and gene activation has been mainly from ex-vivo models and is very helpful.
- The future research needs to bring these ex-vivo models to in-vivo and then after large-scale prospective human trials of vitamin D supplementation in different disease states as well as predisposed individuals in their preclinical stage to assess the role of vitamin D supplementation in prevention and amelioration of extraskeletal diseases.

References

1. Weisberg P, Scanlon KS, Li R, Cogswell ME. Nutritional rickets among children in the United States: review of cases reported between 1986 and 2003. Am J Clin Nutr. 2004;80(6 Suppl):1697S–705S. https://doi.org/10.1093/ajcn/80.6.1697S.
2. Saintonge S, Bang H, Gerber LM. Implications of a new definition of vitamin D deficiency in a multiracial us adolescent population: the National Health and Nutrition Examination Survey III. Pediatrics. 2009;123(3):797–803. https://doi.org/10.1542/peds.2008-1195.
3. Institute of Medicine (US) Committee to review dietary reference intakes for Vitamin D and Calcium; Ross AC, Taylor CL, Yaktine AL, et al., editors. Dietary reference intakes for calcium and Vitamin D. Washington: National Academies Press/Dietary reference intakes for adequacy: calcium and Vitamin D; 2011. 5. Available from: https://www.ncbi.nlm.nih.gov/books/NBK56056/
4. Misra M, Pacaud D, Petryk A, Collett-Solberg PF, Kappy M. Drug and therapeutics Committee of the Lawson Wilkins Pediatric Endocrine Society. Vitamin D deficiency in children and its management: review of

current knowledge and recommendations. Pediatrics. 2008;122(2):398–417. https://doi.org/10.1542/peds.2007-1894.

5. Munns CF, Shaw N, Butler G, Högler W, et al. Global consensus recommendations on prevention and management of nutritional rickets. J Clin Endocrinol Metab. 2016;101(2):394–415. https://doi.org/10.1210/jc.2015-2175. Epub 2016 Jan 8. PMID: 26745253. PMCID: PMC4880117
6. Carlberg C. Vitamin D and its target genes. Nutrients. 2022;14(7):1354. https://doi.org/10.3390/nu14071354. PMID: 35405966. PMCID: PMC9003440

Vitamin E

33

Sanu Raja Yadav

Introduction

- Vitamin E is a group of lipid-soluble vitamins that consists of a family of eight structurally related molecules with a common chromanol ring head and variable side chains—namely, four tocopherols (alpha, beta, delta, and gamma analogs) and four tocotrienols (alpha, beta, delta, and gamma analogs). The RRR-alpha-tocopherol (R configuration at all three chiral centers) is the vitamin E isomer with the most biological activity [1].
- The other naturally occurring forms of Vitamin E (beta, delta, and gamma-tocopherol and all tocotrienols) are not converted to alpha-tocopherol by humans and are also poorly recognized by alpha-tocopherol transfer protein. Hence, they do not significantly contribute to bodily vitamin E requirements.
- Vitamin E was discovered as an "anti-sterility factor" that prevented fetal resorption in rats by Evans and Bishop in 1922—deficient in rats fed rancid lard, while replenished with plant-based wheat germ oil—leading to the name tocopherol ("tocos" for fetus and "pheros" for bearing in Greek) [2].

S. R. Yadav (✉)
Division of Pediatric Gastroenterology, Department of Pediatrics,
University of Missouri School of Medicine, Columbia, MO, USA
e-mail: srymb5@health.missouri.edu

K. Radhakrishnan (ed.), *Handbook of Clinical and Practical Pediatric Nutrition*, https://doi.org/10.1007/978-3-031-97759-6_33

Table 33.1 Common dietary sources of vitamin E

Sunflower seeds	Safflower oil	Soybean and corn oil
Almonds	Hazelnuts	Peanuts
Wheat germ oil	Spinach	Broccoli

Natural Sources and Vitamin E supplements

- Vitamin E is primarily present in plant-based lipids such as seed/nuts and vegetable oils - alpha-tocopherol in olive oil, sunflower oil, almond oil, and gamma-tocopherol in soybean and corn oils. Significant amounts can also be present in green leafy foods and fortified cereals (Table 33.1).
- Dietary supplements contain alpha-tocopheryl esters such as acetate and succinate for stability and require digestion by pancreatic esterases and bile acid.
- Recommended daily allowance for vitamin E is 15 mg daily for adults while 4–7 mg in infancy/early childhood. Tolerable upper limit of intake is reported to be 1000 mg daily [3]. Higher than upper limits can potentially lead to hemorrhagic complications.

Metabolism and Transport

- Vitamin E is absorbed in the small intestine after esterified forms (natural or supplements) are hydrolyzed by pancreatic carboxyl ester hydrolases in the presence of bile acids. The absorbed alpha-tocopherol is secreted by the enterocytes into chylomicrons and transported through lymphatic pathway to systemic circulation and eventually to the liver, where chylomicron remnants are taken up, and the alpha-tocopherol is packaged into VLDL and released into circulation, subsequently metabolized to LDL and HDLs for delivery to peripheral tissues [4].
- The uptake of alpha-tocopherol into hepatocytes is facilitated by alpha-tocopherol transport protein (αTTP), which has significantly preferential binding of alpha-tocopherol than other vitamin E isomers. αTTP is a cytosolic protein of the cellular

retinaldehyde binding protein (CRAL-BP) family. It helps with cytosolic transport of alpha-tocopherol from chylomicron remnants to the plasma membrane in hepatocytes where it is incorporated into nascent VLDL.

Physiological Functions of Vitamin E

- Alpha-tocopherol is a potent lipid-soluble antioxidant and in vivo reacts with fatty acid peroxyl radicals, generated by lipid peroxidation, to break the chain reaction of fatty acid auto-oxidation process. This autooxidation (esp. of LDL) is postulated to underlie some of the major degenerative health conditions such as aging, atherosclerosis, cardiovascular diseases, and Alzheimer's disease. Paradoxically, vitamin E can also be a pro-oxidant in certain environments.
- After oxidation, alpha-tocopherol may be regenerated by reduction of the tocopheroxyl radical by either vitamin C at the aqueous cytosolic interface or with ubiquinol-10 within the cell membrane.
- Vitamin E also possesses multiple nonantioxidant actions [5]—such as modulation of inflammation through inhibition of protein kinase C and upregulation of cytosolic phospholipase A2 and cyclo-oxygenase activities; inhibition of cellular proliferation in cancer; and regulation of various gene expressions including xanthine oxidase, scavenger receptors SR-A and CD36, and tropomyosin and collagenase, among others.

Vitamin E Deficiency

- Vitamin E deficiency is uncommon except in conditions that lead to fat malabsorption—exocrine pancreatic insufficiency, cholestatic conditions, and short bowel syndrome with significant ileal resections or loss of function. Clinical manifestations can include neuropathies (spinocerebellar dysfunction with ataxia, low or absent reflexes, loss of touch/proprioception), skeletal myopathy, retinal degeneration, hemolytic anemia, and intestinal lipofuscinosis [6].

- Rare genetic conditions can also present with manifestations of vitamin E deficiency such as Ataxia with vitamin E deficiency (AVED) caused by mutation of hepatic α-TTP proteins. This autosomal recessive neurodegenerative disease is characterized by spinocerebellar ataxia and retinal degeneration by adolescence. High-dose supplementation of vitamin E has been shown to overcome or halt the progression of disease in this condition.
- Abetalipoproteinemia (mutations in microsomal triglyceride transfer proteins) or hypobetalipoproteinemia (mutations involving apolipoprotein B) can also lead to varying severity of chylomicron/LDL and fat-soluble vitamin deficiencies, presenting with progressive ataxia and sensory-motor neuropathy. Chylomicron retention disease (mutations in SAR1b protein blocking ApoB48 and chylomicron formation) can similarly produce sequela of severe vitamin E deficiency.
- Premature and very low birth weight babies can be at risk for vitamin E deficiency, if they are on high PUFA diet without appropriate vitamin E supplementation. Babies can present with severe hemolytic anemia with edema in such conditions. Although high vitamin E supplementation has been shown to be protective against retinopathy and intraventricular hemorrhage, it can also lead to increased risk for sepsis and necrotizing colitis, and routine supplementation is not recommended [7] (Table 33.2).

Table 33.2 Etiologies of vitamin E deficiency

Exocrine pancreatic insufficiency—cystic Fibrosis, Shwachman Diamond syndrome, chronic pancreatitis
Cholestatic conditions—biliary atresia, primary sclerosing cholangitis, familial intrahepatic cholestasis, primary biliary cholangitis
Loss of ileal absorptive area—short bowel syndrome, severe Crohn's disease, congenital intestinal lymphangiectasia
Ataxia with Vitamin E deficiency—genetic mutations in hepatic alpha-tocopherol transfer protein
Abetalipoproteinemia and hypobetalipoproteinemia, chylomicron retention disease
Premature and LBW infants on high PUFA diet

Measurements and Dosing

- Vitamin E dosing is often measured as equivalents of the most active isomer which is RRR-alpha-tocopherol. One mg of RRR-alpha-tocopherol equivalent is found in 2.22 international units (IU) of synthetic vitamin E and 1.49 international units (IU) of natural source vitamin E [1].
- Normal serum concentrations of alpha-tocopherol are typically around 1 mg/dL for alpha-tocopherol and values below 0.5 mg/dL are considered deficient. For conversion, 1 mg/dL of alpha-tocopherol is equal to 23.2 μmol/L. Although both alpha and gamma-tocopherols are measured at most commercial assays—alpha-tocopherol is the most important component for nutritional assessment.
- Serum concentrations of alpha-tocopherol may be affected by hyperlipidemia (falsely high) and hypoproteinemia (falsely low) and need caution for interpretation.

Treatment of Vitamin E Deficiency

- Treatment dosing for repletion in pediatric population with cholestasis is approx. 25–50 IU/kg/day of alpha-tocopherol equivalent. Adult doses for repletion are often between 75 and 800 IU daily.
- Typical recommended dosing in children with pancreatic insufficiency as in cystic fibrosis is as follows:
  - Less than 1 year—40–50 IU.
  - 1–3 years—80–150 IU
  - 4–8 years—100–200 IU
  - >8 years—200–400 IU.
- Much higher doses of Vitamin E administration are recommended in management of abetalipoproteinemia to prevent and/or partially reverse the neurological consequences—doses in the range of 75–250 IU/kg/day are often necessary.
- Water-soluble vitamin E formulations (alpha-tocopherol PEG succinate) are available for better absorption in malabsorptive

conditions including cholestasis. These are available as over the counter supplements, no FDA-approved product is available in the United States.

Vitamin E Toxicity

- Vitamin E toxicity is rare and significantly higher doses (>1000 mg alpha-tocopherol equivalent per day) can predispose to hemorrhagic effects, hypothesized to occur through inhibition of platelet aggregation and adhesion. Few studies have also raised concern for increased risk of prostate cancer and all-cause mortality with long-term use of high doses of Vitamin E. Milder forms of adverse effects such as muscle weakness, fatigue, nausea, and diarrhea may be possible. In infants, high-dose supplementations have been associated with increased sepsis and necrotizing enterocolitis.

Future Research Possibilities

- Molecular mechanisms behind the oxidant and nonoxidant properties of Vitamin E molecules are largely unknown and further studies are needed to learn about them, specifically its role in modulating signal transduction at cellular level and in influencing various gene transcriptions, in both health and disease.

References

1. Schneider C. Chemistry and biology of vitamin E. Mol Nutr Food Res. 2005;49:7–30.
2. Evans HM, Bishop KS. On the existence of a hitherto unrecognized dietary factor essential for reproduction. Science. 1922;56:650–1.

3. Compounds I of M (US) P on DA and R (2000) Dietary reference intakes for Vitamin C, Vitamin E, selenium, and carotenoids. diet ref intakes Vitamin C, Vitamin E, selenium, carotenoids. https://doi.org/10.17226/9810.
4. Rigotti A. Absorption, transport, and tissue delivery of vitamin E. Mol Asp Med. 2007;28:423–36.
5. Jiang Q. Metabolism of natural forms of vitamin E and biological actions of vitamin E metabolites. Free Radic Biol Med. 2021;179:375.
6. Eggermont E. Recent advances in vitamin E metabolism and deficiency. Eur J Pediatr. 2006;165:429–34.
7. Xiong Z, Liu L, Jian Z, Ma Y, Li H, Jin X, Liao B, Wang K. Vitamin E and multiple health outcomes: an umbrella review of meta-analyses. Nutrients. 2023;15:3301.

Vitamin K

34

Supraja Swamy,
Senthilkumar Sankararaman,
and Kadakkal Radhakrishnan

History of Vitamin K

- Vitamin K was discovered in the 1930s while Carl Peter Henrik Dam was researching cholesterol metabolism in chickens. He observed spontaneous hemorrhage for chickens fed a fat-free diet, postulating the role of fat-soluble vitamins in coagulation (K refers to Koagulation in *German* language) [1].
- By the 1970s, the mechanism action of vitamin K was more comprehensively understood with regard to gamma-carboxyglutamic acid, prothrombin, and later the discovery of vitamin K-dependent proteins and their role in hemostasis [2].

S. Swamy (✉)
Department of Pediatric Gastroenterology, Wake Forest University, Winston Salem, NC, USA
e-mail: sswamy@wakehealth.edu

S. Sankararaman · K. Radhakrishnan
Division of Pediatric Gastroenterology Hepatology and Nutrition, Cleveland Clinic Children's Hospital, Cleveland, OH, USA
e-mail: SANKARS6@ccf.org; radhakk@ccf.org

K. Radhakrishnan (ed.), *Handbook of Clinical and Practical Pediatric Nutrition*, https://doi.org/10.1007/978-3-031-97759-6_34

Table 34.1 Recommended dietary allowance for vitamin K (table adapted from National Institutes of Health) [5]

Age	Male	Female
Birth to 6 months	2 mcg	2 mcg
7–12 months	2.5 mcg	2.5 mcg
1–3 years	30 mcg	30 mcg
4–8 years	55 mcg	55 mcg
9–13 years	60 mcg	60 mcg
14–18 years	75 mcg	75 mcg
19+ years	120 mcg	90 mcg

Vitamin K Forms

- There are three forms of Vitamin K: K1, K2, K3.
- Vitamin K1, or phylloquinone, is found in leafy green vegetables and is a product of photosynthesis. This form is used for therapy [3].
- Vitamin K2, or menaquinone, is created when the intestinal flora converts Vitamin K1 to K2. Dietary sources include fermented products, egg yolks, chicken, beef, and liver [3].
- Vitamin K3, or menadione, is a synthetic form of vitamin K, which can be a structural precursor to K1 or K2 in the liver. It is no longer used for supplementation in humans due to potential toxicity in infants with glucose-6-phosphate dehydrogenase deficiency. Synthetic vitamin K1 is preferred [4].
- **Recommended dietary allowance** for vitamin K is noted in Table 34.1.

Vitamin K Physiology

- Vitamin K is a fat-soluble vitamin required for the gamma-carboxylation of coagulation factors II, VII, IX, X, proteins C and S [3].
- Vitamin K1 is more concentrated in the liver while K2 has increased extrahepatic bioavailability.

- Osteocalcin is a bone vitamin K-dependent protein that acts as a regulator for bone formation. Adequate vitamin K status has therefore been associated with lower risk of fracture and better bone mineral density [2].
- Matrix Gla-protein is another vitamin K-dependent protein that plays an important role in preventing arterial and cartilage calcification.

Vitamin K Cycle [6]

- Vitamin K is reduced intracellularly to vitamin K hydroquinone via vitamin K epoxide reductase (Fig. 34.1).
- Vitamin K hydroquinone gets oxidized by gamma-glutamyl carboxylase subsequently creating vitamin K epoxide.
- Vitamin K epoxide is reconverted to vitamin K by vitamin K epoxide reductase.

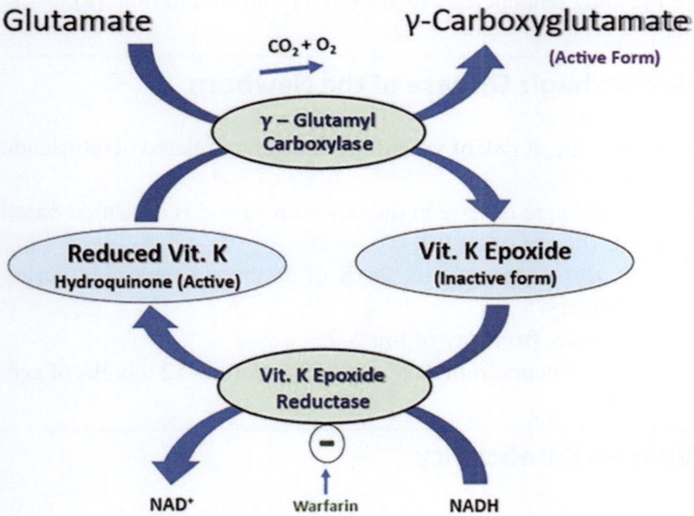

Fig. 34.1 Vitamin K metabolic cycle

Vitamin K Status in Newborns

- Vitamin K minimally crosses the placental barrier, leading to newborns having physiologically low stores of vitamin K and vitamin K-dependent clotting factors [7].
- Prenatal maternal vitamin K supplementation therefore does not prevent neonatal vitamin K deficiency.
- The American Academy of Pediatrics (AAP) recommends administering 1 mg of intramuscular (IM) vitamin K prophylactically to all neonates regardless of gestational age. IM vitamin K within 6 h of birth has been shown to be more effective at preventing vitamin K deficiency bleeding than parenteral supplementation [8].
- For preterm infants less than 1500 mg, the AAP recommends weight-dependent dosing of 0.3–0.5 mg/kg [8].
- Breastmilk contains minimal quantities of vitamin K; therefore, vitamin K deficiency bleeding should be considered in exclusively breastfed infants under 6 months with bruising or bleeding tendencies with elevated prothrombin time [8].

Hemorrhagic Disease of the Newborn

- Infants are at risk of vitamin K deficiency-related hemorrhagic disease.
- Hemorrhagic disease in the newborn period is classified based off of time of onset [9].
  - Early: occurs within 24 h of birth or sometimes during delivery.
  - Classic: from day of life 2–7.
  - Late: occurs from 8 days of life up until 6–12 months of age.

Vitamin K Deficiency

- Presentation:
  - Patients may present with spontaneous bleeding after minor trauma or hemorrhage. These patients may have a history of taking anticonvulsants, anticoagulants, or antibiotics.

Patients with fat malabsorptive disorders including cystic fibrosis, celiac disease, or inflammatory bowel disease may be at risk as well. [4]

- Physical exams can be notable for ecchymosis, petechiae, mucosal bleeding, or easy bruising and intracranial bleed.

- Evaluation
  - Prothrombin time (PT) is typically significantly elevated in advanced stages of vitamin K deficiency. However, elevated PT is also indicative of decompensated liver disease. Assuming normal liver function, a raising PT, indicates that total body vitamin K is less than 50%. Normalization of PT after administration of vitamin K is indicative of vitamin K deficiency bleeding.
  - Low serum vitamin K level is indicative of vitamin K deficiency, but recent ingestion of vitamin K may impact the serum levels.
  - Measuring elevations in proteins induced by vitamin K absence or antagonism (PIVKA) by quantitative assay is a sensitive way of evaluating vitamin K deficiency [10]. Des-gamma-carboxy prothrombin, also referred to as PIVKA-II, is often used in research studies to evaluate vitamin K status. It is secreted by tumor cells in primary hepatocellular carcinoma and is also utilized as a tumor marker [10].
- Other vitamin K deficiency states:
  - Pancreatic insufficiency-exocrine pancreatic insufficiency states such as cystic fibrosis or chronic pancreatitis are associated with fat-soluble vitamin depletion, including vitamins A, D, E, and K [11].
  - Cholestatic liver disease, including progressive familial intrahepatic cholestasis and primary biliary cirrhosis [12].

    Patients with vitamin K deficiency in cholestatic liver disease often also have deficiencies in vitamins A and E as well [12].

    Patients with vitamin K deficiency secondary to cholestatic liver disease may not respond to oral supplementation due to impaired intestinal absorption [12].

- Rare disorders of vitamin K metabolism.

  Hereditary combined deficiency of vitamin K-dependent clotting factors.

  This is a rare form of congenital bleeding with low levels of coagulation factors II, VII, IX, X, and proteins C and S [13].
- Management of deficiency and dose recommendation [4]·
  - Vitamin K deficiency: 1–2 mg of vitamin K given orally, with a maximum oral dose of 25 mg.
  - Newborn prophylaxis: 0.5 to 1 mg intramuscular injection of vitamin K.
  - Neonatal vitamin K deficiency bleeding: 1–2 mg intramuscular or intravenous vitamin K.

Toxicity of Vitamin K

- Vitamin K toxicity is rare with few reported cases in literature. Reported side effects of vitamin K administration include gastrointestinal complaints or injection site injection [14].

Future Directions

- Research regarding vitamin K, diet, and its impact on the gut microbiome with regard to health outcomes are to be evaluated [15]. Its role in systemic diseases (specifically vitamin K2) beyond hepatology is also being explored including diabetes, cardiovascular disease, bone fractures, kidney disease, immune function, and obesity [16].

References

1. Gröber U, Reichrath J, Holick MF, Kisters K. Vitamin K: an old vitamin in a new perspective. Dermatoendocrinol. 2014;6(1):e968490. https://doi.org/10.4161/19381972.2014.968490.
2. Ferland G. The discovery of vitamin K and its clinical applications. Ann Nutr Metab. 2012;61(3):213–8. https://doi.org/10.1159/000343108.

3. Mihatsch WA, Braegger C, Bronsky J, et al. Prevention of Vitamin K deficiency bleeding in newborn infants: a position paper by the ESPGHAN Committee on nutrition. J Pediatr Gastroenterol Nutr. 2016;63(1):123–9. https://doi.org/10.1097/MPG.0000000000001232.
4. Eden Rina E DSFCJM. Vitamin K deficiency. StatPearls.
5. Vitamin K: fact sheet for health professionals.
6. Imbrescia K, Moszcynski Z. Vitamin K. StatPearls.
7. Shearer MJ. Vitamin K metabolism and nutriture. Blood Rev. 1992;6(2):92–104. https://doi.org/10.1016/0268-960x(92)90011-e.
8. Hand I, Noble L, Abrams SA, Committee on Fetus and Newborn Committee on Nutrition SONB. Vitamin K and the newborn Infant. Pediatrics. 2022;149(3):e2021056036. https://doi.org/10.1542/peds.2021-056036.
9. Kher P, Verma R. Hemorrhagic disease of the newborn. StatPearls.
10. Dong L, Qiu X, Gao F, Wang K, Xu X. Protein induced by vitamin K absence or antagonisII: experience to date and future directions. Biochim Biophys Acta Rev Cancer. 2023;1878(6):189016. https://doi.org/10.1016/j.bbcan.2023.189016.
11. Estes-Doetsch H, Roberts K, Newkirk M, Parker A. Fat-soluble vitamin deficiency and exocrine pancreatic insufficiency among adults with chronic pancreatitis: Is routine monitoring necessary for all patients? Nutr Clin Pract. 2024;39(1):129–40. https://doi.org/10.1002/ncp.11082.
12. Sultana H, Komai M, Shirakawa H. The role of vitamin K in cholestatic liver disease. Nutrients. 2021;13(8) https://doi.org/10.3390/nu13082515.
13. Napolitano M, Mariani G, Lapecorella M. Hereditary combined deficiency of the vitamin K-dependent clotting factors. Orphanet J Rare Dis. 2010;5:21. https://doi.org/10.1186/1750-1172-5-21.
14. Mladěnka P, Macáková K, Kujovská Krčmová L, et al. Vitamin K – sources, physiological role, kinetics, deficiency, detection, therapeutic use, and toxicity. Nutr Rev. 2022;80(4):677–98. https://doi.org/10.1093/nutrit/nuab061.
15. Dai L, Mafra D, Shiels PG, Hackeng TM, Stenvinkel P, Schurgers LJ. Vitamin K and hallmarks of ageing: focus on diet and gut microbiome. Nutrients. 2023;15(12) https://doi.org/10.3390/nu15122727.
16. Halder M, Petsophonsakul P, Akbulut AC, et al. Vitamin K: double bonds beyond coagulation insights into differences between vitamin K1 and K2 in health and disease. Int J Mol Sci. 2019;20(4) https://doi.org/10.3390/ijms20040896.

Part VI

Medical Nutrition Therapy

35 Congenital Heart Disease: Nutritional Considerations

Rukmini Komarlu and Christina DeTallo

Background

Congenital heart disease (CHD) is one of the most common congenital disorders in newborns and a frequent cause of infant mortality. Congenital heart disease was defined by Mitchell and colleagues as a "gross structural abnormality of the heart or intrathoracic great vessels that is actually or possibly of functional significance," with an overall incidence of 8.14/1000 total births [1].

- There has however been an increasing prevalence of CHD, with Hoffman and Kaplan estimating the birth prevalence to be ~9–10/1000 live births with other studies varying from 3 to 6/1000 live births [2, 3].

R. Komarlu (✉)
Division of Pediatric Cardiology and Cardiovascular Medicine, Department of Heart, Vascular and Thoracic Cleveland Clinic, Children's Institute, Cleveland, OH, USA
e-mail: KOMARLR@ccf.org

C. DeTallo
Pediatric Nutrition Support, Department of Pediatric Gastroenterology, Hepatology, and Nutrition, Cleveland Clinic, Children's Hospital, Cleveland, OH, USA
e-mail: DETALLC@ccf.org

K. Radhakrishnan (ed.), *Handbook of Clinical and Practical Pediatric Nutrition*, https://doi.org/10.1007/978-3-031-97759-6_35

- The ACC/AHA guidelines for management of congenital heart disease classified CHD anatomy into simple, moderate, and severe complexity lesions as outlined in Table 35.1 [4].
- Moderate to severe CHD has a more consistent birth prevalence of ~1.5/1000 live births [2].
- CHD is likely multifactorial in etiology due to the interplay between genetic and environmental factors.

Table 35.1 Stratification of congenital heart disease based on complexity

Type of heart disease	Lesions
Simple	Isolated small atrial septal defect Isolated small ventricular septal defect Mild pulmonary valve stenosis
Moderate complexity	Partial anomalous pulmonary venous connection Moderate and large secundum atrial septal defect Ostium primum atrial septal defect Sinus venosus defect Moderate and large patent ductus arteriosus Atrioventricular septal defect Ebstein anomaly Straddling atrioventricular valve Congenital mitral valve disease Congenital aortic valve disease Subvalvar aortic stenosis Supravalvar aortic stenosis Sinus of Valsalva fistula/aneurysm Aorto to left ventricular fistula Coarctation of the aorta Moderate or greater pulmonary valve stenosis Moderate or greater pulmonary valve regurgitation Peripheral pulmonary stenosis Infundibular right ventricular outflow tract obstruction Ventricular septal defect with associated abnormality or moderate or greater shunt Anomalous origin of the coronary artery from pulmonary artery Anomalous aortic origin of coronary artery from the opposite sinus

(continued)

Table 35.1 (continued)

Type of heart disease	Lesions
Great complexity	Single ventricle defects Ductal-dependent systemic blood flow Hypoplastic left heart syndrome and variants Coarctation of the aorta Interrupted aortic arch Ductal-dependent pulmonary blood flow Pulmonary atresia with intact ventricular septum Tricuspid atresia with pulmonary atresia/pulmonary stenosis Tetralogy of Fallot pulmonary atresia with ventricular septal defect/Tetralogy of Fallot with multiple aortopulmonary collaterals Transposition of the great arteries Total anomalous pulmonary venous connection Truncus arteriosus Double outlet right ventricle Mitral atresia Other: isomerism, heterotaxy syndromes, crisscross heart

- Several chromosomal aneuploidies (Down syndrome, Turner syndrome, DiGeorge syndrome, Trisomy 13, Trisomy 18) contribute to 8–10% of CHD, and single gene defects account for 3–5% of cases [5].
- Advances in technology have enabled increased fetal diagnosis with approximately one-third of all cardiac malformations and 57–83% of critical CHD being detected prenatally [6, 7]. With resulting terminations in severe cases, there could be a reduction in birth prevalence of CHD.
- Similarly, advances in diagnosis and medical and surgical management have resulted in increased survival into adulthood. Depending on the defect, the mortality among patients with CHD has declined by ~50–70% with the greatest reduction for moderate and severe defects [5] (Table 35.1).

Common Cyanotic Lesions

- Single ventricle defects.
  - Ductal-dependent systemic blood flow.
    Hypoplastic left heart syndrome and variants.
    Coarctation of the aorta.
    Interrupted aortic arch.
  - Ductal-dependent pulmonary blood flow.
    Pulmonary atresia with intact ventricular septum.
    Tricuspid atresia with pulmonary atresia/pulmonary stenosis.
- Tetralogy of Fallot/double outlet right ventricle.
- Transposition of the great arteries.
- Total anomalous pulmonary venous connection.
- Truncus arteriosus.

Common Acyanotic Lesions

- Atrial septal defect +/– partial anomalous pulmonary venous return.
- Ventricular septal defect.
- Atrioventricular septal defect.
- Patent ductus arteriosus.
- Ebstein's anomaly.
- Heart failure (dilated cardiomyopathy, ALCAPA).

Management and Outcomes of Congenital Heart Disease

- Many simple isolated small atrial and ventricular septal defects resolve spontaneously and do not warrant surgical intervention.
- Patients with hemodynamically significant shunt lesions (moderate or large atrial and ventricular septal defects, atrioventricular septal defect, patent ductus arteriosus) will manifest with symptoms of pulmonary overcirculation as the pulmonary vascular resistance drops over the first 6 to 10 weeks of life.

- While the simple lesions may not warrant any intervention, surgical intervention is usually warranted in the moderate and severe complexity CHD with variable timing depending on the severity and type of lesion, accounting for ~40% of all surgical interventions in children aged <1 year [8].
- Cyanotic and greater complexity CHD usually warrants intervention in the first few months of life, with surgery ranging from complete repair to palliation.
- Surgical strategy varies among lesions (complete surgical repair in one procedure for atrioventricular septal defect vs staged repair in hypoplastic left heart syndrome) with most moderate and severe complexity lesions undergoing surgery in the first few months of life [8].
- Pre- and post-operatively, these patients may face additional complications such as infections, arrhythmias, heart failure, pulmonary hypertension, and multi-organ involvement, sometimes contributing to prolonged length of hospital stay. In one study, postoperative complications occurred in 43% of pediatric cardiac surgeries performed with and without cardiopulmonary bypass, resulting in longer mechanical ventilation and cardiac ICU and length of hospital stay [9]. Additionally patients may need hemodynamic support with Extracorporeal Membrane Oxygenator (ECMO) or Ventricular Assist Device (VAD) transiently or for extended period of time prior to either decannulation or listing for transplant with one study finding that 16% had ECMO and 7% had VAD at time of listing for transplant [10]. Outcomes of ECMO versus VAD in Children with Congenital Heart Disease as a Bridge to Transplant in Recent Era: Analysis from United Network for Organ Sharing Database [11].
- The highest-risk population is the cohort of patients with hypoplastic left heart syndrome (HLHS). These patients undergo a series of palliative procedures starting with either the Stage 1 Norwood procedure or hybrid procedure in the neonatal period, followed by the Glenn procedure commonly performed between 4 and 6 months of age.
- Interstage death occurs in 2–16% of patients with restrictive atrial septum and remains at 12% overall in the multicenter Single Ventricle Reconstruction Trial, Shunt, conduit, branch

pulmonary artery, and aortic arch stenosis, as well as tricuspid regurgitation can additionally be contributory [10, 12].
- Post-Glenn procedure, SVC syndrome, pleural effusions, arrhythmias, pulmonary hypertension, and phrenic nerve injury can contribute to prolonged length of stay [10].
- The final surgical palliation is the Fontan procedure performed between 3 and 5 years of age with postoperative pleural effusions, arrhythmias, hypoxemia, impaired systolic and diastolic ventricular function, elevated pulmonary vascular resistance, thromboembolism, and hepatic dysfunction contributing to morbidity and mortality.
- A failing Fontan patient can demonstrate plastic bronchitis and protein-losing enteropathy with potential need for heart transplant [10]. Therefore, neonates, infants, and children with CHD are prone to nutritional deficits with multifactorial cause.

Nutrition Management in Congenital Heart Disease

Nutrition Assessment and Malnutrition

Neonates and children born with CHD often require surgical intervention within the first few weeks of life.

- Although survival rates have improved, clinicians and parents are left dealing with nutritional challenges including growth faltering, malnutrition, and feeding difficulties [13]. There are risks and clinical findings impacting the nutritional status for this group that the medical team should consider when managing preoperatively and postoperatively (Table 35.2).
- Accurate nutrition assessment includes review of the above considerations, as well as the individual's feeding history, biochemical data, and visual and anthropometric evaluation.
- Despite normal birth anthropometrics for this population, neonates demonstrate nutrition challenges quickly with

Table 35.2 Clinical risks and considerations with CHD [1]

Risks	Considerations
Poor weight gain	Total caloric intake
	Tachypnea
	Metabolic demand
Feeding difficulties	Gastrointestinal health (reflux, early satiety)
	Oral-motor (poor coordination, vocal cord injury)
	Feeding intolerance
	Genetic factors
Malnutrition	Fluid limitations
	Fluid, electrolyte, and nutrient losses
	Frequency of nutrient intake disruption
	Poor perfusion (systemic, gut)
	Necrotizing enterocolitis (NEC)
Energy estimation inaccuracy	Over or underestimation with predictive equations
	Evidenced-based literature often excludes term infants or includes infants without CHD (SCCM/ASPEN; ESPNIC)

15–41% developing malnutrition in the first few months of life placing them at high risk for short-term and long-term comorbidities [14].

- Increased metabolic demand results from increased resting energy expenditure, increased cardiac output, pulmonary hypertension (PH), and increased nutrient losses including electrolytes and minerals from diuretic therapies [15].

The impact on nutritional status varies with the type of cardiac lesion.

- Malnutrition in CHD is associated with poor clinical outcomes with the most significant malnutrition occurring in conditions associated with increased pulmonary blood flow, cyanosis severity, and pulmonary hypertension [16, 17].
- Critical brain development occurs within the first 1000 days and inadequate nutritional support leads to cognitive develop-

mental delays, decreased growth potential, and decreased immune function [18].

- Ross et al. found lower length for age (HAZ) and weight for age z-scores (WAZ) were associated with increased mortality, infection, longer hospitalizations, and adverse surgical outcomes [19].
- Cyanotic heart disorders and PH lead to stunting in children whereas acyanotic heart disorders are associated with wasting [15].
- Children with cyanotic heart disorders may have higher total energy expenditure warranting higher caloric intake owing to underlying tissue hypoxia; this could be offset by their relative lack of activity [34].
- Increased morbidity and mortality are associated with HLHS and other single ventricle defect variants, as these infants undergo a series of surgical procedures and demonstrate poor weight gain interstage [20, 21].

Feeding Practices, Protocols, and Nutritional Needs

Variations in nutrition practice exist across heart centers and a lack of standardized enteral feeding practices in this population makes it difficult to study outcomes.

- There are several causes for delayed enteral nutrition and centers remain in disagreement regarding early nutritional practices.
- Concern for poor gut perfusion frequently leads to prohibited feeding approaches despite evidence indicating enteral feeding is safe and should be provided to patients with critical CHD with close monitoring [22].
- Evidence also supports that stable low-dose vasoactives, prostaglandin (PGE) infusions, and umbilical lines are not contraindications to oral and enteral feeding for these infants [23].
- Standard feeding protocols improve clinical outcomes by reducing variability, severity of NEC, time for PN therapy,

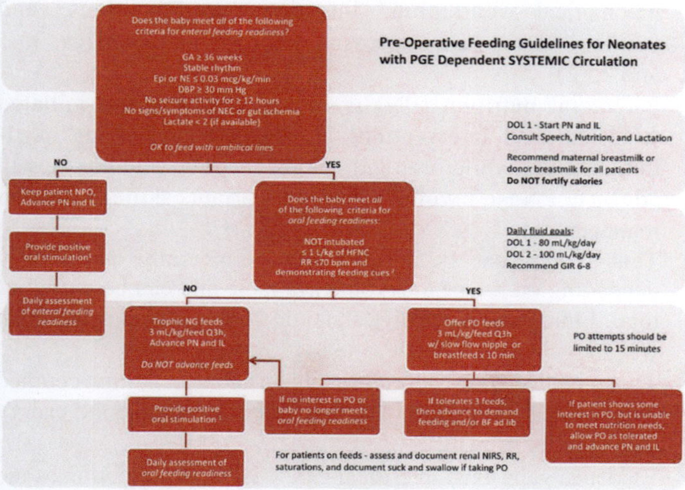

Fig. 35.1 Algorithm for ductal-dependent systemic blood flow

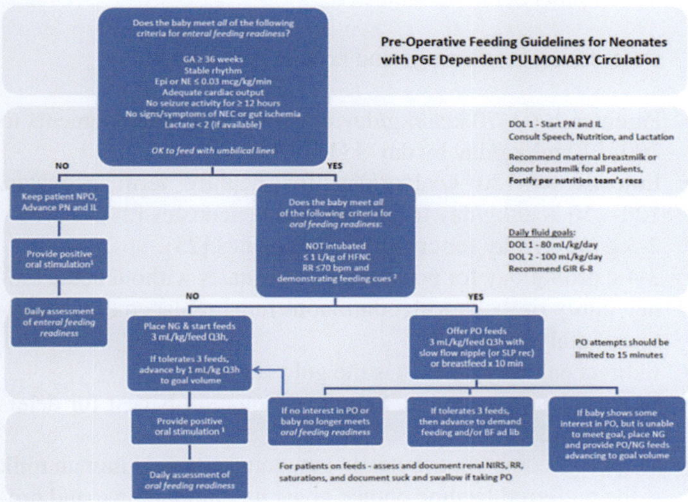

Fig. 35.2 Algorithm for ductal-dependent pulmonary blood flow

mechanical ventilation, infectious complications, and length of stay while improving anthropometrics (Figs. 35.1 and 35.2).

- Parenteral nutrition (PN) is often warranted and initiated when surgical interventions are delayed optimizing nutritional intake while oral and enteral feeding volumes slowly advance. PN isn't without risk and warrants skilled clinician management.
- This therapy can be administered peripherally or centrally depending on the venous route available and can be partial or total. Fluids and electrolytes should be calculated using birth weight.
- The imbalance between caloric intake and expenditure coupled with feeding difficulties and intolerances decrease the energy available for growth.
- Evidence gaps exist in critical care CHD representation as the 2017 SCCM/ASPEN guidelines include critically ill children, but not term infants and the 2020 ESPNIC guidelines included term infants but none with CHD.

Determination of energy and protein requirements

- Parenteral: 60–70 kcal/kg/day on day 1 with advancements to 100–120 ml/kg/day by day 3 [15].
- Enteral: 90–120 kcal/kg/day for healthy term neonates, 120–150 kcal/kg/day for postoperative neonates [24].
- 2-3 g pro/kg/day for critically ill neonates [25].
- 3-4 g pro/kg/day for postoperative neonates without acute kidney injury or those with continuous renal replacement or peritoneal dialysis [26].
- Indirect calorimetry (IC) is the gold standard [25].
- When IC isn't available, Schofield Equation is best for determination [25].
- Trophic feeding contributes to gut maturation and human milk is the preferred feeding choice given its immunologic and protective benefits [27].

- There are a variety of commercially prepared formulas also available for feeding when human or donor milk isn't available, which can be concentrated.
- Nutrient-dense feeds are a standard of practice. Breastmilk fortification or formula concentration is necessary to optimize nutritional intake when fluid intake is limited, or weight gain velocity is below expected.
- High-calorie feedings of 24, 27, or 30 calories per ounce are routinely incorporated into the daily nutrition care plan to support optimal intake to promote expected weight gain velocities. These feeding adjustments can be accomplished by reducing the standard water ratio for powder and liquid concentrate commercial formulas or by adding powdered formulas or modulars to breastmilk or formulas.
- It is important for medical providers to have up-to-date product information to prevent fortification or concentration errors which could lead to dehydration and electrolyte abnormalities.
- Initiation at and advancement by 10–20 ml/kg/day is considered safe practice.
- Implementing standard protocols for enteral initiation, advancement including the feeding choice, feeding mode, and other considerations, provides clear guidance to the bedside care team. Including members from the medical care team to develop, implement, and monitor compliance with these guidelines leads to improved outcomes [15].
- Children with CHD who cannot meet their nutritional needs orally often require feeding devices for optimal nutritional

intake due to congestive heart failure, reflux, swallowing dysfunction, and other endocrine and genetic factors.

- The inability to feed without an assistive device may be an indicator of immature feeding skills and predict developmental progress [28].
- There are several feeding methods used for those with CHD including the short-term modalities of oral and nasogastric feedings or nasoduodenal and jejunal feeding tubes. Surgically placed gastrostomy and jejunostomy feeding tubes are also options.
- Nutrient-dense feeds can be administered via continuous infusion or intermittent bolus feeding.

Nutrition Monitoring and Evaluation

- Growth measurements and weight gain velocity are associated with clinical outcomes.
- Weight for Age Z-score (WAZ), Height for Age Z-score (HAZ), and Weight for Height Z-score (WHZ) deficiencies increase the risk of mortality in CHD [15]. Postoperative measurements at 3, 6, and 12 months are predictors of cognitive and motor outcomes [29].
- Comprehensive multi-disciplinary clinics involving developmental pediatricians, registered dietitians, feeding therapists, and medical experts allow developmental assessment and evaluation providing insight into the presence and magnitude of neurodevelopmental impairment. These assessments lead to decision-making for early interventions (Table 35.3).

Table 35.3 Frequency of monitoring of anthropometric measurements

Anthropometric measurement	Frequency while hospitalized
Weight	Daily when hemodynamically stable
Length	Weekly
Head circumference	Monthly

Nutritional Management with CHD Complications

There are well-identified complications following cardiac surgeries including vocal cord injury, chylothorax, and protein-losing enteropathy. All these conditions impact nutritional intake.

- Vocal cord impairment is the result of laryngeal nerve manipulation and injury to the vagus nerve [30]. This injury leads to increased aspiration rates.
- Swallow evaluations are highly recommended to evaluate aspiration and the need for dietary modification.
- Thickened feeds may be warranted for safe oral feeding or nutrition support with tube feeding when severe impairment is detected. There are a variety of commercial thickeners available, each with specific age and weight requirements warranting collaboration with speech and language pathology, occupational therapy, and the registered dietitian for correct mixing and preparation without disruption to the nutrient balance of the feeding therapy.

Chylothorax is an accumulation of chyle within the pleural space and is prevalent (3.8%) following cardiac surgery [31].

- Injury to the thoracic duct, accessory lymphatics, or increased systemic venous pressure leads to chyle leaks which are associated with malnutrition and immune compromise [31].
- Persistent effusions and loss of fat, cholesterol, electrolytes, protein, and lymphocytes leads to increased morbidity and mortality following cardiac surgery [32].
- Dietary therapy for chylothorax management involves strict intake with a low-fat diet.
- When formula or enteral nutrition is required, specialty formulas containing minimal long-chain fat and high medium-chain fat (medium chain triglycerides - MCT) are prescribed. These therapies tend to be prescribed over a 4–6-week period but there is inconsistency across heart centers.
- Individuals following a low-fat diet for extended periods of time are at risk for essential fatty acid deficiency (EFA). Intake should include 2–4% of their total energy intake from linoleic sources with 0.25–0.5% from linolenic sources to reduce risk of EFA [30].

Protein-losing enteropathy is common after the Fontan procedure.

- This complication is characterized by the loss of proteins, particularly, albumin, through the gastrointestinal tract. These losses accumulate causing abdominal distention from ascites, malabsorption, diarrhea, and electrolyte abnormalities [13].
- Dietary management includes a high protein diet with fat intake transitioned to medium-chain fats versus long-chain fat. Similarly to chylothorax management, those individuals requiring specialized formula or enteral nutrition should receive high MCT-containing formulas (Table 35.4).

Table 35.4 Types of commercially available MCT formulas

Commercially available MCT formulas	Age Indication	Manufacturer	Ratio
Monogen	>1 year	Nutricia	93:7
Portagen	>1 year	Mead Johnson	87:13
Enfaport (infant)	<1 year	Mead Johnson	83:17
Vivonex pediatric	>1 year	Nestle	70:30
Alfamino junior	>1 year	Nestle	65:35
Pediasure peptide	>1 year	Abbott	60:40
Pediasure peptide 1.5	>1 year	Abbott	60:40
Pregestimil	<1 year	Mead Johnson	55:45
Gerber extensive HA	<1 year	Nestle	49:51
Alfamino	<1 year	Nestle	43:57
Kate farms standard 1.5	>1 year	Kate Farms	40:60
Neocate junior	>1 year	Nutricia	35:65
Alimentum	<1 year	Abbott	33:67
Elecare	<1 year	Abbott	33:67
Elecare junior	>1 year	Abbott	33:67
Neocate	<1 year	Nutricia	33:67

Nutritional Management in Heart Failure and Transplantation

As mentioned previously, malnutrition, feeding difficulties, and increased energy demand are nutrition-related complications associated with heart failure. These complications worsen through the transplant waitlist period.

- Clinical considerations when determining nutrition needs for the pediatric heart failure patient include a full understanding of the limitations with weight-based measurements. This is common practice; however, the data is misleading with inconsistent fluid status.
- Identifying an accurate dry weight is necessary for accurately assessing nutrition status [33].

- In addition, weight and BMI measures poorly represent accurate fat and muscle mass composition warranting additional anthropometric review including mid-upper arm circumference and triceps skin fold measurements [33].
- Ventricular assist device (VAD) placement improves anthropometrics compared to routine nutrition therapies alone likely due to the hemo-dynamic and neuro-hormonal improvements [33].
- In addition, studies have shown VADs improve cachexia, weight, frailty, and handgrip strength [33].
- Enteral, parenteral, and a combination of nutrition support therapies are commonly prescribed for pediatric patients with VAD placement.
- As identified above, nutrition protocols for VAD patients are recommended for improved outcomes and consistency.

Transplantation is a treatment for end-stage heart failure and requires optimized nutrition pre-transplant and post-transplant for successful graft survival.

- Nutritional requirements for children undergoing evaluation for transplantation involve dietary reference intakes for age with adjustments based on growth requirements.
- Poor nutritional status pre-transplant increases postoperative risk and complication including poor wound healing, prolonged hospitalization, and increased risk for infection [30].
- Nutritional lab surveillance is helpful to identify nutrient adequacy and deficiencies for nutrition prescription.
- Oral supplementation in addition to planned meals offers additional calories and protein optimizing nutritional intake.
- For those requiring nutrition support, standard formulas are appropriate and can be administered as intermittent bolus feeds or overnight supplementing the individual's overall nutritional intake.
- PN therapy is also an option for those who demonstrate malnutrition despite adequate oral/enteral nutrition support.

References

1. Mitchell SC, Korones SB, Berendes HW. Congenital heart disease in 56,109 births. Incidence and natural history. Circulation. 1971;43(3):323–32. https://doi.org/10.1161/01.cir.43.3.323. PMID: 5102136
2. Hoffman JI, Kaplan S. The incidence of congenital heart disease. J Am Coll Cardiol. 2002;39(12):1890–900. https://doi.org/10.1016/s0735-1097(02)01886-7. PMID: 12084585
3. van der Linde D, Konings EE, Slager MA, Witsenburg M, Helbing WA, Takkenberg JJ, Roos-Hesselink JW. Birth prevalence of congenital heart disease worldwide: a systematic review and meta-analysis. J Am Coll Cardiol. 2011;58(21):2241–7. https://doi.org/10.1016/j.jacc.2011.08.025. PMID: 22078432
4. Stout KK, Daniels CJ, Aboulhosn JA, Bozkurt B, Broberg CS, Colman JM, Crumb SR, Dearani JA, Fuller S, Gurvitz M, Khairy P, Landzberg MJ, Saidi A, Valente AM, Van Hare GF. 2018 AHA/ACC guideline for the management of adults with congenital heart disease: executive summary: a report of the American College of Cardiology/American Heart Association Task Force on Clinical Practice Guidelines. Circulation. 2019;139(14):e637–97. https://doi.org/10.1161/CIR.0000000000000602. Erratum in: Circulation. 2019 Apr 2;139(14): e831-e832. doi: 10.1161/CIR.0000000000000684. PMID: 30586768
5. van der Bom T, Zomer AC, Zwinderman AH, Meijboom FJ, Bouma BJ, Mulder BJ. The changing epidemiology of congenital heart disease. Nat Rev Cardiol. 2011;8(1):50–60. https://doi.org/10.1038/nrcardio.2010.166. Epub 2010 Nov 2. PMID: 21045784
6. Tegnander E, Williams W, Johansen OJ, Blaas HG, Eik-Nes SH. Prenatal detection of heart defects in a non-selected population of 30,149 fetuses–detection rates and outcome. Ultrasound Obstet Gynecol. 2006;27(3):252–65. https://doi.org/10.1002/uog.2710. PMID: 16456842
7. Tomek V, Marek J, Jičínská H, Škovránek J. Fetal cardiology in the Czech Republic: current management of prenatally diagnosed congenital heart diseases and arrhythmias. Physiol Res. 2009;58(Suppl 2):S159–66. https://doi.org/10.33549/physiolres.931912. PMID: 20131933
8. Damkjær M, Garne E, Loane M, Urhoj SK, Ballardini E, Cavero-Carbonell C, Coi A, García-Villodre L, Given J, Gissler M, Heino A, Jordan S, Limb E, Neville AJ, Pierini A, Rissmann A, Tan J, Scanlon I, Morris JK. Timing of cardiac surgical interventions and postoperative mortality in children with severe congenital heart defects across Europe: data from the EUROlinkCAT study. J Am Heart Assoc. 2023;12(24):e029871. https://doi.org/10.1161/JAHA.122.029871. Epub 2023 Dec 18. Erratum in: J Am Heart Assoc. 2024 Mar 19;13(6):e027766. doi: 10.1161/JAHA.122.027766. PMID: 38108249; PMCID: PMC10863769
9. Agarwal HS, Wolfram KB, Saville BR, Donahue BS, Bichell DP. Postoperative complications and association with outcomes in pedi-

atric cardiac surgery. J Thorac Cardiovasc Surg. 2014;148(2):609–16.e1. https://doi.org/10.1016/j.jtcvs.2013.10.031. Epub 2013 Nov 23. PMID: 24280709
10. Feinstein JA, Benson DW, Dubin AM, Cohen MS, Maxey DM, Mahle WT, Pahl E, Villafañe J, Bhatt AB, Peng LF, Johnson BA, Marsden AL, Daniels CJ, Rudd NA, Caldarone CA, Mussatto KA, Morales DL, Ivy DD, Gaynor JW, Tweddell JS, Deal BJ, Furck AK, Rosenthal GL, Ohye RG, Ghanayem NS, Cheatham JP, Tworetzky W, Martin GR. Hypoplastic left heart syndrome: current considerations and expectations. J Am Coll Cardiol. 2012;59(1 Suppl):S1–42. https://doi.org/10.1016/j.jacc.2011.09.022. Erratum in: J Am Coll Cardiol. 2012 Jan 31;59(5):544. PMID: 22192720; PMCID: PMC6110391
11. Trivedi J et al. Outcomes of ECMO versus VAD in Children with Congenital Heart Disease as a Bridge to Transplant in Recent Era: Analysis from United Network for Organ Sharing Database. J Heart Lung Transplant. 40(4):S8–9.
12. Ghanayem NS, Allen KR, Tabbutt S, Atz AM, Clabby ML, Cooper DS, Eghtesady P, Frommelt PC, Gruber PJ, Hill KD, Kaltman JR, Laussen PC, Lewis AB, Lurito KJ, Minich LL, Ohye RG, Schonbeck JV, Schwartz SM, Singh RK, Goldberg CS; Pediatric Heart Network Investigators. Interstage mortality after the Norwood procedure: Results of the multicenter Single Ventricle Reconstruction trial. J Thorac Cardiovasc Surg. 2012;144(4):896-906. https://doi.org/10.1016/j.jtcvs.2012.05.020. Epub 2012 Jul 11. PMID: 22795436; PMCID: PMC3985484.
13. Sullivan E, Irving S, Srinivasan V, Ravishankar C, editors. The A.S.P.E.N. pediatric and neonatal nutrition support handbook. 3rd ed. Silver Springs: American Society for Parenteral and Enteral Nutrition; 2024. p. 257–68.
14. Martini S, Beghetti I, Annunziata M, et al. Enteral nutrition in term infants with congenital heart disease: knowledge gaps and future directions to improve clinical practice. Nutrients. 2021;13(3):932.
15. Luca A, Miron I, Mindru D, et al. Optimizing nutrition parameters for neonates and infants with congenital heart disease. Nutrients. 2022:1–11.
16. Toole B, Toole L, Kyle U, et al. Perioperative nutritional support and malnutrition in infants and children with congenital heart disease. Congenit Heart Dis. 2014;9(1):15–25.
17. Wong J, Cheifetz I, Nakao M, et al. Nutrition support for children undergoing congenital heart surgeries: a narrative review. World J Pediatr Congenit Heart Surg. 2015;6(3):443–54.
18. Georgieff M, Ramel S, Cusick S. Nutritional influences on brain development. Acta Paediatr. 2018;107(8):1310–21.
19. Ross F, Radman M, Jacobs M, et al. Associations between anthropometric indices and outcomes of congenital heart operations in infants and young children: an analysis of data from the Society of Thoracic Surgeons Database. Am Heart J. 2020;224:85–97.
20. Slicker J, Sables-Baus S, Lambert L, et al. Perioperative feeding approaches in single ventricle infants: a survey of 46 centers. Congenit Heart Dis. 2016;11:707–15.

21. Menon S, McCandless R, Mack G, et al. Clinical outcomes and resource use for infants with hypoplastic left heart syndrome during bidirectional Glenn: summary from the Joint Council for Congenital Heart Disease National Cardiology Quality Collaborative registry. Pediatr Cardiol. 2013;34:143–8.
22. Shine A, Foyle L, Gentles E, et al. Growth and nutritional intake of infants with univentricular circulation. J Pediatr. 2021;237:79–82.
23. Sagiv E, Tjoeng Y, Davis M, et al. Assessing the association between pre-operative feeding and the development of oral feeding skills in infants with single ventricle heart disease: an analysis of the NPC-QIC dataset. Pediatr Cardiol. 2022;43(5):1141–55.
24. Mills KI, Kim JH, Fogg K, et al. Nutritional considerations for the neonate with congenital heart disease. Pediatrics. 2022;150(2):1–20.
25. Mehta N, Skillman H, Irving S, et al. Guidelines for the provision and assessment of nutrition support therapy in the pediatric critically Ill patient: Society of Critical Care Medicine and American Society for Parenteral and Enteral Nutrition. Pediatr Crit Care Med. 2017;18(7):675–715.
26. Owens J, Musa N. Nutrition support after neonatal surgery. Nutr Clin Pract. 2009;24(2):242–9.
27. Cognata A, Kataria-Hale J, Giffiths P, et al. Human milk use in the preoperative period is associated with a lower risk for necrotizing enterocolitis in neonates with complex congenital heart disease. J Pediatr. 2019;215:11–6.
28. Medoff-Cooper B, Irving S, Hanlon A, et al. The association among feeding mode, growth, and developmental outcomes in infants with complex congenital heart disease at 6 and 12 months of age. J Pediatr. 2016;169:154–9.
29. Holst, L, Serrano, F, Shekerdemian, L, et al. Impact of feeding mode on neurodevelopmental outcome in infants and children with congenital heart disease.
30. Antino J, Freudenberg M, Chawla A, editors. The A.S.P.E.N. pediatric nutrition support care curriculum. 2nd ed. Silver Springs: American Society for Parenteral and Enteral Nutrition; 2015. p. 337–50.
31. Lion R, Winder M, Amirnovin R, et al. Development of consensus recommendations for the management of post-operative chylothorax in paediatric CHD. Cardiol Young. 2022;32:1202–9.
32. Raatz A, Schober M, Zant R, et al. Risk factors for chylothorax and persistent serous effusions after congenital heart surgery. Eur J Cardiothorac Surg. 2019;56:1162–9.
33. Horsly M, Pathak S, Morales D, et al. Nutritional outcomes of patients with pediatric and congenital heart disease requiring ventricular assist devices. JPEN. 2022;46(7):1553–8.
34. Leitch CA, Karn CA, Peppard RJ, Granger D, Liechty EA, Ensing GJ, Denne SC. Increased energy expenditure in infants with cyanotic congenital heart disease. J Pediatr. 1998;133(6):755–60. https://doi.org/10.1016/s0022-3476(98)70146-5. PMID: 9842039

Diabetes in Children: Nutritional Considerations

36

Sumana Narasimhan
and Jennifer Hyland

The most common cause of diabetes in pediatric age group (< 18 years of age) is Type 1 diabetes (US Incidence 1 in 400) [1]. Type 2 diabetes is now increasingly prevalent in youth [2]. It is important to know the accepted diagnostic criteria for diabetes. Fingerstick glucose measurements cannot be used to diagnose diabetes and must be confirmed by plasma glucose measurement.

S. Narasimhan (✉)
Cleveland Clinic Lerner College of Medicine, Case Western Reserve University, Cleveland, OH, USA

Section of Pediatric Endocrinology, Cleveland Clinic Children's Hospital, Cleveland, OH, USA
e-mail: NARASIS@ccf.org

J. Hyland
Pediatric Nutrition Support , Division of Pediatric Gastroenterology, Hepatology and Nutrition, Cleveland Clinic Children's Hospital, Cleveland, OH, USA
e-mail: HYLANDJ2@ccf.org

K. Radhakrishnan (ed.), *Handbook of Clinical and Practical Pediatric Nutrition*, https://doi.org/10.1007/978-3-031-97759-6_36

Diagnostic Criteria for Diabetes [3]

A1C ≥6.5% (≥48 mmol/mol).

OR

Fasting plasma glucose ≥126 mg/dL (≥7.0 mmol/L)*.

OR

Oral glucose tolerance test: 2-h plasma glucose ≥200 mg/dL (≥11.1 mmol/L) using glucose load.

OR

In an individual with classic symptoms of hyperglycemia or hyperglycemic crisis, a random plasma glucose ≥200 mg/dL (≥11.1 mmol/L). Random is any time of the day without regard to time since previous meal.

* Fasting is defined as no caloric intake for at least 8 h.*.

**To convert mg/dl to mmol/l, divide the mg/dl value by 18 (Table 36.1).

Table 36.1 Etiology of diabetes in children

		Comments
Beta cell destruction		
Immune mediated	Type 1 diabetes	Insulin deficiency
Insulin resistance	Type 2 diabetes	
Drug induced	Glucocorticoids	Insulin resistance
	L-asparaginase	
	Vacor Beta blockers	
	Cyclosporine, sirolimus	
	Diazoxide	
Diseases of exocrine pancreas		
	Cystic fibrosis-related diabetes	
	Abdominal trauma	
	Chronic pancreatitis	
	Ionizing radiation	
Infections		
	Congenital rubella	
	Cytomegalovirus	
Other diseases associated with diabetes		
	Cushings	
	Pheochromocytoma	
	Endocrine tumors	

Types of Diabetes

- Type 1 diabetes (T1D) is characterized by destruction of beta cells, usually caused by an autoimmune process, resulting in loss of endogenous insulin production.
- Type 2 diabetes (T2D) is characterized by insulin resistance and lack of adequate insulin response.
- Diabetes can also present due to genetic mutations. Neonatal diabetes can result from any of >20 different genetic mutations. MODY is the abbreviation for monogenic diabetes (aka maturity onset diabetes of the Young), caused by various mutations in genes involved in glucose sensing or beta cell function (Table 36.2).

Table 36.2 Genetic causes of diabetes

Genetic defects of beta cell function		
MODY 1	Chromosome 20	HNF 4A
MODY 2	Chromosome 7	Glucokinase
MODY 3	Chromosome 12	HNF 1A
MODY 4	Chromosome 13	IPF-1
MODY 5	Chromosome 17	HNF-1beta
MODY 6	Chromosome 2q32	Neuro-D1/beta2
MODY 7–14		
Mitochondrial DNA mutations		
	Pearson syndrome Kearns Sayre	
Wolfram syndrome	DIDMOAD (Chromosome 4p)	WFS-1
Neonatal diabetes		
	Transient	KCNJ11, ABCC8, INS, HNF1beta
	Permanent	Agenesis of pancreas Glucokinase deficiency Homozygous KCNJ11 ABCC8

(continued)

Table 36.2 (continued)

Genetic defects of beta cell function		
Genetic defects of insulin action		
	Rabson-Mendenhall	
	Leprechaunism	
	Type A insulin resistance	
Genetic syndromes		
Prader Willi syndrome	Chromosome 15	
Down syndrome	Chromosome 21	
Klinefelter syndrome	XXY	

- Diabetes can also be secondary to medications (transient: thiazides, corticosteroids, isoniazid, theophylline, nalidixic acid or permanent: streptozotocin, alloxan, rodenticide vacor).
- Destruction of pancreas as in chronic pancreatitis, rare cases of abdominal trauma, radiation damage, or after surgical removal of the pancreas can also lead to development of diabetes.

Type 1 Diabetes

Stages of Type 1 Diabetes [4]

- Type 1A diabetes (T1D) results from decreased insulin secretion due to autoimmune destruction of beta cells in pancreatic islets of Langerhans. Circulating autoantibodies to pancreatic islet antigens are detectable long before the onset of symptoms. Autoantibodies commonly found in T1D are glutamic acid decarboxylase antibody (GAD-65), tyrosine phosphatase-like protein (IA-2), Insulin autoantibody (IAA), and Zinc transporter antibody (ZnT8).
- Children may be euglycemic for many months while autoantibodies destroy the beta cells (Stage 1 diabetes).
- Glucose intolerance may be detectable on oral glucose tolerance test before symptoms appear (Stage 2 diabetes) but this is

rarely detected as patients are still asymptomatic despite ongoing beta cell destruction.
- Symptoms typically present when beta cell function is reduced by 80% (Stage 3 diabetes) [4].

Clinical Presentation of T1D
- Progressive loss of beta cell function leads to hyperglycemia, glucosuria, and osmotic diuresis, resulting in polyuria, polydipsia, and nocturnal enuresis.
- Lack of Insulin triggers lipolysis, leading to ketones as a byproduct of fatty acid breakdown.
- Weight loss and ketonemia ensue; if insulin deficiency goes untreated, the child may present with classic signs of diabetic ketoacidosis: vomiting, abdominal pain, Kussmaul breathing, hyperglycemia, ketonemia, dehydration, and metabolic acidosis.

Laboratory Evaluation in Diabetes
- Venous glucose level > 126 mg/dl (fasting) or > 200 mg/dl (random/ 2 h post-oral glucose load) is diagnostic of diabetes.
- HbA1C > 6.5% is supportive of but not a diagnostic criterion in children and adolescents, as HbA1C can be variable (Table 36.3).
- Diagnostic criteria for diabetes were described earlier in the chapter.
- Glucose in urine can also be supportive of the diagnosis of T1D, although glucosuria can be seen in other conditions such as stress or renal glucosuria.
- Autoantibodies, as previously described, are positive in approximately 90% of patients with T1D, confirming the autoimmune etiology of T1D.
- Autoantibodies may be positive in up to 10% of patients with Type 2 diabetes [5].

Table 36.3 HbA1C and average blood glucose

A1C (%)	Estimated average glucose (mg/dl)	Estimated average glucose (mmol/l)
< 5.7	<117	6.5
5.7–6.4	117–137	6.5–7.6
6.5	140	7.8
7.0	154	8.6
7.5	169	9.4
8.0	183	10.1
8.5	197	10.9
9.0	212	11.8
9.5	226	12.6
10	240	13.4

Management of Type 1 Diabetes

- The cornerstones of management of T1D in children are-.
  - Subcutaneous insulin dosing based on blood glucose measurement and.
  - Accurate carbohydrate counting.
- It is important to have a "whole family" approach to a child with T1D, involving parents as well as extended family and childcare providers in the education process. The social history and activities of the child before, during, and after school will also impact diabetes management. At diagnosis, a coordinated team approach involving diabetes educator, nutritionist, and pediatric endocrinologist, with input from pediatric psychology (if available) can help the family and child adjust to this new life-altering diagnosis.
- Diabetes education at time of diagnosis focuses on "survival skills": the mechanics of blood glucose checking, carbohydrate counting (covered in section on nutrition), calculation and administration of Insulin, recognition, and treatment of hypoglycemia and "sick day" management for intercurrent illness to recognize early symptoms of diabetic ketoacidosis.

Nutrition management of Type 1 and Type 2 diabetes is covered in the latter part of this chapter.

- Self-monitoring of blood glucose level (SMBG) is essential to the management of diabetes and must be performed at least before meals/snacks and at bedtime.
- Glucometers have evolved to use minimal amounts of blood, using lancets that are more comfortable than in years past.
- Glucometers are less accurate in the extremes of blood glucose measurement and can also be affected by technical issues such as inadequate blood volume on strip, expired strip, presence of sugar on the finger, hematocrit of the patient, poor perfusion, high triglyceride level, medications such as acetaminophen [6] and ambient conditions such as extremes of temperature and high altitude.
- The recent evolution and refinement in continuous glucose monitoring (CGM) has revolutionized the management of diabetes by providing painless, real time glucose levels for the user (see section on technology).

Insulin Therapy

Therapy with insulin is key to managing diabetes.

Multiple daily injection (MDI) regimens most commonly involve a long-acting (basal) insulin analog such as Insulin Glargine along with short-acting (bolus) insulin analogs to cover carbohydrates at mealtimes or correct high blood glucose levels. The total daily dose is calculated based on the child's age and can vary between 0.2 units/kg/day in very young children to 1–1.2 Units/kg/day in adolescents.

The dose of long-acting insulin (Glargine/ Detemir) is 50% of the total daily dose and is administered once a day via subcutaneous injection. The current long-acting analogs (Glargine/Detemir) are "peakless" and provide a stable level of Insulin in the body for approximately 24 h; newer analogs such as Degludec can last for up to 36 h. Long-acting Insulin is administered at the same time every day.

At mealtimes, the family is instructed to count carbohydrates (in grams) to calculate the insulin dose. Mealtime coverage for carbohydrates consumed (food bolus) is calculated using "carbohydrate ratio." The "carb ratio" is estimated by dividing the number 500 by the total daily dose of insulin. The "carb ratio" may vary depending on time of day (nighttime vs daytime meals) or type of meal (different carb ratios for meals vs snacks). The "food bolus" dose is calculated by dividing the carbohydrates consumed by the "carb ratio."

The dose of short-acting insulin also depends on the blood glucose level (by fingerstick/CGM) checked prior to the meal. This is referred to as "Correction factor or Insulin Sensitivity Factor (ISF)" and is typically calculated by dividing the number 1800 by total daily dose of insulin. The dose of insulin to "correct" the blood glucose to target (correction bolus) is calculated as follows: Actual blood glucose minus Target blood glucose divided by ISF.

The dose for food bolus is added to the dose for correction bolus to calculate the total dose of short acting insulin. It is best to take insulin for a meal 15 min prior to eating.

Diabetes Technology

The past decade has seen great advances in diabetes technology

- Blood glucose monitoring: Blood glucose monitors are now more advanced with greater accuracy, requiring a smaller volume of blood for testing. Some monitors have "smart" features that link with apps to help monitor trends to help with diabetes management.
- Continuous glucose monitors (CGM): Most CGM systems involve the temporary insertion of a tiny sensor in the subcutaneous tissue that communicates the glucose reading from the interstitial tissue to a reader device or an app on a smartphone. A detailed discussion of CGM systems is beyond the scope of this chapter. The reader is directed to the websites of various manufacturers of CGM systems for details of each brand.
- Insulin Pens and "smart Insulin pens": Insulin pens have made it easier to administer insulin, obviating the need to carry vials and syringes. Smart Insulin pens may have features that help

with dosing as well as recording doses to help improve compliance with diabetes management.
- Insulin pumps have come a long way since they were first introduced in 1974 as a large bedside device. Most Insulin pumps use one type of Insulin (short-acting Insulin, Lispro/ Aspart) delivered via a needle/ cannula that stays in the subcutaneous tissue and delivers insulin at a preset rate. Modern pumps offer "closed loop" systems, where the CGM communicates with the pump that adjusts the rate of insulin delivery based on the blood glucose and the carbohydrate grams entered by the user.

The reader is also referred to website of the American Diabetes Association (www.diabetes.org).

Treatment of Type 2 Diabetes (T2D)

T2D in youth is managed by diet and exercise combined with medications. **Nutrition management is covered in the chapter's latter part and Chapter on Obesity (Chap. 37).**

Medications Used to Manage T2D
- Metformin reduces gluconeogenesis and reduces insulin resistance. Metformin is the initial choice for youth with T2D in youth who are metabolically stable or asymptomatic. Glucagon-like-peptide-1 (GLP-1) agonists are efficacious in reducing body weight as well as lowering HbA1C in children with T2D [8]. These medications may be considered if glycemic goals are no longer met with metformin and lifestyle change. Sodium-glucose cotransporter 2 (SGLT2) inhibitors work by increasing the amount of glucose excreted in urine, thus lowering blood glucose levels. Empagliflozin and Dapagliflozin are approved for children with T2D 10 years and older in combination with metformin, diet and exercise. Non-insulin therapies should be maximized before re-initiating or intensifying insulin therapy in established patients with diabetes who are not meeting glycemic goals.

Insulin in T2D

- Subcutaneous insulin is the initial treatment of choice along with metformin for youth with T2D who present with marked hyperglycemia (Blood glucose >250 mg/dl (> 13.9 mmol/L) or HbA1C > 8.5% (>/= 69 mmol/mol) without ketosis and who are symptomatic at diagnosis. Insulin dose can be tapered over 2–6 weeks if glucose goals are met in patients. Intravenous insulin may be required to correct ketosis and/or ketoacidosis in some children with Type 2 diabetes who present with acute metabolic decompensation. Once acidosis is resolved, metformin therapy may be initiated.

Adverse Events in Diabetes

Hypoglycemia

- Blood glucose level < 70 mg/dl can manifest as fast heartbeat, anxiety, sweating, irritability, and hunger. If untreated, blood glucose can fall further and lead to neuroglycopenic symptoms such as dizziness, headache, and even seizures.
- Children and youth with diabetes can develop hypoglycemia that can be caused by carbohydrate/insulin mismatch, after physical activity, acute illness with poor oral intake, or from consumption of alcohol. The American Diabetes Association recommends the "rule of 15" (15 g fast-acting glucose by mouth, recheck in 15 min) for mild to moderate hypoglycemia where the patient is awake and able to take by mouth.
- For severe hypoglycemia/seizure, the use of glucagon (Intramuscular injection of 0.5–1 mg or intranasal glucagon) is recommended.

Hyperglycemia

- Blood glucose levels above 250 mg/dl can manifest as increased thirst, increased urination, headache, blurry vision, dry mouth, and be caused by inadequate insulin dosing, missed insulin dose, acute illness, medications (steroids) or sometimes as a response to exercise.

- It is important to recognize the cause of high blood glucose and check for development of ketones by urine or blood ketone measurement.
- Treatment of hyperglycemia usually requires extra insulin dose for correction and fluids to help correct dehydration from osmotic diuresis.

Diabetic Ketoacidosis (DKA)

- DKA is a serious condition of hyperglycemia, ketosis, and metabolic acidosis that can occur due to absolute or relative insulin deficiency.
- DKA can occur in youth with Type as well as Type 2 diabetes. Insulin deficiency leads to hyperglycemia (blood glucose > 200 mg/dl) and lipolysis that leads to ketonemia (serum beta-hydroxybutyrate>3 mmol/L) and ketonuria; dehydration and metabolic acidosis (Venous pH < 7.3 or bicarb <15 mmol/L).
- A full discussion of DKA and its management are beyond the scope of this chapter.
- The management of DKA in children includes judicious use of fluids, as excess fluid boluses can precipitate cerebral edema. Intravenous insulin (1 unit/kg/hr) along with fluids gradually corrects metabolic acidosis and reduces ketonemia.
- Concurrent electrolyte imbalances need to be corrected appropriately; hypokalemia can occur once insulin infusion is initiated, hypophosphatemia, hypocalcemia, and acute kidney injury (AKI) can also complicate the picture.
- Frequent neurologic checks are necessary to monitor for cerebral edema.
- Once DKA is resolved, the child can be transitioned to subcutaneous insulin, allowed to eat, and switched to a diabetes plan suitable for homegoing.

Hyperglycemic Hyperosmolar State (HHS)

- HHS is a serious complication that can occur in patients with Type 2 diabetes, characterized by profound hyperglycemia (blood glucose > 600 mg/dl), glycosuria, hyperosmolarity (serum osmolarity >320 mmol/L), prerenal azotemia and absence of ketosis or acidosis.

- The patient may present with altered mental status due to hyperosmolarity.
- Treatment involves careful hydration with isotonic fluids and electrolyte in ICU setting, while maintaining serum glucose around 250–300 mg/dl to avoid rapid changes in serum osmolarity.

Nutrition Assessment in Pediatric Diabetes [7]

- Nutrition assessment is essential for all patients with diabetes. Patients with newly diagnosed Type 1 diabetes will likely present with weight loss due to the body's inability to get glucose into the cells and convert to energy. The body breaks down fat and muscle for energy, contributing to rapid weight loss. Weight should return to baseline with insulin initiation.
- Energy needs: Energy needs for pediatric patients with Type 1 diabetes are similar to the energy needs of children and adolescents of the same age without diabetes.
- Energy needs for pediatric patients with Type 2 diabetes are similar to the energy needs of children who are overweight or obese.
- Protein Needs: Protein needs are calculated according to the dietary reference intake (DRI).

Principles of Nutrition Management in Pediatric Diabetes

- Provide individualized medical nutrition therapy as an essential component of the overall treatment plan.
- Recommend a cardioprotective dietary pattern, within the total energy requirement to maintain normal growth and development.
- No ideal distribution of macronutrients for diabetes nutrition therapy has been identified, therefore use of the Dietary Reference Intakes is routinely recommended45–65% of calories coming from carbohydrate-containing foods.

Carbohydrates are an important source of fiber, vitamins, and minerals and should not be removed or restricted from the diet of a growing child or teenager. Instead, the family should be taught how to manage intake appropriately (Table 36.4).

Goals of nutrition therapy for patients with prediabetes and diabetes [10].

Table 36.4 Nutrition management in diabetes [7, 9]

Type 1 diabetes	Type 2 diabetes
Educate families on carbohydrate counting for insulin to carbohydrate ratio specific to patient Provide guidelines for how to integrate meal patterns and insulin therapy with an individual's food and physical activity preferences Do not typically limit carbohydrate intake for children Promote intake from whole grains, fruits, and dairy products Carbohydrate-free foods are not unlimited, portion sizes should be monitored Meal composition impacts postprandial glucose patterns. Education on the impact of high fat and high protein meals and adjustment of insulin is recommended Recommend limit/avoid sugar-sweetened beverages to avoid glucose spikes Review strategies for the prevention of dyslipidemia, cardiovascular disease, hypertension and nephropathy	Youth with overweight/obesity and type 2 diabetes should be provided with developmentally and culturally appropriate lifestyle programs that are integrated with diabetes management, with a goal to achieve a 7–10% decrease in excess weight If patient is started on mealtime insulin therapy, provide education on full carbohydrate counting similar to Type 1 patients If not on insulin, educate on role of carbohydrates in blood glucose management, and provide further education on general healthy eating patterns (USDA myplate.gov, Mediterranean diet, or any meal pattern suitable to patient and lifestyle) Attention to total energy intake is important, as excessive energy intake may lead to weight gain even if glycemic control is achieved; while inadequate energy intake can also lead to complications and nutrient deficiencies. Lifestyle modifications should be based on chronic care model Recommend avoid sugar-sweetened beverages to reduce the risk of further weight gain and metabolic conditions Weight loss maybe recommended, depending on patient's age (see *** chapter for obesity guidelines

- Emphasize selecting non-starchy vegetables and lean protein options.
- Emphasize choosing, when selected, quality carbohydrate foods.
- Focus on starchy vegetables, legumes, peas and lentils, whole grains, fruits, and milk.
- Minimize added sugars and refined grains and associated foods.
- Choose whole and minimally processed foods.
- Minimize added saturated fat and added sodium.
- Emphasize choosing foods to support dietary fiber requirements.

Carbohydrate Counting

- Most children with Type 1 diabetes use carbohydrate counting as a method of estimating carbohydrates consumed to dose rapid-acting mealtime insulin.
- Carbohydrate counting allows individuals to have a flexible eating pattern, and administer insulin based on the total amount of carbohydrates eaten at each meal and snack.

Goals for the Registered Dietitian

- Educate families on carbohydrate vs noncarbohydrate foods.
- Teach families to read food labels. Attention to serving size and total carbohydrates.
- Teach families to use measuring cups and food scales.
- Identify reliable websites and phone applications for carbohydrate counting (Tables 36.5 and 36.6).

Table 36.5 Carbohydrate needs [7]

Average carbohydrate recommendations per meal for optimal growth and development			
Gender	Age < 5 years	Age 5–12 years	Teens
Girls	30–45 g	45–60 g	45–75 g
Boys	30–45 g	45–60 g	45–75+ g

Carbohydrate amounts must be individualized based on energy needs and activity levels

Table 36.6 Nutrient impact on blood glucose levels

Protein	Studies have found that a high protein intake (>75 g alone) can significantly impact blood glucose levels hours after eating. The American Diabetes Association recommends people who take mealtime insulin take additional insulin for high-protein meals. Intake of >75 g is unlikely in a pediatric patient; therefore, it is rare that protein needs to be accounted while counting carbohydrates. Recommendations should be individualized. https://www.diabetes.org
Fat	Studies have found that meals with a high-fat content led to a delayed and prolonged increase in blood glucose levels, from 2 to 6 h after the meal. An additive effect takes place when consuming high-fat and high-protein meals together. As of the print of this textbook, further studies are needed to formulate appropriate recommendations for accounting for this postprandial effect[18]. Patients with Type 1 diabetes can work closely with their medical team on potential strategies to limit this extended postprandial rise with high-fat meals.
Fiber	Dietary fiber is not completely digested and absorbed; therefore, it does not cause the blood glucose levels to rise in the same way that other carbohydrates do. It is important to educate families on the role of fiber in the diet and recommend consumption of fiber-containing foods at all meals; however, we do not routinely recommend counting carbohydrates any differently for those foods that are higher in fiber. The term "net carbs" does not have a legal definition and is not used by the Food and Drug Administration or recognized by American Diabetes Association. Once a family is more well established in diabetes care, a trial of adjusting for fiber can be attempted. However, results are seen on an individualized basis, as this is not a routine recommendation by the American Diabetes Association. It is important to monitor blood glucose trends to see if this method is beneficial. Ref: https://www.diabetes.org
Artificial sweeteners	There is insufficient evidence about non-nutritive sweeteners affecting hemoglobin A1C, fasting glucose levels or insulin levels. It is important to inform families that "sugar free" does not always mean "carbohydrate free." These foods are not necessarily lower in carbohydrate than the original version of the food [11].

Poor Weight Gain with Type 1 Diabetes

- If a patient with Type 1 diabetes is not exhibiting appropriate weight gain, recommend increasing calories, while continuing to use carbohydrate counting to manage diabetes while optimizing insulin therapy.
- It is often beneficial to increase unsaturated fatty acids in the diet.
- If patient requires a nutrition supplement recommend a low glucose-containing product (Boost Glucose Control, Glucerna).

Diabetes Away from Home

School/Daycare

- Children spend a large amount of time in daycare/ school. Hence it is extremely important to develop a "school plan" for diabetes care so that the child can safely attend school.
- School plans typically include the details of the child's insulin plan, frequency of blood glucose monitoring and guidelines on management of hypoglycemia, emergency contacts, and phone number for physician.
- It is important for the physician, family, and school nurse to work together to provide a safe, effective diabetes management plan. (The family should be made aware of laws that protect children with diabetes (Ref: https://diabetes.org/advocacy/safe-at-school-state-laws).

College

- Transitioning to college is a big step for youth with diabetes and this can be accomplished by gradually allowing the adolescent to manage his/her diabetes, schedule appointments, manage prescriptions and supplies prior to the final step of matriculating to college and dorm life.
- Resources such as the College Diabetes Network https://www.collegediabetesnetwork.org/ have local chapters in various universities to help young people navigate college and be successful while controlling their diabetes.

Sports [9]

- It is important to maintain physical activity in children with T1D and T2D, as exercise positively affects insulin sensitivity, physical fitness, weight management, social interaction, and mood.
- Recommended goal for physical activity is 60 minutes daily, with vigorous muscle-strengthening and bone-strengthening activities at least 3 days per week.
- For children with T1D, it is important to closely monitor blood glucose levels before, during, and after exercise and plan for carbohydrate intake prior to and during exercise if required. Insulin doses may need to be adjusted in anticipation of and following exercise [12].
- Patients and their parents should be educated on goals and management of glycemia before, during, and after activity; based on their individualized patterns and level of activity.
  - If blood glucose is <100 mg/dL before a workout, recommend consumption of 15 grams of carbohydrate, without insulin coverage, for every 30–60 minutes of physical activity.
  - Children may require more carbohydrates with higher intensity activities, and activities of longer duration. This should be assessed through analyzing glucose trends.
  - The prevention and treatment of hypoglycemia associated with physical activity includes decreasing the prandial insulin for the meal/snack before exercise and/or increasing food intake. Patients with insulin pumps may choose to lower their basal rate during activity.

Telehealth and Diabetes

- Modern technology allows for telehealth that increases access, saves time, and improves patient satisfaction in pediatric T1D [12].
- Telehealth for diabetes offers a great way to optimize glycemic control when alternated with in-person visits. Diabetes tech-

nology allows for uploading CGM and pump data to cloud based applications that the treating physician can use to adjust insulin doses and management tailored to the patient's needs.

Surveillance for Diabetes Complications

- The goal for diabetes management is to maintain glycemic targets and prevent diabetes-related complications by timely screening, early detection, and treatment [9].
- Glycemic control is monitored by Hemoglobin A1C, glycosylated Hb or "Time in Range." The HbA1C goal for youth with T1D is <7.5% and T2D is <7%.
- Monitoring for autoimmune conditions such as Celiac disease and autoimmune thyroid disease is recommended for youth with T1D. Celiac disease affects the diet of a child with T1D, hence close follow-up with nutritionist is essential.
- Youth with diabetes should be monitored periodically for microvascular complications (retinopathy, nephropathy, and neuropathy) and undergo cardiovascular risk screening for hypertension and dyslipidemia. The rate of development of these complications is higher in youth with T2D [13].

Advocacy and Diabetes

- Diabetes is a challenging disease that demands a lot from the child and their family. It is important for children and youth with diabetes to have the legal protections that allow them to safely attend day-care, school, participate in sports, and work. Organizations such as the American Diabetes Association https://www.diabetes.org have published numerous advocacy statements that are important tools in helping educate schools, daycare providers, and employers and provide a framework to help policymakers pass laws to protect people with chronic illnesses such as diabetes. Parents of children with diabetes should be made aware of 504 plans (based on Section 504,

Rehabilitation Act of 1973) that outline accommodations that a school must provide for a child with diabetes.

- The Americans with Disabilities Act (ADA) protects people with diabetes as people with disabilities and is an important law for the workplace to prevent discrimination against people with diabetes.

References

1. National Diabetes Statistics Report, May 2024. https://www.cdc.gov/diabetes/php/data-research/index.html
2. Wagenknecht LE, Lawrence JM, Isom S, et al. Trends in incidence of youth-onset type 1 and type 2 diabetes in the USA, 2002-18: results from the population-based SEARCH for Diabetes in Youth study. Lancet Diabetes Endocrinol. 2023;11(4):242–50. https://doi.org/10.1016/S2213-8587(23)00025-6.
3. American Diabetes Association Professional Practice C.2. Diagnosis and classification of diabetes: standards of care in diabetes-2024. Diabetes Care. 2024;47(Suppl 1):S20–42. https://doi.org/10.2337/dc24-S002.
4. Insel RA, Dunne JL, Atkinson MA, et al. Staging presymptomatic type 1 diabetes: a scientific statement of JDRF, the Endocrine Society, and the American Diabetes Association. Diabetes Care. 2015;38(10):1964–74. https://doi.org/10.2337/dc15-1419.
5. Klingensmith GJ, Pyle L, Arslanian S, et al. The presence of GAD and IA-2 antibodies in youth with a type 2 diabetes phenotype: results from the TODAY study. Diabetes Care. 2010;33(9):1970–5. https://doi.org/10.2337/dc10-0373.
6. Maahs DM, DeSalvo D, Pyle L, et al. Effect of acetaminophen on CGM glucose in an outpatient setting. Diabetes Care. 2015;38(10):e158–9. https://doi.org/10.2337/dc15-1096.
7. American Dietetic Association. Pediatric nutrition care manual®. Diabetes Mellitus. https://www.nutritioncaremanual.org/
8. Chadda KR, Cheng TS, Ong KK. GLP-1 agonists for obesity and type 2 diabetes in children: Systematic review and meta-analysis. Obes Rev. 2021;22(6):e13177. https://doi.org/10.1111/obr.13177.
9. American Diabetes Association Professional Practice. C.14. Children and adolescents: standards of care in diabetes-2024. Diabetes Care. 2024;47(Suppl 1):S258–81. https://doi.org/10.2337/dc24-S014.
10. Evert AB, Dennison M, Gardner CD, et al. Nutrition therapy for adults with diabetes or prediabetes: a consensus report. Diabetes Care. 2019;42(5):731–54. https://doi.org/10.2337/dci19-0014.

11. Lohner S, Kuellenberg de Gaudry D, Toews I, Ferenci T, Meerpohl JJ. Non-nutritive sweeteners for diabetes mellitus. Cochrane Database Syst Rev. 2020;5(5):CD012885. https://doi.org/10.1002/14651858.CD012885.pub2.
12. Fogel JL, Raymond JK. Implementing telehealth in pediatric type 1 diabetes mellitus. Pediatr Clin N Am. 2020;67(4):661–4. https://doi.org/10.1016/j.pcl.2020.04.009.
13. TODAY Study Group, Bjornstad P, Drews KL, et al. Long-term complications in youth-onset type 2 diabetes. N Engl J Med. 2021;385(5):416–26. https://doi.org/10.1056/NEJMoa2100165.

Pediatric Obesity

37

Roy Kim and Evelyn Benden

Obesity is a condition of excessive body fat that poses a health risk [1]. For children, obesity is defined as having a body mass index (BMI) at or above the 95th percentile for age and sex. Approximately one in five U.S. children and adolescents have obesity [2].

Obesity severity can be expressed as BMI percentage of the 95%ile for age and sex (Table 37.1).

Extended BMI-for-Age Growth Charts for children and adolescents can be used to monitor children with a BMI up to 60 kg/m^2 [3].

R. Kim (✉)
Section for Pediatric Endocrinology, Cleveland Clinic Children's Hospital, Cleveland, OH, USA
e-mail: KIMR@ccf.org

E. Benden
Cleveland Clinic, Cleveland, OH, USA

Pediatric Nutrition Support, Division of Pediatric Gastroenterology, Hepatology, and Nutrition, Cleveland Clinic Children's Hospital, Cleveland, OH, USA
e-mail: BENDENE@ccf.org

K. Radhakrishnan (ed.), *Handbook of Clinical and Practical Pediatric Nutrition*, https://doi.org/10.1007/978-3-031-97759-6_37

Table 37.1 Classification of overweight and obesity in children

Classification	BMI for age
Overweight	85-94th%ile
Obesity	≥95th%ile
Class I obesity	At 100% of the 95th%ile to <120% of the 95th%ile
Class II obesity	120% to <140% of the 95th percentile
Class III obesity	≥140% of the 95th percentile

Etiology

Obesity is a complex disorder that is multifactorial in etiology. Table 37.2 highlights known risk factors for pediatric obesity.

Comorbidities and Medical Complications Caused by Obesity

- Dyslipidemia/hypercholesterolemia
- Hypertension
- Prediabetes or Type 2 diabetes mellitus
- Metabolic dysfunction associated fatty liver disease (MAFLD) and nonalcoholic steatohepatitis (NASH)
- Obstructive sleep apnea
- Polycystic ovarian syndrome
- Orthopedic comorbidities (slipped capital femoral epiphysis, Blount's disease)
- Idiopathic intracranial hypertension
- Depression
- Cancer

Table 37.2 Childhood obesity risk factors: [4]

Policy	Marketing of unhealthy foods Underserved communities, communities of lower socioeconomic status Children in families that have immigrated Food insecurity
Community	School environment (quality of meal programs, vending machine offerings, proximity to convenience stores) Lack of access to fresh food Fast food restaurants Limited access to safe locations for physical activity Environmental health/chemical exposure
Family/home environment	Parenting feeding styles and home environment (routines, limit setting, etc.) Sugar-sweetened beverages Larger portion sizes Consumption of ultra-processed foods Frequency of eating outside the home Screen time and increased sedentary behavior Sleep duration Environmental smoke exposure Psychosocial stress/adverse childhood experiences
Individual level	*Genetic factors*: Prader–Willi syndrome, Bardet Biedl syndrome, leptin deficiency, MC4R mutation, other monogenic and syndromic conditions *Prenatal risk factors*: Parental obesity, maternal weight gain, gestational diabetes, maternal smoking, placental insufficiency *Postnatal risk factors*: Low or high birth weight, early breastfeeding cessation, and formula feeding, earlier start of complementary feeding, rapid weight gain during infancy/early childhood, early use of antibiotics *Childhood risk factors*: Endocrine disorders, children with developmental/physical disabilities or special healthcare needs impacting nutrition or physical activity (ex. autism spectrum disorder, myelomeningocele, ADHD), appetitive traits such as eating quickly or eating in absence of hunger, medication use, altered microbiome

Clinical Assessment of Childhood Obesity

- History: age of onset of obesity, diet history, food acceptance, hyperphagia, developmental milestones.
- Medications: steroids, antipsychotics, paroxetine, valproic acid, insulin, others.
- Physical Exam: Vital signs, tonsil size, thyroid, cardiorespiratory systems, skin: acanthosis nigricans; Short stature: may suggest an endocrine or genetic cause.
- Lab values to assess
  - Lipid Panel
  - HgbA1C and fasting glucose
  - Liver function tests (ALT/AST)
  - Complete metabolic panel
  - Full vitamin profile for patients being considered for bariatric surgery
  - Genetic and endocrine testing if suggestive features

How Is Pediatric Obesity Treated?

Children with obesity should receive intensive health behavior and lifestyle treatment (IHBLT) that is child-focused, family-centered, longitudinal, and coordinated through a child's medical home. Programs that reach 26 contact hours are more effective, but shorter programs are also beneficial. Treatment should include nutrition counseling and promote increased physical activity [4].

The treatment team may include:

- Medical: Primary Care Physician, Pediatrician/Nurse Practitioner, Nurse, Physician Subspecialists and Surgeons
- Nutrition: Registered Dietitian Nutritionist (Table 37.3)
- Physical Therapist or Exercise Physiologist
- Psychosocial: Psychologist, Social Worker

Table 37.3 Nutrition management approaches to pediatric obesity

Diet plan [5]	General Features *	Appropriate Candidates	Other considerations
General healthy eating plan	Avoid skipping meals and set meal/snack schedule Limit grazing and choose healthy snacks Education on MyPlate, balanced meals, and age-appropriate portion sizes Increasing fruit/vegetable intake Increasing protein intake/adding protein source to meals and snacks Decrease or eliminate sugar-sweetened beverages Increase home-prepared meals (limit fast food/restaurants) Vitamin/mineral supplementation based on intake/labs	Initial treatment for all ages	
Low carbohydrate or low glycemic load	Controls total carbohydrates (carbs) and/or glycemic load Limits intake of added sugars, refined grains, and starchy vegetables Encourages carbohydrate intake to be fruits, whole grains, legumes, dairy and non-starchy vegetables	Tanner stage 5 or patients with MAFLD, insulin resistance, PCOS, or metabolic syndrome;	Amount of weight loss not shown to be superior to low fat diet [10]
Partial liquid/meal replacement	Low calorie, adequate/high protein 2–3 meal replacements such as shake/bar with <250 calories and > 10 grams of protein Supplement each meal replacement with a fruit/veg and add 1 balanced meal per day	Tanner stage 5 BMI >97%ile Strong family support; ability to purchase meal replacements	Useful to achieve early weight reduction however effects wane over time [11]

(continued)

Table 37.3 (continued)

Diet plan [5]	General Features *	Appropriate Candidates	Other considerations
Protein-sparing modified fast [9]	Very low calorie and very low carbohydrate Induces fat burning and ketosis Not nutritionally complete; requires supplementation of minerals and daily multivitamin Requires medical monitoring, daily ketone checks, frequent lab tests	Tanner stage 5 BMI >97%ile Strong family support Ability to adhere to stringent plan	Refeeding phase requires monitoring, limited data on long-term benefits
Mediterranean [7]	Increased whole grains, fruits, vegetables, nuts, legumes, oily fish, healthy fats Lower processed foods, red meat, added sugars	Insulin resistance Dyslipidemia Metabolic syndrome	Provides more metabolic benefit than weight loss benefit
DASH (dietary approaches to stop hypertension) [8]	Promotes fruits, vegetables and whole grains Includes low-fat dairy, fish, poultry, beans and nuts Focuses on reducing sodium, saturated fat and sweets	High blood pressure High cholesterol	
Time-limited eating	Minimal studies available in youth Limiting daily intake to certain time frame (usually 8–12 h)	May decrease late-night eating behaviors	Limited data on efficacy and safety

[a]Nutrition interventions should be part of a *multidisciplinary team approach*. Treatment will also require environmental, behavioral, and medical interventions. There are limited long-term data on nutritional approaches to childhood obesity. Most trials are limited to 3–12 months. Lifestyle interventions can lower BMI z-score by 0.2, an amount sufficient to improve obesity-related comorbidities. Due to the chronicity and relapsing nature of obesity, sustaining these benefits requires longitudinal care

General Weight Loss Goals

Children 2–5 years
BMI percentile
85–94%ile maintain weight until BMI <85%ile or slowed weight gain
≥ 95%ile maintain weight until BMI <85%ile or slowed weight gain
Weight loss ≤1 lb./month loss recommended if BMI >21 kg/m2
Children 6–11 years
BMI percentile
85–94%ile maintain weight until BMI <85%ile or slowed weight gain
95–98%ile maintain weight until BMI <85%ile or weight loss ~1 lb./month
> 99%ile weight loss ~2lbs/month
Children 12–18 years
BMI percentile
85–94%ile maintain weight until BMI <85%ile or slowed weight gain
≥ 95%ile weight loss ≤2 lbs./week

[a]To be used as a general guideline. Specific weight loss goals should be individualized for each patient

Medical and Surgical Management

Sleep: Inadequate sleep is associated with increased appetite, weight gain, and insulin resistance. Therefore, ensuring adequate restful sleep each night is important for the treatment of obesity. This should include evaluation and treatment for obstructive sleep apnea or other sleep disorders.

Behavioral Health Assessment: Children with obesity are more likely to have depression and anxiety. They may be bullied or teased or have low self-image due to social media messaging or stigmatizing experiences in the healthcare system. Disordered eating behaviors may be present. Evaluation by a psychologist or licensed counselor is essential for comprehensive care.

Physical Activity: At least one hour per day of active moderate to vigorous physical activity is recommended for all children over age 5 years.

Pharmacotherapy and Bariatric Surgery: Adolescents (12 years and older) with obesity should be offered weight loss pharmacotherapy as an adjunct to health behavior and lifestyle treatment (Table 37.4). Teens (13 years and older) with severe obesity, should be evaluated for metabolic and bariatric surgery [4, 6].

Table 37.4 Pharmacologic treatments

	Benefit	Side effects	Comments
GLP1RA (liraglutide, semaglutide) [12, 13]	6–16% decrease in BMI	GI side effects are common; nausea, vomiting, dizziness	Age 12y+; given by daily or weekly subcutaneous injection; initiate with low dose to lower risk of side effects
Orlistat	Modest weight reduction	Diarrhea, soiling, vitamin deficiency	Age 12y+; inhibits fat absorption; patients should take fat-soluble vitamin supplement; available over the counter
Phentermine/topiramate extended release [14]	8–10% decrease in BMI	Topiramate: Kidney stones, acidosis, birth defects, cognitive slowing	Age 12y+; females should be on contraceptive; should be weaned off
Phentermine	Amount weight loss varies	Can increase heart rate and blood pressure, other cardiovascular effects, dry mouth	Age 17y+; controlled substance; requires frequent monitoring

Monitoring and supplements are needed after bariatric surgery to prevent vitamin deficiencies and refeeding syndrome.

References

1. World Health Organization. Obesity. World Health Organization. Published 2024. https://www.who.int/health-topics/obesity#tab=tab_1.

2. Centers for Disease Control and Prevention. Childhood Obesity Facts. Obesity. Published April 2, 2024. https://www.cdc.gov/obesity/php/data-research/childhood-obesity-facts.html.
3. Reference Population | Overview CDC Growth Charts | Growth Chart Training | Nutrition | DNPAO | CDC. www.cdc.gov. Published January 23, 2019. https://www.cdc.gov/nccdphp/dnpao/growthcharts/training/overview/page4.html
4. Hampl SE, Hassink SG, Skinner AC, et al. Clinical practice guideline for the evaluation and treatment of children and adolescents with obesity. Pediatrics. 2023;151(2) https://doi.org/10.1542/peds.2022-060640.
5. Kirk S, Ogata B, Wichert E, Handu D, Rozga M. Treatment of pediatric overweight and obesity: position of the academy of nutrition and dietetics based on an umbrella review of systematic reviews. Journal of the academy of Nutr Diet 2022;122(4). doi:https://doi.org/10.1016/j.jand.2022.01.008, 848.
6. National Institute of Diabetes and Digestive and Kidney Diseases. Helping your child who is overweight | NIDDK. National Institute of Diabetes and Digestive and Kidney Diseases Published March 22, 2019. https://www.niddk.nih.gov/health-information/weight-management/helping-your-child-who-is-overweight.
7. Muscogiuri G, Verde L, Sulu C, et al. Mediterranean diet and obesity-related disorders: what is the evidence? Curr Obes Rep. 2022;11 https://doi.org/10.1007/s13679-022-00481-1.
8. National Heart, Lung, and Blood Institute. DASH eating plan. Nih.gov. Published December 29, 2021. https://www.nhlbi.nih.gov/education/dash-eating-plan.
9. Zhong Y, Chen X, Huang C, et al. The effects of a low carbohydrate diet combined with partial meal replacement on obese individuals. Nutrition & Metabolism. 2023;20(1):18. https://doi.org/10.1186/s12986-023-00740-5.
10. Mirza NM, et al. Effects of a low glycemic load or a low-fat dietary intervention on body weight in obese Hispanic American children and adolescents: a randomized controlled trial. Am J Clin Nutr. 2013;97:276.
11. Berkowitz RI, et al. Obesity. 2011;19:1193–9. https://doi.org/10.1038/oby.2010.288.
12. Kelly AS, et al. A randomized, controlled trial of Liraglutide for adolescents with obesity. N Engl J Med. 2020;382:2117–28. https://doi.org/10.1056/NEJMoa1916038.
13. Weghuber et al Once-weekly Semaglutide in adolescents with obesity N Engl J Med 2022; DOI:https://doi.org/10.1056/NEJMoa2208601
14. Kelly AS, et al. Phentermine/topiramate for the treatment of adolescent obesity. NEJM Evidence. 2022;1:6. https://doi.org/10.1056/EVIDoa2200014.

Nutrition and Inflammatory Bowel Disease

38

Diana Schnee, Maria Haught,
Jacob A. Kurowski, and Sandra C. Kim

Background

Inflammatory bowel diseases (IBD) are chronic, relapsing, and remitting inflammatory diseases affecting the gastrointestinal tract and can also involve other organ systems. There are three major categories of IBD: Crohn's disease (CD), ulcerative colitis (UC), and IBD unclassified (IBD-U); however, it can be difficult to utilize these three classifications at times given that IBD can be heterogeneous. Up to 25% of all patients living with IBD are diagnosed in childhood, imposing a lifelong chronic disease with a significant impact on a child's nutritional status,

D. Schnee · M. Haught
Pediatric Nutrition Support, Pediatric Gastroenterology, Hepatology, and Nutrition, Children's Institute, Cleveland Clinic Children's Hospital, Cleveland, OH, USA
e-mail: SCHNEED2@ccf.org; HAUGHTM4@ccf.org

J. A. Kurowski
Pediatric Inflammatory Bowel Diseases, Division of Pediatric Gastroenterology, Hepatology & Nutrition, Cleveland Clinic Children's Hospital, Cleveland Clinic, Cleveland, OH, USA

S. C. Kim (✉)
Division of Pediatric Gastroenterology, Hepatology and Nutrition, Cleveland Clinic Children's Hospital, Cleveland, OH, USA
e-mail: KIMS23@ccf.org

K. Radhakrishnan (ed.), *Handbook of Clinical and Practical Pediatric Nutrition*, https://doi.org/10.1007/978-3-031-97759-6_38

and as a result, growth, and bone health. To date, over three hundred genetic polymorphisms have been identified as risk factors for the development of IBD. Furthermore, many patients in childhood present with a colitis-predominant phenotype and go on to develop small bowel CD later in life. While there is no single, accepted diagnostic criteria for IBD, it is widely recognized that histologic chronicity is an absolute requirement for the diagnosis.

Crohn's Disease

- **Crohn's disease (CD)** is characterized by the presence of chronic intestinal inflammation identified in any location from the mouth to the anus, often in a patchy distribution.
- CD is classified by the location and phenotypical behavior of the disease. Up to 90% of patients will have terminal ileal involvement at some point in their disease course and may include the colon and proximal small intestine.
- CD is a transmural, full-thickness inflammatory process that can lead to fibrosis in some patients, along with stricturing and/or internal penetrating disease phenotypes when patients develop more complicated disease.
- Early and effective control of inflammation is particularly important to reduce the risk of disease progression to these complication forms of CD that often result in significant complications, including obstruction, abscesses, perforation, and surgery.
- While the rectum is often spared in CD patients with colitis, up to 30% of patients will develop perianal disease (fistulas, inflamed tags, structuring) which, are particularly difficult complications to treat.
- A considerable proportion of prepubertal patients (over a third of all patients based on existing studies) with CD will have impairments in growth and malnutrition.

Ulcerative Colitis

- **Ulcerative colitis (UC)** involves the surface epithelium and submucosa without transmural inflammation of the colon. It is, however, recognized that fibrosis may still develop.
- In UC, inflammation typically starts in the rectum and evolves proximally with locations classified as either proctitis, proctosigmoiditis, left-sided colitis, or extensive/pancolitis. Isolated right-sided colitis is less common and often associated with primary sclerosing cholangitis (PSC).
- Macroscopically, the disease is confluent and lacks deep ulcerations that are often seen in CD.
- Malnutrition may result from anorexia and significant gastrointestinal losses with fluid imbalances, as opposed to the significant malabsorption noted in CD malabsorption given the small intestine is not involved. Furthermore, growth failure is noted in less than 10% of UC patients and should raise suspicion for CD if the nutrition and growth impairments do not match what would be expected.

IBD-Unclassified

- IBD-U is a designation for patients with chronic inflammation in the colon that cannot be classified into UC or CD due to an uncharacteristic pattern of colitis or question of small intestine involvement either in the proximal or distal small intestines.
- Less than 10% of patients carry a designation of IBD-U, historically referred to as indeterminate colitis, and many will be reclassified as the disease declares itself over time. If a patient with IBD-U has growth failure that cannot be attributed to another cause, a diagnosis of CD may be highly suspected.

Nutrition and IBD

- Nutrition plays a vital role in the treatment of both patients with both active disease/inflammation and those with disease in remission (where it is helpful to decrease the likelihood of future disease exacerbations). This highlights the importance of nutritional screening at the time of diagnosis and as part of routine health maintenance on a semiannual basis. Malnutrition in IBD results from malabsorption, decreased enteral intake, and increased metabolic demand with a subsequent catabolic state. Nutritional failure and growth failure are both also markers of disease activity and they are endpoints in treatment targets [1, 2].
- Patients with CD are particularly at risk for malnutrition due to small intestinal inflammation which can impact oral intake. Furthermore, there are caloric deficits due to inflammation-induced catabolic state and intestinal tract losses from malabsorption.
- In severe to extensive UC, there is significant protein loss (reflected in serum albumin) which may also result in malnutrition though typically less severe than noted in patients with severe CD.
- Early assessment by a dietitian with expertise in pediatric gastroenterology and IBD is critical to appropriately characterize the degree of malnutrition and implement a plan that will facilitate healing.
- Nutritional failure in IBD is defined as weight percentile changed lower by two isobars, weight loss ≥10% or weight < 3rd % for age.
- Growth failure is defined as height percentile changed lower by two isobars, height velocity < 3rd %, or height percentile <3rd % for age.
- Enteral interventions to treat malnutrition are always preferential to parenteral nutrition except when enteral is contraindicated at the discretion of the treating physician.
- Nutritional interventions for patients with active CD include either exclusive enteral nutrition (EEN) or partial enteral nutri-

tion (PEN) when clinically indicated. EEN is defined as 90–100% medically complete formula with the 0–10% regular (typically lower residue solids) diet. Formula can be polymeric rather than a hydrolyzed or elemental formula.

- EEN utilization leads to similar/better outcomes to corticosteroids, in patients with mild-moderate inflammatory Crohn's disease (especially small intestinal). EEN is associated with induction of clinical remission, normalization of inflammatory markers, improved quality of life, and avoiding the side effects of steroids. Induction is given for 8–12 weeks with the possibility of continuing longer as part of maintenance therapy based on tolerance and response.
- EEN also may be of particular benefit in the preoperative state for nutritional rehabilitation and is associated with improved surgical outcomes compared to total parenteral nutrition or no nutrition interventions [5, 6].
- PEN can be given as part of induction therapy with the Crohn's disease exclusion diet (CDED) or alone as adjuvant therapy to prednisone or biologic also has significant benefits in improving nutritional status and inflammation [3, 4]. PEN is defined as anything less than 90% of calories from formula.
- For long-term maintenance of remission, no diet has shown to have superior efficacy to current biologics.
- However, diets high in fiber and low in ultra-processed foods with particular emphasis on the Mediterranean diet have been shown to reduce the risk of disease exacerbations and improve long-term outcomes in IBD [7]. Intake of ultra-processed foods may also increase the risk of development of CD [8].

Diet and Dietary Interventions IN IBD

This section of the chapter will review the practical clinical aspect of implementing dietary interventions and other nutritional considerations:

Healthy Eating/Mediterranean Diet

Used as an adjunct therapy and recommended long term to support remission for both Crohn's Disease and Ulcerative Colitis.

Overall Themes

- Avoid/minimize: Processed food/added sugars, red meat, convenience foods/fast food [1].
- Focus on: Whole foods including produce, legumes, whole grains, lean meats, fish, nuts, and healthy fats (avocado, olive oil) [1].
- Diet often includes the Mediterranean diet or a whole foods diet (Table 38.1).

Some patients may identify trigger foods that aggravate their IBD (often seeds, simple sugars, spicy food, caffeine, and acidic food) which they should continue to avoid.

Caution with soluble fiber intake is primarily warranted in the presence of strictures, intestinal narrowing, or general intolerance in the case of a flare. Fiber does play a key role in intestinal mucosal healing and should be gradually introduced as tolerated [2].

During an Exacerbation

- Limit fiber with strictures or intestinal narrowing (allow canned fruits with no skins, well-cooked vegetables).
- Focus on protein for healing and to fight inflammation.
- No concentrated sweets including candy, juice, sugar, and high fructose corn syrups.
- Small, frequent meals.
- Drink adequate fluids and chew food thoroughly.
- No caffeine or alcohol.
- Possible lactose intolerance.
- Use nutritionally complete medical formula as needed to sustain weight/nutritional status.

Table 38.1 Mediterranean diet/real foods diet

Summary	Use of whole foods to support a healthy gut microbiome, reduce symptoms, and support remission.
Foods allowed	Fresh fruits/vegetables, lean protein, healthy fats. Limiting red meat. When in remission: Nuts, seeds, legumes, potatoes with skin, whole grains
Foods to avoid	Greasy/fatty foods, acidic foods, lactose, emulsifiers, proceed foods, added sugars/sugar alcohols. During flare: Lactose, nuts, seeds, high fiber
Induction vs maintenance therapy	Maintenance therapy

Dietary Therapies

Induction/Maintenance Therapy

The diets discussed below are those most frequently used for induction/maintenance therapy for Crohn's Disease. Nutrition therapy is most effective in mild/moderate disease although can be considered in severe disease as an adjunct therapy [3, 4]. (Table 38.2).

Additional diets including the specific carbohydrate diet, IBD anti-inflammatory diet, the auto immune protocol, and the low-FODMAP diet have limited conclusive evidence on effectiveness for treatment of IBD. These diets may be utilized as adjunctive therapy for symptom management but are not common practice [2, 3].

- **Specific Carbohydrate Diet (SCD)** [7].
  - Diet intended to alter intestinal flora and heal the GI tract by removing fermentable carbohydrates that cause an overgrowth of bad bacteria and impair intestinal absorption.
  - Depending on GI symptoms a stepwise approach may be used to advance diet.
  - Lifelong diet if used for disease management.

Table 38.2 Nutritional therapies for inflammatory bowel disease

Exclusive enteral nutrition therapy (EEN) [5]	
Summary	Use of nutritional oral supplement drinks (polymeric, nutritionally complete) to help heal the intestinal tract and induce remission over about 8 weeks.
Foods allowed	Nutrition shakes/oral supplements to meet 90–100% of energy needs plus 0–10% of total calories from solid foods. Fluids allowed: Nutrition shakes, water, dextrose-based sports drinks (amount may be limited), broth
Foods to avoid	Most food should be avoided except the amount which is allowed while on the diet (up to 10% of total calories). Avoid high-fiber foods (whole grains, beans), and nuts/seeds in the presence of stricture. Lactose and high-fat foods may also not be tolerated.
Induction vs maintenance therapy	Typically used for induction therapy. May be used in combination with medication or as pre-operative nutritional rehabilitation. Can be used for maintenance therapy by working up to one free eating day per week, however long-term adherence is difficult.
Crohn's disease exclusion diet (CDED) [6]	
Summary	Partial enteral nutrition therapy (PEN) + CDED complaint foods. Uses nutritional oral supplement drinks (polymeric, nutritionally complete) for PEN. Removes harmful food products that negatively change gut bacteria and cause inflammation. Includes three phases: Weeks 0–6: 50% of calories from oral supplements +50% of calories from CDED compliant foods Weeks 7–12: 25% of calories from oral supplements +75% of calories from CDED compliant foods Weeks 13+ maintenance. Includes all CDED-compliant foods, 25% of calories from oral supplements 5 days/week; liberalized diet 2 days per week.

(continued)

Table 38.2 (continued)

Foods allowed	For each phase, there are mandatory foods: Chicken, eggs, potato, banana, apple. Additionally, there are allowed foods that gradually expand with each phase (portion sizes are specified). Examples: Fresh fish, white rice, rice noodles, rice flour, avocado, strawberries, melon, tomato, cucumber, carrot, fresh herbs/spices, olive oil, limited honey/sugar, herbal tea, fresh orange juice.
Foods to avoid	Processed meats, dairy, soy, milk alternatives, corn, wheat products, dried fruit, frozen vegetables, condiments, all processed/packaged snack foods
Induction vs maintenance therapy	Full plan includes induction and maintenance therapy. Can be used for induction. No fixed dietary restrictions for life (after ~9 months on diet). Limited research has been conducted on use of CDED for maintenance therapy.

- Allows for consumption of:
  - Meat, poultry, eggs, fish/shellfish without additives.
  - Some legumes include all-natural peanut butter, navy beans, lentils, and peas.
  - Most fresh/frozen/raw/cooked vegetables.
  - Most fresh/frozen/raw/cooked/dried fruits without added sugar.
  - Most nuts/nut flours.
  - Honey, dates, butter, some hard cheeses, and homemade yogurt.
- Strict avoidance of:
  - All forms of sugar except honey and dates.
  - All grains.
  - Some legumes (e.g.: chickpeas, soybeans).
  - Starchy vegetables (potatoes).
  - All milk/milk products high in lactose.
  - Most commercially prepared food due to additives.

- **Modified SCD (mSCD)** [7].
  - A modification of the SCD with some liberalization of certain carbohydrates and starches to ease the rigidity of the diet without the onset of GI symptoms.
    - Typical modifications include the addition of oats, rice, sweet potato, 100% cocoa, and pure maple syrup.
  - Patients may start with SCD and then transition to mSCD once in remission.
- **IBD Anti-Inflammatory Diet (IBD-AID)** [8–9].
  - Diet intended to balance the gut microbiome and reduce inflammation.
  - Focus on pre- and probiotic-containing foods (e.g., plain yogurt, fermented vegetables, oats, ground flax seed).
  - Avoidance of lactose, wheat, refined sugar, corn, and processed food.
  - Consists of three phases of advancing texture/fiber content of foods, which are utilized during various stages of inflammation/healing. Advancement through stages depends on symptoms.
  - Continues to focus on specific sources of carbohydrates, legumes/legume flours, fruits, vegetables, lean meats, and omega-3 fatty acids.
- **Autoimmune Protocol Diet (AIP)** [10].
  - Consists of three phases: elimination, reintroduction, maintenance.
  - Mimics a Paleolithic diet with the focus on non-processed meats/poultry, fish, eggs, fruits in moderation, and specific vegetables (no nightshades).
- **Semi-vegetarian Diet** [11].
  - Focuses on consumption of whole foods, eggs, yogurt, produce, legumes, brown rice, pickled vegetables, and limited animal proteins.
  - May be helpful in preventing relapse of Crohn's disease although this has not been well evaluated in children.
- **Low FODMAP Diet** [3].
  - See Chap. 52 for more information on dietary components.
  - May be helpful with symptom resolution but has not been found to have an impact on disease state.

- Some patients may have a component of irritable bowel syndrome (IBS) associated with IBD, despite optimal disease control. They may benefit from FODMAP diet.

Other Nutrition Considerations in IBD Management

Estimated Energy/Protein Needs

- Energy needs increase during a flare especially in the setting of weight loss/malnutrition.
- Protein: during a flare, protein needs may increase to 150% of the DRI due to inflammation.
- Fluids: maintenance fluids are generally appropriate; possible increased needs based on GI output.
- If a flare or patient has large sweat loss from heat/activity, an oral rehydration solution or low-sugar beverage with electrolytes may be needed.

Nutrition Supplementation

Supplements: *not all may be warranted*

- Daily multivitamin.
- Folate (if on a 5-ASA and/or methotrexate).
- Calcium (depending on dietary intake and chronic steroid use, to optimize bone strength/development).
- Vitamin D.
- Iron.
- Zinc, magnesium if levels are low/chronic diarrhea.
- Vitamin B12 in patients with ileal Crohn's disease with/without resection.
- Omega 3 fatty acids and turmeric may be recommended to help with inflammation.

Total parenteral nutrition may be utilized in the setting of:

- Severe disease necessitating complete bowel rest.
- Poor outcomes following enteral nutrition or diet adjustments.
- Intestinal failure, bowel obstructions, inability to place tube feed.

Social/Environmental

- The elimination of "trigger" foods may lead to malnutrition, food aversions/fears, and disordered eating such as ARFID (please refer to Chap. 51 on eating disorders).
- Strongly consider patient/family buy-in when choosing a course of therapy as there are significant social and financial impacts.

Future Research in Diet and IBD

There is significant need for ongoing research in diet and IBD. With an increased demand for more natural means to manage IBD-related symptoms and for long-term treatment, patients and providers are hoping to find sustainable diet therapies. At present, many of the IBD diets, while effective, are not always feasible for families due to cost and/or commitment. Continued evaluation of the effect of certain foods on the immune system and microbiome will be an essential part on ongoing research.

References

1. Mediterranean diet for IBD—dietary options [internet]. Nutritionaltherapyforibd.org. 2021. Available from: https://www.nutritionaltherapyforibd.org/dietary-options/mediterranean-diet.
2. Hashash JG, Elkins J, Lewis JD, Binion DG. AGA clinical practice update on diet and nutritional therapies in patients with inflammatory bowel disease: expert review. Gastroenterology. 2024;166(3):521.
3. Reznikov EA, Suskind DL. Current nutritional therapies in inflammatory bowel disease: improving clinical remission rates and sustainability of

long-term dietary therapies. Nutrients [Internet]. 2023;15(3):668. Available from: https://www.ncbi.nlm.nih.gov/pmc/articles/PMC9920576/.
4. Manski S, Noverati N, Policarpo T, Rubin E, Shivashankar R. Diet and nutrition in inflammatory bowel disease: a review of the literature. Crohn's Colitis 360 [Internet]. 2023;6(1):otad077. Available from: https://www.ncbi.nlm.nih.gov/pmc/articles/PMC10782214/.
5. Critch J, Day AS, Otley A, King-Moore C, Teitelbaum JE, Shashidhar H. Use of enteral nutrition for the control of intestinal inflammation in pediatric Crohn disease. J Pediatr Gastroenterol Nutr. 2012;54(2):298–305.
6. Levine A, Wine E, Assa A, Sigall Boneh R, Shaoul R, Kori M, et al. Crohn's disease exclusion diet plus partial enteral nutrition induces sustained remission in a randomized controlled trial. Gastroenterology. 2019;157(2):440–450.e8.
7. Suskind DL. Nutrition in immune balance (NIMBAL) therapy. Nimbal Publishing; 2015.
8. Olendzki BC, Silverstein TD, Persuitte GM, Ma Y, Baldwin KR, Cave D. An anti-inflammatory diet as treatment for inflammatory bowel disease: a case series report. Nutr J. 2014;13(1):5.
9. IBD Anti-Inflammatory Diet [Internet]. University of Massachusetts Medical School. 2015. Available from: https://www.umassmed.edu/nutrition/ibd/ibdaid/.
10. Konijeti GG, Kim N, Lewis JD, Groven S, Chandrasekaran A, Grandhe S, et al. Efficacy of the autoimmune protocol diet for inflammatory bowel disease. Inflamm Bowel Dis [Internet]. 2017;23(11):2054–60. Available from: https://www.ncbi.nlm.nih.gov/pmc/articles/PMC5647120/.
11. Chiba M. Lifestyle-related disease in Crohn's disease: relapse prevention by a semi-vegetarian diet. World J Gastroenterol [Internet]. 2010;16(20):2484. Available from: https://www.ncbi.nlm.nih.gov/pmc/articles/PMC2877178/.

Failure to Thrive and Feeding Problems

39

Jessica Barry, Evelyn Benden, and Christine Bowen

Failure to Thrive

Definition

Failure to thrive (FTT), also known as faltering growth, indicates insufficient weight gain or absence of appropriate physical growth in children [1].

Diagnosis

Relies on plotting of weight and height/length on the appropriate growth chart (WHO for birth to 24 months, CDC for 2 to 20 years). WHO and CDC growth charts are sex- and age-specific (corrected age if born prematurely).

J. Barry (✉) · E. Benden · C. Bowen
Division of Pediatric Gastroenterology, Hepatology, & Nutrition, Cleveland Clinic Children's, Cleveland, OH, USA
e-mail: BARRYJ4@ccf.org; BENDENE@ccf.org; BOWENC@ccf.org

K. Radhakrishnan (ed.), *Handbook of Clinical and Practical Pediatric Nutrition*, https://doi.org/10.1007/978-3-031-97759-6_39

Acceptable criteria for diagnosing FTT [2]:

- Weight-for-length <5th%ile
- BMI/age <5th%ile
- Weight for age dropping by at least 2 major percentiles on a growth chart after having previously achieved a stable growth pattern.

Etiology

The evaluation of FTT can be approached in an organized manner to help determine the underlying etiology. Asking six questions below can provide good insight into the different causes of FTT. These questions provide a practical approach to FTT.

1. Insufficient calorie intake: this is by far the most common cause of FTT. This may be due to poor access to food, improper feeding choices or poor desire to eat, poor mixing of formula, and occasionally, emotional neglect.
2. Difficulty with swallowing: It is important to recognize that the causes leading to swallow dysfunction can be varied; anatomic as in cleft palate and lip, behavioral (as in children with sensory issues as in autism), neurologic (as in children with cerebral palsy and neuromuscular disorders with swallowing dysfunction/risk of aspiration).
3. Increased gastric losses: from emesis—i.e., in children with severe gastroesophageal reflux disorder seen with neuromuscular disorders as in cerebral palsy, or pyloric stenosis.
4. Pancreatic/biliary malabsorption: This would be seen in children with exocrine pancreatic insufficiency (for example cystic fibrosis), or hepatobiliary disorders leading to poor bile acid secretion and fat malabsorption.
5. Mucosal/intestinal disorders leading to increased losses and insufficient absorption of provided calories, (diarrhea (autoimmune enteropathies, inflammatory, infectious, enzyme deficiencies)), emesis (obstructive/anatomical, infectious).

6. Metabolic:
   (a) Increased metabolic needs for calorie consumption (increased cardiac demand (i.e., congenital or acquired), pulmonary (i.e., chronic illness, cystic fibrosis), chronic illness, malignancy, or competition for calories from gastrointestinal (GI) parasitic infections).
   (b) Metabolic Disorders leading to poor generation of energy-mitochondrial disorders or congenital disorders of glycosylation
   (c) Renal disorders leading to acidosis—seen in end-stage renal disorders or renal tubular acidosis

Answer to one or more of the questions above can contribute to failure to thrive in an individual patient. For example, an infant with congenital heart disease like a ventricular septal defect in congestive heart failure will have increased energy needs from increased cardiac work, increased work of breathing, but also from poor oral intake secondary to increased respiratory efforts.

An evaluation pertaining to these most commonly considered etiologies will allow the provider to plan imaging and or laboratory assessment to ensure all aspects are considered and evaluated. Once areas are excluded or ruled in, this will allow for planning and management to optimize nutritional rehabilitation for the patient.

It is important to continue to evaluate response to nutritional interventions including but not limited to follow-up laboratory assessments when indicated.

Treatment

Nutrition interventions:

- Increased caloric intake via nutrient-rich foods
- Increased caloric intake via oral supplementation/high-calorie fluid
- Structured meal and snack schedule

Medical Interventions: A few examples

1. Appetite stimulants:
   (a) Cyproheptadine: stimulates appetite, increases gastric fundic accommodation, thus leading to increased caloric intake
   (b) Other options like Megesterol, Dronabinol, etc. may be used in unique situations, like post-chemotherapy anorexia. The practitioner will need to familiarize themselves with these medications and their potential side effects.
2. Discontinuation of stimulants, i.e., (ADHD medications) which may lessen appetite and thus decrease caloric intake.
3. Anti-emetics: Zofran may be used to counteract nausea symptoms and enhance oral intake where pertinent, i.e., consider in patients on medications increasing nausea symptoms such as chemotherapeutics.

Feeding Disorders

Pediatric Feeding Disorder

ICD Codes—Published in 2022 ICD-10-CM

R63.31 Pediatric feeding disorder, acute
R63.32 Pediatric feeding disorder, chronic

Definition

Pediatric Feeding Disorder (PFD) is defined as impaired oral intake that is not age-appropriate and is associated with medical, nutritional, feeding skill, and/or psychosocial dysfunction [3].

Pediatric feeding disorders are commonly associated with:

- Autism
- Other developmental disabilities (cerebral palsy, down syndrome, etc.)
- Prematurity

- Delayed oral motor skills
- Medical conditions (ex. GI disorders, food allergies, cardiac disorders, pulmonary disease)
- Malnutrition

  A child with a feeding disorder may have some degree of malnutrition. However, a diagnosis of malnutrition is not required for a child to be diagnosed with a pediatric feeding disorder. Refer to nutrition assessment section (Chap. 2) for more information on malnutrition.

Possible Signs of a Pediatric Feeding Disorder:

- Coughing, choking, labored breathing with eating or drinking.
- Crying, arching, grimacing with eating or drinking.
- Oral motor/oral sensory concerns-
- Dysphagia, drooling, gagging, spitting/vomiting, difficulty chewing, pocketing food in checks, overstuffing mouth, preference for certain texture.
- Delayed feeding skill development-
- Prolonged use of bottle, use of inappropriate utensils/feeding tools, or drinking system.
- Need for oral formula supplement or enteral nutrition (usually NG-Tube or G-Tube).
- Inadequate or excessive consumption of a particular food group/nutrient.
- Excessively long or short mealtimes or grazing on food throughout the day.
- Requires distraction, bribes/rewards, or threats to eat.
- Disruptive mealtime behaviors.
- Child and/or caregiver stress with eating/mealtimes.

Avoidant Restrictive Food Intake Disorder (ARFID)

Diagnostic and Statistical Manual of Mental Disorders, Fifth Edition

F50.82 Avoidant-restrictive food intake disorder

Definition

Avoidant Restrictive Food Intake Disorder is defined as an eating or feeding disturbance (e.g., apparent lack of interest in eating or food; avoidance based on the sensory characteristics of food; concern about the aversive consequences of eating) as associated by persistent failure to meet appropriate nutritional and/or energy needs associated with one or more of the following:

- Significant weight loss (or failure to achieve expected weight gain or faltering growth in children)
- Significant nutritional deficiency
- Dependence on enteral feeding or oral nutritional supplements
- Marked interference with psycho-social functioning [4]

Presentation Sub-types of ARFID:

- Sensory Sensitivity—aversion to various sensory properties of food
- Fear of Aversive Consequences—concern (real or imagined) for choking, vomiting, GI distress, etc.
- Apparent Lack of Interest in Eating/Food—physiologic lack of hunger, does not find food rewarding [5]

Pediatric populations at increased risk for developing ARFID:

- Medical complications at birth and/or in early childhood that impact ability to tolerate food or liquid by mouth and/or make eating uncomfortable.
- Children who don't outgrow developmentally normal picky eating or those with severe picky eating.
- Autism spectrum disorder.
- Children with sensory processing difficulties/oral hypersensitivity.
- Picky eaters with over-accommodating parents.
- Heightened parental and family anxiety around food/mealtimes.

ARFID vs PFD

Similarities:	Differences:
Patients often enter care for their feeding problem between ages 4 and 13 (may be earlier for PFD) Feeding problem is often related to sensory characteristics of food/food rituals. Lack of body image/weight gain concern	Patients with PFD often have an underlying medical complexity Patients with PFD often also have some level of oral motor deficit and/or oral aversion

*For information on ARFID in adolescents and overlap with Anorexia Nervosa, refer to Eating Disorders chapter (Chap. 51) for more information

Treatment

PFD and ARFID can be complex and typically require a multidisciplinary team approach

- Medical: Primary Care Physician or Nurse Practitioner, Gastroenterologist, Developmental Pediatrician, etc.
- Nutrition: Registered Dietitian Nutritionist.
- Therapist: Occupational Therapist, Speech Language Pathologist.
- Psychosocial: Psychologist, Behavioral Health Clinician, Social Worker [6, 7]

Common Nutrition Concerns:

- Malnutrition or delayed weight gain/growth
- Overweight/obesity
- Limited diet variety and/or inadequate nutrient intake (ex. protein, fiber)
- Vitamin/mineral deficiencies (vitamin D, vitamin C, vitamin A, iron, zinc, calcium)
- Excessive milk/fluid consumption
- Reliance on oral supplement or enteral nutrition
- Disordered eating pattern (grazing, eating overnight, only eating in certain settings, etc.)

Nutrition Interventions:

- Set meal/snack schedule
- Assist in creating menu to rotate all comfortably eaten foods
- Educate caregivers on food groups and age-appropriate portion sizes
- Limit fluids to appropriate volume and/or replace with nutritive beverages
- Initiate an oral supplement and manage intake
- Recommend enteral nutrition (when appropriate) and manage feeding regimen
- Recommend nutritional labs to order
- Recommend vitamin/mineral supplementation based on intake or labs

For patients who are underweight/malnourished, improvement of nutrition status should be a priority. However, nutrition interventions are ideally part of a multidisciplinary team approach as treatment will also likely require environmental, therapeutic and behavioral interventions

References

1. Goh LH, How CH, Ng KH. Failure to thrive in babies and toddlers. Singapore Med J. 2016;57(6):287–91.
2. Lezo A, Baldini L, Asteggiano M. Failure to thrive in the outpatient clinic: a new insight. Nutrients. 2020;12(8):2202. https://doi.org/10.3390/nu12082202. PMID: 32722001; PMCID: PMC7468984
3. Goday PS, Huh SY, Silverman A, et al. Pediatric feeding disorder. J Pediatr Gastroenterol Nutr. 2019;68(1):124–9. https://doi.org/10.1097/MPG.0000000000002188.
4. American Psychiatric Association. Diagnostic and statistical manual of mental disorders. 5th ed. American Psychiatric Publishing; 2013.

5. Thomas JJ, Eddy K. Cognitive-behavioral therapy for avoidant/restrictive food intake disorder: children, adolescents, and adults. Cambridge University Press; 2019.
6. Pediatric Feeding and Swallowing. American Speech-Language-Hearing Association. https://www.asha.org/practice-portal/clinical-topics/pediatric-feeding-and-swallowing/
7. What is Pediatric Feeding Disorder? Feeding Matters. https://www.feedingmatters.org/what-is-pfd/

Nutritional Considerations in Pediatric Liver Disease

40

Vera Hupertz and Andrea Adler

Patients with chronic liver disease require special attention to their nutritional needs. They are at risk for significant malnutrition and subsequent frailty and sarcopenia that can result in poor long-term outcomes.

Chronic Liver Disease

Why are patients with liver disease at risk [1–3]?

1. Poor intake
   (a) Disease-related anorexia, delayed gastric emptying, nausea/vomiting, abdominal distension (secondary to ascites and/or organomegaly), fluid-restriction.
   (b) Comorbidity related: dysgeusia secondary to nutritional deficiencies, poor dentition, depression, dietary modifications in the context of renal or heart impairment.
   (c) Iatrogenic: enteral feeding cessation for procedures, lack of early nutrition re-initiation post procedures, subopti-

V. Hupertz · A. Adler (✉)
Division of Pediatric Gastroenterology, Hepatology, and Nutrition, Cleveland Clinic Children's Hospital, Cleveland, OH, USA
e-mail: HUPERTV@ccf.org; adlera@ccf.org

K. Radhakrishnan (ed.), *Handbook of Clinical and Practical Pediatric Nutrition*, https://doi.org/10.1007/978-3-031-97759-6_40

mal/inappropriate feeding approaches (e.g., restricting protein intake in acute liver failure), and medication side effects.

2. Altered nutrient metabolism
   (a) Increased energy expenditure: futile metabolic cycles (e.g. lipolysis of triglycerides to free fatty acids with subsequent re-esterification to triglycerides), recurrent infections, medications, altered bile acid signaling.
   (b) Insulin resistance: peripheral lipolysis and suboptimal protein synthesis in liver and muscle.
   (c) Abnormal Growth Hormone (GH) signaling: GH resistance, limited insulin-like growth factor 1 release following GH signaling.
   (d) Abnormal oxidation of macronutrients: e.g., increased leucine oxidation, which further limits protein synthesis; fat oxidation even if in fasted state.
   (e) Other: Limited glycogen stores
3. Maldigestion and/or malabsorption
   (a) Maldigestion: limited intraluminal bile acids (e.g. in cholestasis or biliary diversion), pancreatic insufficiency (primary or secondary, depending on underlying liver disease), rapid transit through the gastrointestinal tract.
   (b) Malabsorption: portal hypertension-related enteropathy, medication-related
   (c) Increased losses: diarrhea, electrolytes, and minerals lost in renal impairment

Evaluation of the Nutritional Status of a Child with Chronic Liver Disease

History and Physical Exam

- It is important to start with the basics when evaluating a child with liver disease for nutritional deficiencies. Intake can be affected by numerous factors (see above) and should be evaluated.

- Medications may have side effects causing anorexia or nausea and should be reviewed.
- In addition, financial and social access to food, vitamins, and/or supplements should be explored.
- On physical exam, anthropometric measurements including height/length, mid-upper arm circumference (MUAC), and triceps skin fold thickness are better markers of nutritional sufficiency than weight.
- Weight may be affected inappropriately by organomegaly, ascites, edema, and anasarca and could normalize a body mass index (BMI) or weight for length measurement [3].
- MUAC helps assess body status as it is not influenced by ascites as it reflects muscle mass and fat stores [1, 3]. There are published Z-score for 6 months to 18.5 years and then standardized percentiles for those over 18.5 years. Please see Chap. 2 for reference standards for the MUAC Z-score. Typically, MUAC is obtained with the dietitian monthly assessments; however, if the patient is severely malnourished, monitoring more frequently may be advisable [1]. See Chap. 2 for assessment of growth and anthropometric measurements.
- All children with liver disease should be monitored for growth on age-appropriate growth charts. Linear growth improves after transplant, however long-term use of medications like corticosteroids may cause linear growth to still be below normative standards [1].
- In addition, a Nutrition Focused Physical Exam (NFPE) should be completed. See Chap. 2 for general information on completing the NFPE. Key items on the NFPE to watch for, especially if the patient has ascites:
  - On the front of the body, are the ribs visible?
  - On the back of the body, are the ribs, vertebrae, or the scapulas visible?
  - Are the clavicles protruding?

    If the answer is yes to any of the above, there are depleted or absent fat and or muscle stores.

- Functional measurement of muscle mass can be done using various techniques. Lurz et al. measured frailty in children with end-stage liver disease (ESLD) compared to those with compensated chronic liver disease and found that patients with ESLD had higher frailty scores overall [4]. Testing included -
  - Standardized measurements of grip strength for evaluation of weakness
  - 6-min walk distance for evaluation of slowness
  - Triceps skinfold (TSF) thickness for evaluation of shrinkage, and
  - Patient/parental questionnaires for exhaustion and physical activity evaluation.

Metabolic Risks and Evaluation (Table 40.1)

- Electrolytes, glucose, and albumin can be easily measured on routine blood work. Hypoalbuminemia can also be secondary to losses through the gut as well as loss of functional hepatic cell mass.
- Coagulation factors, which have a lower half-life than albumin, are useful for monitoring protein production. Because they can be affected by malabsorption of vitamin K, vitamin K deficiency needs to be monitored and treated.

Table 40.1 Recommendations for laboratory evaluation and interpretation for nutrient deficiencies in liver failure [1, 3, 5]

Laboratory finding	Causes
Hyper- and hypoglycemia	Hyperinsulinemia and insulin resistance, low glycogen stores
Hyponatremia	Total body free water and sodium retention
Hypoalbuminemia	Loss of functional capacity of the liver
Prolonged prothrombin time (PT)	Loss of functional capacity of the liver and/or malabsorption of vitamin K
Essential fatty acid deficiency (EFA)	Fat malabsorption and inadequate intake of EFA due to high ratio of medium-chain triglycerides
Fat-soluble vitamin deficiencies	Fat malabsorption

- Essential fatty acid deficiency can be monitored by measuring appropriate levels. Low levels of linoleic acid, alpha-linolenic acid, eicosapentanoic acid, and/or docosahexanoic acid while the patient has clinical signs of essential fatty acid deficiency or severe fat-soluble vitamin deficiency [1].
- It is recommended that fat-soluble vitamins (vitamin A, D, E, K) be checked every 1–3 months based on severity until normal then can space out to every 3–6 months [1, 3].
- Sarcopenia (severe muscle depletion) has been associated with impaired growth and outcomes in several pediatric chronic conditions. A few reports of the effect of sarcopenia in pediatric patients suggest that there was a higher transplant waitlist mortality in patients with ESLD and longer ICU stays post-transplant [6, 7].
- A marker of sarcopenia that has been used in pediatric patients is the total psoas muscle surface area at intervertebral lumbar spaces of L3-4 and L4-5. Z-scores have been established and scores less than −2 are consistent with sarcopenia. Unfortunately, it relies on getting imaging specifically for this area though it might be found on cross-sectional imaging done for other reasons.

Dietary Recommendations

- Children with ESLD require increased energy, and their diet should supply about 130% of the predicted equations (typically using the DRI); use indirect calorimetry if available. If providing parenteral nutrition, limit to the DRI to prevent overfeeding as it is directly absorbed and isn't affected by malabsorption. Use these as starting points and monitor closely.
- Protein intake should be minimum of the DRI for age but may need 2–3 g/kg to promote growth; if having hepatic encephalopathy, consider a lower protein diet for a short period of time. Once the encephalopathy is controlled, resume the regular protein intake as much as practically possible [1]. Some children may intermittently over ingest protein (especially true for teenagers eating "double meat" subs or meals). This can result in intermittent encephalopathy despite ongoing medical therapy. Close investigation into the dietary habits can successfully reveal these dietary misadventures.

- With regards to fluids in acute liver failure, it is important to supply adequate electrolytes and fluid without overhydration.
- In addition, close monitoring of glucose levels to maintain normal glucose levels needs to be done. Glucose infusions of 4–8 mg/kg/min to keep euglycemic but may need 10–15 mg/kg/min to maintain normal glucose levels.
- In infants, in order to supply adequate energy and nutrient sources [3, 5, 8, 9], feeds may need to be concentrated or fortified to promote growth and limit the volume for comfort with ascites and organomegaly.
- Breast milk supplemented with MCT oil or formula high in MCT oil affords additional calories since MCT oil doesn't require bile salts for digestion.
- Feedings can be by mouth or tube feeding and using 1.5 cal/mL products to limit volume especially in children with ascites and organomegaly.
- Care must be taken if the dietary fat is disproportionately high in MCT oil versus long-chain fat, to monitor for essential fatty acid deficiency.
- Baby food may be begun as tolerated at >4–6 months of age (or > 4–6 months corrected age if born prematurely).
- As children get older, it is important to avoid prolonged fasting. Small frequent meals (3 meals and 2–3 snacks) are often better tolerated and focusing on high-calorie, low-sodium foods.
- Sodium restriction (2 mEq/kg/day) may be necessary with ascites and portal hypertension.
- Additional diet modifications are necessary for liver conditions such as Wilson's disease, Glycogen storage disease, Tyrosinemia, Urea cycle defects, Galactosemia, and disorders of amino acid metabolism, however, discussion of these modifications is beyond the scope of this chapter.
- Studies have also shown that parenteral nutrition (PN) support can improve the nutritional state in those who are at risk of worsening malnutrition secondary to intolerance of optimal tube feedings, especially as liver disease worsens. Sullivan et al. showed in biliary atresia patients that PN was not associated with increased risk of infection [10]. The patients on PN did have higher rates of variceal bleeding and ascites which may have been secondary to both progression of the underly-

ing liver disease and increased intravascular volume but yet overall, they had improved MUAC and TSF thickness.
- Fat-soluble vitamins should be monitored regularly due to risk of malabsorption [1, 3].
- Vitamins A, D, E, and K should be given at 2-5 times the recommended dietary allowance and adjusted as needed. It is our practice to monitor at least every 3 months.
- Ca and Mg supplementation should be based on plasma levels and iron supplementation due to chronic blood loss.
- Trace elements like zinc and selenium should be checked every 3 months as well and supplemented based on plasma levels.

Posttransplant

Energy and Protein Needs [11]

Nutrient needs for posttransplant are different for the acute phase versus the chronic/stable phase.

- The acute phase is the first 3 months after transplant and the chronic/stable phase is >3 months after transplant.
- Needs should be adjusted based on patients' growth and nutrition status in addition to medication intake, such as steroids. Energy and protein needs will need to be adjusted from below if the patient is receiving parenteral nutrition.

Energy:
Acute phase: DRI for age (adjusted for wound healing and growth if needed by 10–20%)
Chronic/Stable phase: DRI for age
Protein:
Acute phase: based on age
- Age 0–12 months: 3–3.5 g protein/kg dry body weight
- Age 1–2 years: 2.5–3.5 g protein/kg dry body weight
- Age 3–13 years: 1.5–2.5 g protein/kg dry body weight
- Age + 13 years: 1–1.5 g protein/kg dry body weight

Chronic/Stable phase: DRI for age

Diet/Nutrition Support [1, 11]

- PN may be needed if unable to feed 3–5 days after transplant, depending on the patient's age and nutritional status.
- Enteral Nutrition (EN) may be required if the patient is an infant or has had trouble tolerating feeds. Oral aversion is common in this population, especially if the patient was on tube feeds prior to transplant.
- If the patient is receiving MCT oil-containing products prior to transplant, our practice is to continue the high MCT oil-containing product for 1 month after transplant to let the liver recover, then transition to standard infant/toddler formula either as continued tube feeding or orally.

Laboratory Values

- It is recommended to obtain nutrition laboratory values to assess for nutrient deficiencies posttransplantation. Our standard of practice is to obtain fat-soluble vitamin levels 1 month after transplant to assess liver trends.
- Typically, Vitamin A and E-alpha normalize within 1 month of transplant. Vitamin D typically normalizes but may remain suboptimal based on immune-suppressive medications and long-term usage of corticosteroids. Monitoring Vitamin D 25 hydroxy levels should continue every 3–6 months for the first 2 years posttransplant and then can be spaced out to every 6–12 months [1].
- Anemia may develop due to frequent laboratory studies and attempts should be made to use minimal volumes.
- Electrolyte abnormalities are common with posttransplant immunosuppressive medications and need to be measured chronically such as potassium, calcium, magnesium, and phosphorus [1].

Vitamin Supplementation

- Patients can typically have their aqueous vitamin supplements discontinued 1 month after transplant with resolution of vitamin A and E-alpha deficiencies.

- Vitamin D supplements are typically continued long-term but can be transitioned to standard vitamin D supplements and dosed for maintenance therapy.
- Electrolyte supplements are provided as needed based on serum trends.

References

1. Mouzaki M, Bronsky J, Gupte G, Hojsak I, Jahnel J, Pai N, et al. Nutrition support of children with chronic liver diseases. J Pediatr Gastroenterol Nutr. 2019;69(4):498–511.
2. Carpenter A, Ng VL, Chapman K, Ling SC, Mouzaki M. Predictive equations are inaccurate in the estimation of the resting energy expenditure of children with end-stage liver disease. J Parenter Enter Nutr. 2017;41(3):507–11.
3. Boster J, Kalzckiewicz K, Sundaram S. In: Goday P, Walia C, editors. Chronic liver diseaes. Boca Raton: CRC Press: Taylor & Francis Group; 2022. p. 245–62.
4. Lurz E, Quammie C, Englesbe M, Alonso EM, Lin HC, Hsu EK, et al. Frailty in children with liver disease: a prospective multicenter study. J Pediatr. 2018;194:109–115.e4.
5. Cameron R, Kogan-Liberman D. Nutritional considerations in pediatric liver disease. Pediatr Rev. 2014;35(11):493–6.
6. Boster JM, Browne LP, Pan Z, Zhou W, Ehrlich PF, Sundaram SS. Higher mortality in pediatric liver transplant candidates with sarcopenia. Liver Transplant. 2021;27(6):808–17.
7. Woolfson JP, Perez M, Chavhan GB, Johara FT, Lurz E, Kamath BM, et al. Sarcopenia in children with end-stage liver disease on the transplant waiting list. Liver Transplant. 2021;27(5):641–51.
8. Mouzaki M, Ng V, Kamath BM, Selzner N, Pencharz P, Ling SC. Enteral energy and macronutrients in end-stage liver disease. J Parenter Enter Nutr. 2014;38(6):673–81.
9. Squires JE, Alonso EM, Ibrahim SH, Kasper V, Kehar M, Martinez M, et al. North American Society for Pediatric Gastroenterology, Hepatology, and Nutrition position paper on the diagnosis and management of pediatric acute liver failure. J Pediatr Gastroenterol Nutr. 2022;74(1):138–58.
10. Sullivan JS, Sundaram SS, Pan Z, Sokol RJ. Parenteral nutrition supplementation in biliary atresia patients listed for liver transplantation. Liver Transplant. 2012;18(1):120–8.
11. Asfaw M, Mingle J, Hendricks J, Pharis M, Nucci AM. Nutrition management after pediatric solid organ transplantation. Nutr Clin Pract. 2014;29(2):192–200.

Short Bowel Syndrome and Intestinal Failure

41

Ali Salar Khalili, Nicole Lidyard, and Andrea Adler

Pediatric intestinal failure (PIF) is defined as the reduction of functional intestinal mass below that which can sustain life, resulting in dependence on supplemental parenteral support for a minimum of 60 days within an interval of 74 consecutive days [1]. Short bowel syndrome (SBS) is a subcategory of PIF and is defined as the development of IF secondary to the loss of small bowel due to congenital disease or after surgical resection [1].

A. S. Khalili
Case Western Reserve University School of Medicine, Pediatric Gastroenterology, University Hospitals Cleveland Medical Center, Rainbow Babies and Children's Hospital, Cleveland, OH, USA
e-mail: Ali.Khalili@UHhospitals.org

N. Lidyard
University Hospitals Cleveland Medical Center, Rainbow Babies & Children's Hospital, Department of Pediatric Gastroenterology, Hepatology and Nutrition, Case Western Reserve University, Public Health Nutrition/Dietetics, Cleveland, OH, USA
e-mail: Nicole.Lidyard@UHhospitals.org

A. Adler (✉)
Pediatric Nutrition Support, Division of Pediatric Gastroenterology, Hepatology, and Nutrition, Children's Institute, Cleveland Clinic, Cleveland, OH, USA
e-mail: adlera@ccf.org

K. Radhakrishnan (ed.), *Handbook of Clinical and Practical Pediatric Nutrition*, https://doi.org/10.1007/978-3-031-97759-6_41

The etiology of PIF varies from SBS to motility disorders and enteropathies. SBS is the leading cause of PIF in children with an estimated incidence of 24.5 cases per 100,000 live births, and the incidence is markedly greater in premature live births [2]. The major causes of SBS in children are necrotizing enterocolitis (NEC), midgut volvulus, gastroschisis, intestinal atresia, and extensive Hirschsprung disease.

The goal of therapy in PIF is to achieve weight gain and linear growth, obtain intestinal adaptation, limit parenteral support, and maximized oral and enteral feeding.

Importance of the Anatomical Considerations (Length vs. Location)

The outcome of SBS-related PIF is influenced not just by the length of the remaining bowel after resection but also by its location of lost bowel and age at which there was bowel loss. See Table 41.1 for the areas of nutrient absorption, complications of resection, and results of adaptation.

Table 41.1 Areas of nutrient absorption, complications of resection, and results of adaptation [3]

Bowel	Absorption	Complications of Bowel interruption	Adaptation
Duodenum (D)	*Minerals:* Calcium Phosphorus Magnesium Iron Copper Selenium *Vitamins:* Thiamin Riboflavin Niacin Biotin Folate Vitamins: A, D, E, and K	Macronutrient malabsorption Metabolic acidosis Anemia (iron deficiency anemia) Osteopenia/reduced bone mineral density	Unable to adapt for other intestinal segments

(continued)

Table 41.1 (continued)

Bowel	Absorption	Complications of Bowel interruption	Adaptation
Jejunum (J)	*Minerals:* Calcium Phosphorus Magnesium Iron Zinc Chromium Manganese Pantothenate Molybdenum *Vitamins:* Thiamin Riboflavin Niacin Biotin Folate Vitamin B6 Vitamin C Vitamins: A, D, E, and K	Fluid and electrolyte imbalances Malabsorption of macronutrients Malabsorption of water-soluble vitamin Bacterial overgrowth	Longer villi and an expanded surface area CAN compensate for loss of the I and/or D Cannot absorb bile salts Cannot absorb vitamin B12
Ileum (I) and ICV	*Minerals:* Magnesium *Vitamins:* Folate Vitamin C Vitamin B12 Vitamin D Vitamin K Bile salts	Cannot absorb bile salts Cannot absorb B12 Fat-soluble vitamin loss (A, D, E and K) Increased risk of oxalate stones Bacterial overgrowth (I and ICV) leading to further malabsorption Loss of ICV leads to rapid transit	Ileum can adapt for other intestinal segments (J) ICV function is indispensable and bowel cannot adapt to loss of the ICV
Colon (C)	*Vitamins:* Biotin Vitamin K Sodium Potassium Chloride Water Short chain fatty acids	Reduced ability to absorb water Electrolyte imbalance	

- Small intestine length
  - Remaining portion of the small bowel length is one of the important factors to determine the mortality and independence from parenteral nutrition (PN)

    Intestinal tract approximately doubles in length during the last trimester of normal pregnancy.

    By term, small intestinal length ranges between 200 and250 cm.

    Final length by adulthood ranging from 400 to 700 cm.
- Proximal intestinal loss
  - The clinical impact from the loss of the proximal small bowel (duodenum) is often small and is generally better tolerated.
  - Jejunum is the primary digestive and absorptive site for most macro and micronutrients.
  - Jejunal bowel resection can cause increase in gastric secretions due to the reduction of certain enteric hormones such as somatostatin that inhibit acid production. This can cause malabsorption in some patients and micronutrient deficiencies.
- Distal intestinal Loss
  - Resection of more distal small intestine, especially ileum generally reduces nutrient, fluid and electrolyte absorption more than resection of proximal bowel
  - The distal ileum is more specialized and is the site for selective reabsorption of bile acids.

    If around one-third or more of ileum is lost, the compensatory increase in the hepatic bile acid synthesis will not keep up for increased losses in the stool.

    The proximal bile salt production will be inadequate for efficient lipid emulsification and therefore leads to fat malabsorption, increased long-chain fatty acid (LCFA) concentration in the colon, and fat-soluble vitamin deficiency.
  - The distal ileum is the primary site for absorption of vitamin B12, bound to intrinsic factor. Resection of the terminal

ileum is associated with malabsorption of vitamin B12 and can lead to clinical deficiency unless supplemented.
  - Loss of Ileocecal valve (ICV) adversely affects the motility of proximal gut by removal of the "ileal brake." As a result, it reduces the contact between luminal content and the mucosal surface, worsening the absorption of fluid, electrolytes and nutrients.
- Colon loss
  - The colon plays a crucial role in absorbing water (10–15% of total water absorption), electrolytes, and short-chain fatty acids.
  - In the absence of the colon, patients can experience increase loss of fluid and electrolytes therefore ongoing need for fluid supplementation is commonly required.
  - The colon plays only a secondary role in digestion. Starches that scape absorption in the small intestine and soluble fibers are salvage by bacterial fermentation to short-chain fatty acids.

Intestinal Adaptation

Intestinal adaptation is a compensatory process that begins immediately following massive bowel resection and involves a variety of structural and functional alterations.

- The process may take months to years, and it is believed that children have a greater capacity to adapt and achieve full enteral autonomy compared to adults due to the inherent gut growth potential of young children [4].
- On a macroscopic level, the remaining intestine experiences longitudinal growth in younger children and expands to enhance surface area for absorbing nutrients and fluids.
- On a microscopic level, there is increased villous hyperplasia and deeper crypts. These alterations are more frequently observed in the ileum compared to the jejunum. This leads to increased absorption of nutrients and electrolytes per unit of bowel length.

Clinical Management of SBS-Related IF

- The duration of postoperative ileus typically lasts less than a week, if abdominal sepsis or other complications do not develop. Appropriate replacement of ongoing losses to maintain fluid and electrolyte balance is crucial.
- Due to nature of secretory character of proximal small bowel, patients with high enterostomy can experience increase output (up to 30–50 mL/kg/day) even when they are kept NPO [5].
- Hypersecretion of gastric acid and fluids happens due to the loss of normal hormonal feedback loop with loss of bowel.
- This reduces pH below the optimal level needed for fat absorption (by inactivating pancreatic lipase and de-conjugating bile salts), increases intestinal fluid losses, and alters enteral drug absorption. The use of Histamine-2 receptor antagonist or proton pump inhibitors could help to moderate this effect after massive intestinal resection during the first year of life.

Anthropometrics for IF

See chapters in part 1 of the book for information on normal growth charts, nutrition assessment, nutrition-focused physical exam (NFPE), and mid-upper arm circumference (MUAC). A nutrition assessment should be completed monthly to yearly depending on the age of the patient to assess for growth trends in both weight, and length/height, weight/length or BMI/age, MUAC, and NFPE. The goal is for proportionate growth with weight/length or BMI/age tracks 10–25%ile as linear velocity may not catch-up and lag compared to weight velocity.

Nutrition Intervention

- Macronutrients, micronutrients and fluids: [6]
  - Energy needs

    Parenteral

- Solely parenterally fed patients require 10–15% less energy due to the lack of thermoregulation for digestion/absorption.
- Patients fed as a combination of parenteral and enteral nutrition (assuming absorption) may require 90–95% of the estimated energy requirement (EER).

Enteral/oral

- See Chap. 5 for information on EER guidelines.
- May need up to 150% DRI due to malabsorption

– Protein needs

Parenteral

- ASPEN standards for protein goal are followed while on PN support. See Chap. 6 for information on protein goals while on PN support.

Enteral/oral

- See Chaps. 1 and 8 for information on general protein recommendations.
- Typically 1.5–3.0 g protein/kg/day required to promote growth.

– Fat

Parenteral

- Alterative fat/lipid emulsion should be utilized or limit soy-based lipid emulsions to 1 g/kg/day for those with intestinal failure-associated liver disease (IFALD). See Chap. 6 for information on IV lipid emulsions.

Enteral

- Patients may tolerate products containing medium-chain triglycerides (MCT oil) better than long-chain fats.

Oral

- High fat intake may cause increase in stool output

– Fluids and Electrolytes

Majority of patients initially will require additional fluids, electrolytes, and utilization of PN to maintain adequate hydration, and life-saving treatment.

Typically, at least 120% maintenance fluids are needed.

- Route of Nutrition Intervention [1, 6–8]
  - PN provides complete nutrition. See Chap. 6 for general information on PN.
    - Use American Society for Parenteral and Enteral Nutrition (ASPEN) PN guidelines for PN advancement of macronutrients.
    - Use ASPEN PN guidelines as a start for micronutrient (electrolyte and trace element) dosing.
    - Sodium content in IV fluids or PN support is typically > ½ normal saline.
    - Patients with excessive stool or ostomy output typically have higher zinc and copper needs due to losses from the effluent particularly for jejunostomies.
    - Weaning of PN support
      - As patients tolerate and advance on feeds or diet, it is important to not provide excessive fluid intake and PN volume should be weaned as growth allows.
      - Consider reducing PN calories by 5–10% at a time and monitor weight trends over 1 week to 1 month before making further adjustments.
  - Enteral Nutrition (EN) is the preferred route of nutrition support unless contraindicated. See Chap. 4 for a more comprehensive discussion on infant and pediatric formulas.
    - Infants:
      - Use breastmilk when available.
      - Milk protein intolerance if often common in PIF/SBS infants; elemental/free amino acid infant formula is typically utilized to improve EN tolerance.
    - Children and adolescents:
      - Protein hydrolysate or elemental/free amino acid formulas are typically utilized to improve EN tolerance. Ongoing assessment of tolerance for patient's on standard mixing/dilution of elemental formula is important due to the formula's higher osmolality. Lowering the concentration below the standard mix/dilution could be beneficial.

    - Some older patients may demonstrate optimal tolerance when transitioned to food-based formulas.

  Patients with large output may benefit from addition of soluble fiber, such as liquid pectin, added to formula (oral or by tube feed)

    - Dosage starts at a 1% and increases up to 3% fiber solution.
      - Ex. 1 gram soluble fiber per 100 ml formula = 1% solution.

- Feeding Approaches and Advancement [6, 8, 9]
  - Initially, continuous feeds are the preferred delivery method.
    Increased slow absorption of nutrients continuously over the intestinal villi.
  - Feeds are gradually advanced to avoid issues such as vomiting, distension, and increased output.
    An example of slow advancement: increase feedings by 1-2 ml/hour, 1–3 x per week.
  - Bolus feeds replicate typical eating patterns in infant and children, but intolerance issues, such as dumping syndrome, often arise and are most common in infants. For older children, bolus feeding may be considered.
  - Oral feedings stimulate digestive enzymes and help to prevent oral aversion/pediatric feeding disorder. A combination of both an oral and by tube (EN) regimen should be considered if there is no indication of excess stool output, excessive vomiting, or suspected swallowing concerns.
  - Other general considerations: Utilization of enteral nutrition (oral or by tube feed) and presence of the colon impact adaptation. Additionally, disaccharides over monosaccharides and more whole proteins vs extensively hydrolyzed protein enhance adaptation, however, may not be tolerated.
- Solid Food Introduction Considerations [4, 6, 8]
  - Simple carbohydrates (i.e., fruits, all juices, yogurt with >4 grams sugar per serving) may increase risk of diarrhea. Proteins/meats and vegetables are typically introduced first, followed by starches. Fruit introduction is delayed in this

patient population due to concerns with dumping syndrome/ excessive output.
  - Older children can benefit from ~6 smaller meals rather than three larger meals.
  - Lactose intolerance is often seen in this patient population.
- Micronutrient Deficiencies
  - In general, there is increased risk for vitamin and mineral deficiencies which is increased even further when the patient is weaning off PN.
  - Nutrition deficiencies hinder intestinal adaptation. Deficiencies in vitamins, minerals, and trace elements are associated with IF/SBS patients.
  - General supplementation: Daily MVI with minerals is necessary.
  - Close monitoring, attention, and potential additional supplementation for the following micronutrients: Iron, B12, Fat-soluble vitamins (ADEK), zinc, copper and electrolytes.

Lab Monitoring [6, 8]

- See Chap. 6 for laboratory monitoring while on PN support.
- Routine lab monitoring is essential in patients with PIF. See Table 41.2 for suggested laboratory frequency while on PN support, and for those of specific concern with PIF/SBS.
- Additional laboratory considerations:
  - Methylmalonic Acid (MMA)—used to check for vitamin B12 deficiency
  - Ceruloplasmin (along with serum Cu to assess the estimated free copper value)
    Goal between 10-20ug/dL
  - Fatty Acid Profile for essential fatty acids (see Chap. 6 for PN laboratory monitoring)
  - Vitamin C

Table 41.2 Suggested laboratory monitoring and frequency [6]

	Initially	Follow-up
Metabolic		
Basal metabolic panel	Daily	Included in CMP
Comprehensive metabolic panel	Weekly	Every 1–4 weeks
Magnesium (mg)	Daily to weekly	Every 1–4 weeks
Phosphorus (Phos)	Daily to weekly	Every 1–4 weeks
Triglycerides	Daily to weekly	Monthly
PT/INR	Weekly	Monthly
CBC w/diff	Weekly	Every 1–4 weeks
GGT	Baseline as indicated	Monthly
Nutrition-related		
Iron studies	3 months	Every 3–6 months
Zinc, selenium, manganese, copper, chromium	3 months	Every 3–6 months
Vitamin D	3–6 months	Every 12 months
Vitamin A and E	6 months	Every 12 months
Vitamin B12	6 months	Every 12 months
Folate	6 months	Every 12 months
Carnitine	3–6 months	Every 3–6 months
Thyroid-stimulating hormone (TSH)	Baseline as indicated	Every 12 months

- Urine sodium for those with high ostomy output and/or poor growth

  Goal >20 mEq/L
- Citrulline—marker for remnant bowel mass and function

Pharmacological Therapy

- Antidiarrheal therapy
  - Loperamide: peripheral opioid analog that inhibits small bowel and colonic motility to treat diarrhea and improve nutrient absorption. It is not significantly absorbed, and has no cerebral effects; therefore, high doses can be safely and effectively used to decrease output [10].
  - Antimotility drugs should be avoided in the case of Clostridium difficile-associated diarrhea and used in critically ill patients only in the absence of digestive infection.
- Bile-acid-binding resin
  - Cholestyramine, Colestipol, and colesevelam are options to bind intestinal bile acids.
  - Primary side effects: constipation, heartburn, nausea, vomiting, and stomach pain
  - Used for patients with diarrhea following limited resection of the distal ileum. The diarrhea in these patients may be caused by malabsorbed bile acids entering the colon (bile acid diarrhea), and cholestyramine prevents this process by sequestering bile acids.
- Acid suppression
  - H2 blocker or proton pump inhibitor can reduce the effect of water and sodium losses due to secretory diarrhea associated with gastric hypersecretion.
  - Reduced pH below the optimal level needed for fat absorption by inactivating pancreatic lipase and deconjugating bile salts.
- Antibiotics for small intestinal bacterial overgrowth (SIBO)
  - Several antibiotics can be used including, Metronidazole, Trimethoprim-sulfamethoxazole, Gentamicin (PO), Rifaximin.

    Side effects include diarrhea, headache, nausea, vomiting, and hepatotoxicity among others.
  - Rotating antibiotics may be considered to reduce development of antibiotic resistance. Another rotation is cycling of one antibiotic, alternating one week on and one week off.

- In the setting of candidal central line infection, some center use Nystatin.
- Glucagon-like Peptide-2 (GLP-2)
  - The GLP-2 analog "Teduglutide" has been shown to decrease parenteral nutrition requirements in patients with SBS.
  - Teduglutide is approved in the United States for the treatment of patients 1 year of age (and over 10 kg) with SBS-PIF at a dose of 0.05 mg/kg administered subcutaneously once daily. Real-life response to Teduglutide is highly variable among children with SBS. Most patients reached a primary response of 20% reduction in PN within 6 months of treatment [11]

Complications of Pediatric Intestinal Failure

- Anatomic and Functional Bowel Obstruction
  - Marked dilatation of small bowel that remains after resection is common in SBS especially after jejunal atresia and gastroschisis. This often results in poor peristalsis (dysmotility) that directly contributes to SIBO, malabsorption, and feeding intolerance.
  - Medical therapy is used to treat SIBO and improve motility, but these treatments may have limited efficacy. However, when symptoms are severe or interfere with advancement of EN, surgical interventions may be considered.
- Intestinal failure associated liver disease (IFALD)
  - Etiology is multifactorial and includes sepsis, prematurity, loss of bile acid enterohepatic circulation due to absence of enteral feeding and the components of PN itself (i.e., intravenous lipid emulsions).
  - Prevention strategies [4]
    - Early introduction of enteral feeding
    - Minimizing glucose infusion rate
    - Alternative lipid management in PN

    - Prevention of central line-associated bloodstream infections (CLABSI)
    - Early referral for transplantation assessment
- Central venous catheters (CVC) related complications include:
  - Infection, dislodgement, thrombosis, and decreased quality of life.
  - Sepsis is a risk factor for hepatic dysfunction, death and is a negative predictor of enteral autonomy.
  - The development of central-related thrombosis poses a significant risk for this patient population, and loss of venous access sites may necessitate intestinal transplantation.
- Metabolic bone disease (MBD)
  - It may present in various ways including changes on dual-energy x-ray absorptiometry, pathologic fractures, and bone pain.
  - Multiple factors contribute to MBD
    - Changes in the absorption of key minerals including calcium, magnesium, and phosphorus.
    - Deficiency of vitamin D.
    - High levels of aluminum related to PN.
  - Patients with SBS are prone to hyperoxaluria, which can lead to the formation of calcium oxalate kidney stones.
- Oral aversion and feeding problems
  - Oral aversion and feeding difficulties are common in children with PIF.
  - Some of the challenges that lead to oral aversion are long-term use of nasogastric tubes for feeding, delayed introduction of oral feeding, lack of normalized satiety patterns.
  - Occupational therapists and speech-language pathologists are a key member of the multidisciplinary team and can provide early intervention to improve and prevent the development of oral aversion.
- Micronutrient deficiencies—see chapters on macro/micronutrients and vitamins for information on general nutrient deficiencies.
  - Deficiencies specific to PIF/SBS
    - Zinc

Copper
Carnitine
Fat-soluble vitamins
Essential fatty acid deficiency
Vitamin C deficiency
Electrolytes—specifically Na and Bicarbonate

- SIBO including risk of D-lactic acidosis
- Renal Calculi
- Cholelithiasis and cholecystitis
- Pancreatitis and pancreatic insufficiency
- Enterocolitis—from SIBO
- Long term renal impairment is a concern and not well studied

Surgical Interventions (Non-transplant)

- Consideration for surgical procedures includes inability to advance of enteral nutrition, poor growth, recurrent bacterial infections, market dilation of small bowel, SIBO not responsive to medical therapy.
- Ultimate goals of surgery are to re-establish bowel continuity, maximize intestinal surface area, improvement of motility, and increase transient time.
- Autologous bowel reconstruction surgeries can be divided into three categories:
  - Restoration of intestinal continuity
  - Procedures to improve motility
  - Lengthening and tapering procedures

    Longitudinal intestinal lengthening technique (LILT or Bianchi)

    Serial Transverse Enteroplasty (STEP)
  - Preexisting liver disease especially with portal hypertension increases mortality and is a contraindication for lengthening surgery.

Small Bowel Transplant

Small bowel/multivisceral transplantation in pediatric patients with IF is typically considered when the Intestinal failure cannot be managed through conventional means, such as PN, or when complications from PN threaten the child's life.

Here are the primary indications for transplant in pediatric patients with IF:

1. Progressive and severe intestinal failure-associated liver disease (IFALD)
2. Loss of venous access
3. Recurrent life-threatening central venous catheter-associated bloodstream infections
4. Complete mesenteric thrombosis
5. Severe short bowel syndrome

Posttransplant

There is a lack of evidenced-based standardized protocols for this population due to having too few patients to complete clinical trials. While practices vary for each institution based on their program's experiences, there is often consensus on general nutrition management practices. These include weaning off PN; achieving enteral autonomy which may be oral feeding, EN or both; following appropriate growth patterns and avoiding common posttransplant complications such as diabetes, obesity, kidney disease, rejection, and graft failure requiring the re-initiation of PN support [12].

Anthropometrics

See Chaps. 1 and 2 for information on growth charts, nutrition assessment, NFPE, and MUAC. A nutrition assessment posttransplant should be completed monthly to yearly to assess for growth trends in both weight, and length/height, weight/length or BMI/age, MUAC, and NFPE.

- Despite pretransplant anthropometric status, weight gain and obesity are common posttransplant due to decreased energy needs, long-term steroid usage [13].
- Length or height can take up to 6 months to 2 years to obtain catch-up growth [14].

Estimated Needs

See Chap. 2 for use of predictive equations to determine fluid and energy needs. Protein needs should follow recommendations for PN (see PN Chap. 6). Once transitioned off PN, protein needs should be the DRI with adjustments as needed for growth.

Diet/Nutrition Support

- PN support—See Chap. 6 on PN for general parenteral nutrition information
  - PN order (macronutrients and electrolytes) should be started back at baseline as the patient has had a change in status.
    - Monitor for losses such as Na^+, K^+, Cl^-, Acetate, and Zn from tubes, drains, and ostomy output [15]
    - Monitor glucose trends due to steroid usage
    - Higher doses Mg in the PN may be needed due to drug-nutrient interactions.
    - Higher or lower doses of K^+ and Phos may be needed due to drug-nutrient interactions.
  - Additives in the PN such as MVI, trace elements, carnitine should remain at previous dosages.
  - Fluid volume may be restricted initially after transplant.
  - PN can be weaned as EN is initiated, tolerated, and advanced.

  - Prevent overfeeding by adjusting macronutrients in the PN even if unable to wean PN volume to account for EN support.
  - Goal is to transition to enteral nutrition as soon as clinically possible.
- EN support [12, 15]
  - EN, typically elemental/free amino acid formula, may be started once bowel function returns.
  - Feeds are typically resumed with the pre-transplant formula.

    Must take into consideration the age of the patient along with the age of the donor organs to determine the most appropriate formula.
  - Continuous feeds are preferred over bolus feeds and advanced based on ostomy output.
  - Wean EN as able once a diet is initiated and tolerated.
  - Continue EN until oral intake is sufficient to promote growth.
- Diet
  - Once tolerating EN, a clear liquid diet may be initiated.
  - Diet can be advanced as tolerated. Diet should be:

    low fiber diet

    no concentrated sweets

    no fruit juice; no fruit (except unsweetened apple sauce and bananas)

    low fat

    low lactose
  - Patient's may benefit from oral nutrition supplements.
    - Semi-elemental formulas may be preferred over elemental/free amino acid formulas from a taste perspective.
  - Patients may have an oral aversion, especially if they have had little oral intake prior to transplant.
  - There is risk for new food allergies posttransplant and concern for eosinophilic bowel disease [16].

    Consider avoiding soy, wheat, milk protein, nuts, eggs and seafood for 6 months after transplant.

Vitamin/Mineral Supplements

- Patients may require electrolyte, vitamin, and/or mineral supplements posttransplant once weaned off PN support.
- Sometimes, patient may be weaned off PN support, however, require IV fluids for hydration and electrolyte maintenance or may only require electrolyte supplements orally/enterally.
- Patients may require medication to treat metabolic acidosis (such as a citrate product) due to GI and renal loses.
- Additionally, patients may require a general multivitamin supplement or individual vitamin supplements (i.e., Vitamin A, D, or E) to maintain normal levels.
- Trace elements such as zinc, copper, and selenium may need to be supplemented based on laboratory values. Administration of zinc and copper supplements should be at different times to prevent competing absorption issues.
- Carnitine deficiency can occur and supplements may be required for fat metabolism.

Laboratory Assessment

As with anyone receiving PN support, labs to assess electrolytes should be assessed daily until stable then weekly to ensure appropriate dosages are provided. See PN Chap. 6 which also discusses laboratory monitoring.

- Complete metabolic panel or a hepatic panel should be monitored weekly to assess liver function and more often if concerns about the liver function [17] particularly in multi-visceral transplant patients.
- Posttransplant, patients may have fat malabsorption due to the insufficient function of the lymphatic system and sometimes from pancreatic insufficiency [12].
- Fat-soluble vitamins (vitamin A, E-alpha, D 25 hydroxy) status may be affected.

- A fecal elastae may be evaluated if there are concerns for fat malabsorption and if it is low, pancreatic enzymes should be initiated. If the fecal elastase level is low but there is high stool output, empiric initiation of pancreatic enzymes can be considered as the level may be low due to a dilutional effect of the high stool output.

Additionally, many of the posttransplant medications have known drug-nutrient interactions.

- The medical practitioner should be aware of the side effects of these medications.
- These may include: hyper/hypokalemia, hypophosphatemia, hypomagnesemia, hyperglycemia, hyperglycemia, hyperlipidemia.

Common nutrient deficiencies during the transition phase off of PN onto EN and on exclusive EN include:

- Vitamin A, D, E, copper, selenium, zinc, magnesium, phosphorous, vitamin B12, iron, anemia, and iron deficiency anemia [16, 18, 19].
- Literature varies on how often to obtain nutrition labs after transplant, whether patients are on PN or EN or solid foods.
- See Table 41.3 for suggested laboratory assessment to be obtained every 3–6 months to monitor for trends and more often with abnormal values. These are based on our center's standard of practice and could vary between centers
- In addition, consider obtaining litamin C level every 6 months.

Table 41.3 Micronutrient laboratory assessment posttransplant [8, 12, 20, 21]

Nutrient	How often	Comments
Zinc, copper, Ceruloplasmin, selenium	3–6 months or based on clinical indications	Consider obtaining a C-reactive protein. Ceruloplasmin and copper should be used to calculate a free copper level as serum copper may be bound to albumin and may be artificially low.
Chromium, manganese	Every 6–12 months while on PN; once transitioned off PN, no longer needed	May be elevated even if not added to PN as they are contaminants to other PN additives.
Vitamin A, E-alpha, D-25 hydroxy	Every 3–6 months off PN support or based on clinical indications	
Carnitine profile	Every 6 months while on PN; once transitioned off PN, only if concern for fat metabolism	Patients may require enteral Levocarnitine supplementation
Iron studies	Every 6 months while on PN; once transitioned off PN, based on clinical indiations	
Essential fatty acid profile	Every 3–6 months while on PN; once transitioned off PN, based on clinical indications	Patients may have essential fatty acid deficiency off PN support if they are malabsorbing
Vitamin B12 or Methylmalonic acid (MMA)	Every 6 months	
RBC/serum folate	Every 6 months	

Outcomes

Management of PIF has evolved in recent decades, with improved survival since the advent of specialized multidisciplinary intestinal failure centers, hepatoprotective strategies of PN management, catheter care, and surgical care. Mortality in this population increases by extreme short bowel, IFALD, and recurrent sepsis from CLABSIs. Most centers reported greater than 90% long-term survival, with wide range of mortality rate from 6.4% to 37.5% [22]. However, there are times when intestinal transplantation is the only options for these patients.

Future Research Considerations

- Vitamin C deficiency in PIF
- Pancreatic enzymes supplementation
- Newer GLP-2 analogs
- Newer lock therapies to help with line preservation

References

1. Modi B, Galloway D, Nucci A, Plogsted S, Wales P. ASPEN definitions in pediatric intestinal failure. J Parenter Enter Nutr. 2022;46(1):42–59.
2. Wales PW, de Silva N, Kim J, Lecce L, To T, Moore A. Neonatal short bowel syndrome: population-based estimates of incidence and mortality rates. J Pediatr Surg. 2004;39(5):690–5.
3. Caporilli C, Giannì G, Grassi F, Esposito S. An overview of short-bowel syndrome in pediatric patients: focus on clinical management and prevention of complications. Nutrients. 2023;15(10):2341.
4. Belza C, Wales PW. Management of pediatric intestinal failure related to short bowel syndrome. Semin Pediatr Surg. 2022;31(3):151175.
5. Short KS, Syndrome B. In: Wyllie R, Haymes J, Kay M, editors. Pediatric gastrointestinal and liver disease. 4th ed. Philidelphia: Saunders Elsevier; 2010. p. 374–85.
6. Bashir A, Goday P. Short bowel syndrome. In: Larson-Nath C, editor. ASPEN pediatric and neonatal nutrition support handbook. 3rd ed. Silver Springs: American Society for Parenteral and Enteral Nutrition; 2024.

7. Puoti MG, Köglmeier J. Nutritional management of intestinal failure due to short bowel syndrome in children. Nutrients. 2022;15(1):62.
8. Squires R, Iyer K. Intestinal failure. In: Corkins M, Balint J, Bobo E, Plogsted S, Yaworski J, editors. ASPEN pediatric nutrition support core curriculum. 2nd ed. Silver Springs: American Society for Parenteral and Enteral Nutrition; 2015. p. 427–40.
9. Channabasappa N, Girouard S, Nguyen V, Piper H. Enteral nutrition in pediatric short-bowel syndrome. Nutr Clin Pract. 2020;35(5):848–54.
10. Klek S, Forbes A, Gabe S, Holst M, Wanten G, Irtun Ø, et al. Management of acute intestinal failure: a position paper from the European Society for clinical nutrition and metabolism (ESPEN) special interest group. Clin Nutr. 2016;35(6):1209–18.
11. Kocoshis SA, Merritt RJ, Hill S, Protheroe S, Carter BA, Horslen S, et al. Safety and efficacy of teduglutide in pediatric patients with intestinal failure due to short bowel syndrome: a 24-week, phase III study. JPEN J Parenter Enteral Nutr. 2020;44(4):621–31.
12. Colomb V, Goulet O. Nutrition support after intestinal transplantation: how important is enteral feeding? Curr Opin Clin Nutr Metab Care. 2009;12(2):186–9.
13. Iyer K, Horslen S, Iverson A, Sudan D, Fox I, Shaw B, et al. Nutritional outcome and growth of children after intestinal transplantation. J Pediatr Surg. 2002;37(3):464–6.
14. Venick RS, Wozniak LJ, Colangelo J, Beckwith P, Reyen L, Esmailian YA, et al. Long-term Nutrition and predictors of growth and weight gain following pediatric intestinal transplantation. Transplantation. 2011;92(9):1058–62.
15. Wieman R, Kocoshis SA. Nutrition management of pediatric patients undergoing liver transplantation or intestinal transplantation. In: Goday PS, Mehta NM, editors. Pediatric critical care nutrition [internet]. New York: McGraw-Hill Education; 2015. [cited 2024 Jun 28]. Available from: https://accesspediatrics.mhmedical.com/content.aspx?bookid=1198&sectionid=70672901.
16. Vanderhoof JA, Langnas AN, Pinch LW, Thompson JS, Kaufman SS. Short bowel syndrome. J Pediatr Gastroenterol Nutr. 1992;14(4):359–70.
17. Szeszycki E, Cruse W, Beitzel M. Evaluation and monitoring of pediatric patients receiving specialized nutrition support. In: Corkins M, Balint J, Bobo E, Plogsted S, Yaworski J, editors. The ASPEN pediatric Nutrition support core curriculum. 2nd ed. Chicago: American Society for Parenteral and Enteral Nutrition; 2015. p. 615–39.
18. Yang CF, Duro D, Zurakowski D, Lee M, Jaksic T, Duggan C. High prevalence of multiple micronutrient deficiencies in children with intestinal failure: a longitudinal study. J Pediatr. 2011;159(1):39–44.e1.

19. Ubesie AC, Kocoshis SA, Mezoff AG, Henderson CJ, Helmrath MA, Cole CR. Multiple micronutrient deficiencies among patients with intestinal failure during and after transition to enteral nutrition. J Pediatr. 2013;163(6):1692–6.
20. Youssef NN, Mezoff AG, Carter BA, Cole CR. Medical update and potential advances in the treatment of pediatric intestinal failure. Curr Gastroenterol Rep. 2012;14(3):243–52.
21. Ellsworth K. Nutrition support: vitamin, mineral and trace element management in patients on long-term parenteral nutrition [unpublished lecture notes]. The 9th pediatric intestinal failure and rehabilitation symposium. Los Angeles, CA; Lecture given 2016 Oct 27. In Los Angeles.
22. Fullerton BS, Hong CR, Jaksic T. Long-term outcomes of pediatric intestinal failure. Semin Pediatr Surg. 2017;26(5):328–35.

Food Allergies and Eosinophilic GI Disorders: Nutritional Management

42

Sophia Patel, Brian Schroer, Maria Haught, and Diana Schnee

Allergies are the result of the immune system responding to an external protein that causes inflammation and symptoms [1].

- Allergies occur following a breakdown in tolerance induction, or the prevention of an immune response to the protein, through a mechanism that is not well understood.
- The allergic immune response can come in many forms leading to the need to be clear about what type of immune response is leading to the disease.

S. Patel (✉)
Division of Pediatric Gastroenterology, Cleveland Clinic Children's Hospital, Cleveland, OH, USA
e-mail: PATELS5@ccf.org

B. Schroer
Center of Pediatric Allergy and Immunology, Cleveland Clinic Children's Hospital, Cleveland, OH, USA
e-mail: SCHROEB4@ccf.org

M. Haught · D. Schnee
Pediatric Nutrition Support, Division of of Pediatric Gastroenterology, Hepatology, and Nutrition, Cleveland Clinic Children's Hospital, Cleveland, OH, USA
e-mail: HAUGHTM4@ccf.org; SCHNEED2@ccf.org

K. Radhakrishnan (ed.), *Handbook of Clinical and Practical Pediatric Nutrition*, https://doi.org/10.1007/978-3-031-97759-6_42

- These immune responses can be broken down by whether they are IgE mediated, eosinophilic and IgE mediated (mixed), eosinophilic alone, or T-cell (lymphocytic) mediated.
- A good clinical history is essential to differentiate the type of allergic reaction that is occurring as the nutritional interventions used are different based on the disease.

IgE-Mediated Allergies

- Acute IgE-mediated food allergies can manifest as contact urticaria due to foods due to hives occurring where food touches the skin or as systemic allergic reactions with symptoms including some combination of systemic urticaria where food could not have touched, sneezing, coughing, nausea, vomiting or swelling. These IgE-mediated reactions typically begin soon after ingestion, though some reactions may begin up to 2 hours later. Symptoms such as rashes, vomiting, or coughing rarely last more than 6 hours, though swelling may last longer. Symptoms typically occur every time a food is eaten [1].
- The most common food triggers are milk, egg, peanut, tree nuts, sesame, fish, shellfish, wheat, and soy. The characteristic illness script and timing of symptoms following each exposure makes IgE-mediated food allergies easier to diagnose than most food allergies with the clinical history being the best test for diagnosis. [1]
- Skin prick testing or serum-specific IgE testing to foods are useful at ruling out IgE-mediated food allergies but have a high rate of false positives and should be used to support clinical history or differentiate which food caused a reaction when it is not clear. Oral food challenges are the gold standard diagnostic test [1].
- Unnecessary avoidance of foods such as peanuts and eggs in young infants has been shown to increase the risk for developing IgE-mediated allergy. ([1].

- The dual need to avoid the foods that are causing the symptoms, and to continue ingestion of, or to introduce, potential food allergens to prevent development of allergy drives dietary management of IgE-mediated food allergies [1].

Pollen Food Allergy Syndrome is another acute IgE-mediated food allergy that is found in about one-third of patients with pollen-induced allergic rhinitis [1].

- This disease is characterized by oropharyngeal throat itching immediately after ingestion of mostly plant-based foods such as fresh fruits and vegetables. These symptoms are immediate onset and often resolve quickly after the patient stops eating the food. They only rarely result in severe symptoms.
- Dietary management is patient specific as most patients with mild symptoms can continue to eat the food. Patients who feel the symptoms are not tolerable should avoid the foods that have caused symptoms. Testing for the specific food has false positives and is not always helpful in identifying food triggers.
- Processing the food by heating or peeling the food can eliminate or reduce symptoms, but not in all cases.

IgE Food Allergy Resolution Occurs Frequently to milk and egg. However, many other IgE-mediated food allergies such as peanut and tree nut allergies are not often outgrown naturally [1].

- New food immunotherapies have been used with the goal of protecting patients from reactions due to exposure and may increase the chance of outgrowing the allergy if done at an early age.
- These therapies such as oral immunotherapy and sublingual immunotherapy involve highly controlled exposure to the food allergen, increasing the dose to a daily maintenance dose with continued exposure over many years. They are more effective at younger ages and can cause side effects including acute anaphylaxis and chronic allergic inflammation in the gut.

Mixed (IgE and Non-IgE Mediated) Allergic Disorders

- Eosinophilic Gastrointestinal Disorders (EGIDs) including Eosinophilic Esophagitis (EoE), Eosinophilic Gastritis/ Enteritis, or Eosinophilic Colitis are chronic immune-mediated syndromes with increased incidence in the past 30 years [2].
- This group of disorders is defined by abnormal infiltration of Th2 immune cells including eosinophils into the esophageal, gastric, or intestinal tissue. They occur in an estimated 5/100,000 per year in children, with higher incidence rates in adults [3].
- Non-EoE EGID carries a higher symptom burden and is less likely to be associated with a food trigger [4].
- The etiology of disease process in EGID is multifactorial, with atopic disease being an early risk factor. Impaired epithelial barrier dysfunction in esophageal and gastric tissue causes eosinophil recruitment through a variety of T-helper type 2 (Th2)-mediated pathways [5].
- IgE-mediated symptoms may also occur in patients with EOE suggesting that IgE reactions to foods or other allergens also play a role.
- Over time, this mixed allergic inflammation leads to symptoms of Eosinophilic Esophagitis (EoE), with younger patients experiencing abdominal pain, vomiting, and poor weight gain and older patients experiencing esophageal dysphagia, difficulty swallowing, or food impactions.
- Symptoms of Eosinophilic Gastritis (EoG) and Eosinophilic Enteritis (EoN) include lower gastrointestinal dysfunction with abdominal pain, weight loss, nausea, and vomiting or diarrhea.
- The disease is chronic, and if left untreated, can lead to fibrosis in esophageal tissue, gastric dysmotility, and poor weight gain or failure to thrive.
- EoE is caused by allergic inflammation due to foods [6] with some evidence suggesting aeroallergen sensitivity may also contribute to inflammation. (Dellon PMID: 28774845) [4].

- Diet Elimination options include but are not limited to:
  - Targeted Food Elimination—Food allergen testing could be done via skin prick testing (SPT) and/or atopy patch testing (APT) although some controversy exists on the usefulness of this application (1–3). Any positive test results are avoided as well as cow's milk (due to poor negative predictive value on testing).
  - Empiric Food Elimination—If there are no existing food allergies as identified in the methods listed above (see 'Targeted Food Elimination'), options are to avoid a single food, starting with milk, or to avoid multiple foods at once as specified by the medical team.
    - 4-food elimination diet—avoidance of milk, egg, soy, wheat
    - 6-food elimination diet—avoidance of milk, egg, soy, wheat, peanuts/tree nuts, and fish/shellfish
  - Elemental Diet—Children consume an amino acid-based, hypoallergenic formula exclusively and by effect, remove all allergenic food proteins (1–3). This is not a sustainable treatment option for child who routinely eat a regular diet and should be considered only for those with severe cases or who are chronically tube fed.

- Known mediators of this Th2 inflammation include proteins in food such as cow's milk containing foods, wheat, soy (legumes), eggs, peanut/tree nuts, and fish/shellfish.
- Early studies of EoE determined that a 6-week elemental formula regimen, led to resolution of symptoms and significantly decreased eosinophil count in affected tissue in Ref.6
- As mentioned above, determination of food triggers in EoE is limited by lack of accurate testing for food-related allergens. Skin-based allergen testing including prick and atopy patch testing leads to both false negative and false positives when used to determining which foods are causative in eosinophilic inflammation and are not reliable methods to determine target food eliminations [7–9].

- Therefore, evaluation of inflammation in esophageal tissue before and after food avoidance has become the mainstay of identifying which foods are contributing to the disease.
- Options include avoiding a single food, starting with cow's milk, as the first step.
- Common options for broader elimination include a 2-food elimination (milk and wheat), 4-food elimination diet—avoidance of milk, egg, soy, wheat, or a 6-food elimination diet—avoidance of milk, egg, soy, wheat, peanuts/tree nuts, and fish/shellfish.
- Remission rates following use of the 4-food vs 6-food elimination diet are comparable. Adherence to a single or two food elimination diet is higher than with 4 or 6 food elimination diets.
- A 6-food elimination diet improved symptoms and inflammation in 74% of patients compared with 88% improvement on an elemental diet [10].
- Follow-up studies have reinforced that approximately 25% of patients do not have resolution of inflammation on a 6-food elimination diet suggesting that the more foods that are avoided, the less likely there is an additional benefit [8, 9].
- A 2017 study evaluating a 4-food elimination diet (milk, wheat, egg, soy) in children showed a 64% remission rate in histologic findings of EoE [11].
- Further studies have shown the efficacy in both children and adults in only eliminating a single food, cow's milk, as an equally effective therapy. Milk elimination diet led to a range of 56–64% remission in patients when evaluated in several prospective and retrospective studies [12–15].
- Determination of which foods to eliminate is dependent on the following:
  - Likelihood of benefit to avoidance of the food trigger (noting milk to be the most common trigger).
  - Existing food allergies identified through allergen testing.
  - Ingestion of potential food triggers in current diet.
  - Patient/family buy-in to therapy through shared decision-making.

  - Acceptance of dietary changes especially when considering preexisting feeding difficulties.
  - Socio/economic factors of family/school/childcare to provide appropriate alternatives.
- Reintroduction of single food allergens from a multiple food elimination diet can occur once an endoscopy shows EoE is in remission. Method of food introduction will be directed by a doctor/dietitian and done with a stepwise approach. Repeat endoscopies are likely needed in between each food that is reintroduced [2].
- Endoscopies should be spaced out by at least 8 weeks, preferably 12 weeks, in between food elimination steps.
- Dietary management of food allergies should be driven by the following multiple goals [16].
  - To avoid the least number of foods needed to control the disease.
  - Prevent accidental exposure to the food through hidden sources.
  - Continue ingestion of foods that are not contributing due to the risk of developing allergy/losing tolerance to foods that have been previously tolerated.
  - Adequately replacing the calories and micronutrients that are lost due to food avoidance.
- In the case of malnutrition or poor weight status, catch-up growth may be needed.
- Consider possible nutrient deficiencies depending on the dietary intervention utilized and for how long the patient is on the elimination diet (Table 42.1).
- Patients would benefit from a multidisciplinary approach (gastroenterologist, allergist, and registered dietician with EoE expertise) to therapy to improve the effectiveness of dietary elimination.

Non-IgE-Mediated Allergic Diseases: [17]

- Food protein-induced allergic disease of the gut is common in infancy. Many of these diseases can be misattributed to other conditions such as gastroesophageal reflux disease, lactose intolerance, or intestinal colic.

Table 42.1 Nutrients of concern with dietary elimination

Nutrient considerations	
Elimination of dairy	Calcium, phosphorus, choline, riboflavin, vitamin B12 and vitamin A
Elimination of wheat	Fiber, iron, B vitamins
Elimination of egg	B vitamins, vitamin E
Elimination of soy	No nutrient concerns unless being used to augment a restricted diet
Elimination of peanuts/tree nuts	Folate, niacin, vitamin E, copper, manganese, iron, magnesium, phosphorus
Elimination of fish/shellfish	Omega 3 fatty acids

- Various forms of these immune-mediated gastrointestinal disorders can occur starting around 1–2 months old though possibly earlier.
  - These disorders can manifest in discrete and easy-to-recognize forms such as Food Protein Induced Enterocolitis Syndrome (FPIES) and Food Protein Induced Allergic Proctocolitis syndrome (FPIAP). In chronic FPIES or as early manifestations of EoE, they can lead to chronic non-specific issues such as pain, decreased appetite/poor weight gain, or vomiting present over a long period of time due to chronic FPIES, typically caused by cow milk or soy-based formulas.
- Dietary management of these conditions involves elimination of foods that are the most common triggers from the diet and monitoring for a resolution of symptoms. Reintroduction of the food with a return of symptoms would be needed to confirm the diagnosis to that food.
- Choosing which foods are contributing to the allergy is made difficult by the lack of effective allergy testing to help rule in or rule out any specific food protein as the cause. In addition, at this age, many of these diseases present it is not common to do diagnostic procedures such as an esophagogastroduodenoscopy (EGD) or proctocolonoscopy to make the diagnosis or to monitor for resolution of the inflammation.

- **FPIAP** is caused by an eosinophilic predominant inflammation of the proctocolon that typically leads to acute or chronic symptoms of bloody stools (hematochezia) often associated with abdominal pain, colic, or loose stools that contain mucous due to damage of the distal colon [17].
- This disease typically occurs in young infants and often resolves by 9 months to 1 year old [18].
- The most common triggers in North America are thought to be milk (76%), egg (16%), soy (6%) though there are few updated studies on epidemiology of this disease. Because milk is the most common trigger, this disease has been known as Cow Milk Protein Intolerance. This nomenclature is no longer recommended. [18]
- FPIAP is commonly diagnosed outside the newborn period as the cause of bloody stools. FPIAP has been found to be the cause of bloody stools in 60% of infants. Since 40% of patients with bloody stools do not have FPIAP, clinicians should evaluate alternative causes such as infection, or anal tears before implementing dietary changes. [17, 18]
- **Nutrition management** of FPIAP includes empiric removal of milk protein from maternal diet or changing cow milk-based formula to either a soy-based formula, or a hydrolyzed cow milk formula.
- If cow milk avoidance in maternal diet or extensively hydrolyzed formulas is unsuccessful, then use of an amino acid-based formula can be attempted.
- Reintroduction of milk products can be done as early as 4 weeks2 after exclusion and many societies agree that use of a milk ladder or slow reintroduction of milk is the ideal way to reintroduce to the infant's diet. 19
- Reintroduction of milk or other trigger foods can occur by slow reintroduction and monitoring of symptoms. There is no standard method for reintroduction. For example, a milk ladder starting with baked or cooked dairy in food products such as biscuits or cookies and assessing tolerance, with rapid progression to other less heated forms of milk is an option for reintroducing cow milk and recommended by international gastroenterology societies.

FPIES is thought to be a lymphocytic -mediated disease though the exact immune mechanism is not fully understood. 20

- Symptoms of acute FPIES can be more severe than other non-IgE mediated food allergies and include the onset of profuse vomiting that starts 1–4 h after ingestion and can be associated with lethargy, hypotension, turning pale/grey, or diarrhea starting after the vomiting.
- Acute FPIES is most often caused by solid foods that are introduced at an early age such as rice, oats, egg, milk, soy, or, more recently, peanut.
- Chronic FPIES is becoming less frequent and traditionally presents as recurrent vomiting and diarrhea 1–4 h after ingestion of a formula that is either cow milk or soy based. In chronic FPIES the food is eaten regularly, and it can lead to failure to thrive.
- Patients with FPIES often outgrow the allergy though it may take a number of years to resolve.

Due to the potentially severe reactions, reintroduction of triggering foods should be done in an office setting with clinicians who have experience with food challenges and managing the potentially severe reactions.

References

1. Sicherer SH, Sampson HA. Food allergy: a review and update on epidemiology, pathogenesis, diagnosis, prevention, and management. J Allergy Clin Immunol. 2018;141(1):41–58. https://doi.org/10.1016/j.jaci.2017.11.003. Epub 2017 Nov 21. PMID: 29157945
2. Furuta GT, Katzka DA. Eosinophilic esophagitis. N Engl J Med. 2015;373(17):1640–8. https://doi.org/10.1056/NEJMra1502863. PMID: 26488694
3. Dellon ES, Hirano I. Epidemiology and natural history of eosinophilic esophagitis. Gastroenterology. 2018;154(2):319–332.e3. https://doi.org/10.1053/j.gastro.2017.06.067. Epub 2017 Aug 1. PMID: 28774845

4. Cianferoni A. Eosinophilic esophagitis and other eosinophilic disorders of the gastrointestinal tract. Pediatr Allergy Immunol. 2020;31(Suppl 24):25–7. https://doi.org/10.1111/pai.13153. PMID: 32017217
5. Inage E, Furuta GT, Menard-Katcher C, Masterson JC. Eosinophilic esophagitis: pathophysiology and its clinical implications. Am J Physiol Gastrointest Liver Physiol. 2018;315(5):G879–86. https://doi.org/10.1152/ajpgi.00174.2018. Epub 2018 Sep 13. PMID: 30212252
6. Markowitz JE, Spergel JM, Ruchelli E, Liacouras CA. Elemental diet is an effective treatment for eosinophilic esophagitis in children and adolescents. Am J Gastroenterol. 2003;98(4):777–82. https://doi.org/10.1111/j.1572-0241.2003.07390.x. PMID: 12738455
7. Spergel JM, Brown-Whitehorn T, Beausoleil JL, Shuker M, Liacouras CA. Predictive values for skin prick test and atopy patch test for eosinophilic esophagitis. J Allergy Clin Immunol. 2007;119(2):509–11. https://doi.org/10.1016/j.jaci.2006.11.016. PMID: 17291865
8. Molina-Infante J, Martin-Noguerol E, Alvarado-Arenas M, Porcel-Carreño SL, Jimenez-Timon S, Hernandez-Arbeiza FJ. Selective elimination diet based on skin testing has suboptimal efficacy for adult eosinophilic esophagitis. J Allergy Clin Immunol. 2012;130(5):1200–2. https://doi.org/10.1016/j.jaci.2012.06.027. Epub 2012 Aug 3. PMID: 22867695
9. Philpott H, Thien F. The role of allergy testing in eosinophilic esophagitis: an update of the evidence. Curr Treat Options Gastroenterol. 2017;15(1):26–34. https://doi.org/10.1007/s11938-017-0125-3. PMID: 28124203
10. Kagalwalla AF, Sentongo TA, Ritz S, Hess T, Nelson SP, Emerick KM, Melin-Aldana H, Li BU. Effect of six-food elimination diet on clinical and histologic outcomes in eosinophilic esophagitis. Clin Gastroenterol Hepatol. 2006;4(9):1097–102. https://doi.org/10.1016/j.cgh.2006.05.026. Epub 2006 July 21. PMID: 16860614
11. Kagalwalla AF, Wechsler JB, Amsden K, Schwartz S, Makhija M, Olive A, Davis CM, Manuel-Rubio M, Marcus S, Shaykin R, Sulkowski M, Johnson K, Ross JN, Riffle ME, Groetch M, Melin-Aldana H, Schady D, Palac H, Kim KA, Wershil BK, Collins MH, Chehade M. Efficacy of a 4-food elimination diet for children with eosinophilic esophagitis. Clin Gastroenterol Hepatol. 2017;15(11):1698–1707.e7. https://doi.org/10.1016/j.cgh.2017.05.048. Epub 2017 Jun 8. PMID: 28603055
12. Teoh T, Mill C, Chan E, Zimmer P, Avinashi V. Liberalized versus strict cow's milk elimination for the treatment of children with eosinophilic esophagitis. J Can Assoc Gastroenterol. 2019;2(2):81–5. https://doi.org/10.1093/jcag/gwy030. Epub 2018 Jul 4. PMID: 31294369
13. Kruszewski PG, Russo JM, Franciosi JP, Varni JW, Platts-Mills TA, Erwin EA. Prospective, comparative effectiveness trial of cow's milk elimination and swallowed fluticasone for pediatric eosinophilic esopha-

gitis. Dis Esophagus. 2016;29(4):377–84. https://doi.org/10.1111/dote.12339. Epub 2015 Feb 26. PMID: 25721813

14. Grasso J, Radler DR, Zelig R. Single-food elimination of cow's milk as a treatment for eosinophilic esophagitis in children aged 2-18 years: a review of the literature. Nutr Clin Pract. 2024;39(4):824–36. https://doi.org/10.1002/ncp.11117. Epub 2024 Jan 30. PMID: 38290801
15. Wechsler JB, Schwartz S, Arva NC, Kim KA, Chen L, Makhija M, Amsden K, Keeley K, Mohammed S, Dellon ES, Kagalwalla AF. A single-food Milk elimination diet is effective for treatment of eosinophilic esophagitis in children. Clin Gastroenterol Hepatol. 2022;20(8):1748–1756.e11. https://doi.org/10.1016/j.cgh.2021.03.049. Epub 2021 Apr 3. PMID: 33823291
16. Groetch M, Venter C, Skypala I, Vlieg-Boestra B, et al. American Academy of Allergy, Asthma, and Immunology. Dietary therapy and nutrition management of eosinophilic esophagitis: a work group report of the American Academy of Allergy, Asthma, and Immunology. J All Clin Immunol. 2017;5(2):312–24. PMID:35085004
17. Nowak-Węgrzyn A, Katz Y, Mehr SS, Koletzko S. Non-IgE-mediated gastrointestinal food allergy. J Allergy Clin Immunol. 2015;135(5):1114–24. https://doi.org/10.1016/j.jaci.2015.03.025. PMID: 25956013
18. Lake AM. Food-induced eosinophilic proctocolitis. J Pediatr Gastroenterol Nutr. 2000;30(Suppl):S58–60. https://doi.org/10.1097/00005176-200001001-00009. PMID: 10634300
19. Meyer R, Venter C, Bognanni A, Szajewska H, Shamir R, Nowak-Wegrzyn A, Fiocchi A, Vandenplas Y, WAO DRACMA Guideline Group. World allergy organization (WAO) diagnosis and rationale for action against cow's Milk allergy (DRACMA) guideline update – VII – Milk elimination and reintroduction in the diagnostic process of cow's milk allergy. World Allergy Organ J. 2023;16(7):100785. https://doi.org/10.1016/j.waojou.2023.100785. PMID: 37546235
20. Järvinen KM, Nowak-Węgrzyn A. Food protein-induced enterocolitis syndrome (FPIES): current management strategies and review of the literature. J Allergy Clin Immunol Pract. 2013;1(4):317–22. https://doi.org/10.1016/j.jaip.2013.04.004. Epub 2013 May 31. PMID: 24565536

Nutrition in Pancreatic Disorders

43

Senthilkumar Sankararaman,
Terri Schindler, and Aravind Thavamani

Acute Pancreatitis

Even though most of the management principles of pancreatic disorders were extrapolated from the adult literature, the causes of pancreatic disorders are unique in children and different from the adults [1–4]. The incidence of pancreatic disorders (acute pancreatitis, acute recurrent pancreatitis, and chronic pancreatitis) has been increasing in the pediatric population [2].

S. Sankararaman (✉)
Division of Pediatric Gastroenterology, Hepatology, and Nutrition, Cleveland Clinic Children's Hospital, Cleveland, OH, USA
e-mail: SANKARS6@ccf.org

T. Schindler
Division of Pediatric Pulmonology, University Hospitals Rainbow Babies and Children's Hospital, Cleveland, OH, USA
e-mail: Terri.Schindler@uhhosptials.org

A. Thavamani
Division of Pediatric Gastroenterology, Hepatology, and Nutrition, University Hospitals Rainbow Babies and Children's Hospital, Cleveland, OH, USA
e-mail: Aravind.Thavamani@uhhospitals.org

K. Radhakrishnan (ed.), *Handbook of Clinical and Practical Pediatric Nutrition*, https://doi.org/10.1007/978-3-031-97759-6_43

- **Criteria for Diagnosis**
  - The presence of at least 2/3 criteria: abdominal pain suggestive of pancreatic origin (acute and mostly in the epigastric pain), increased serum amylase and/or lipase (at least three times upper limits of normal), and imaging findings suggestive/compatible with pancreatitis [4, 5]. Lipase is more specific for AP than amylase.
- **Classification**
  - AP is classified as mild, moderate, and severe depending on the presence of complications.
  - Mild AP—The most common type in children and characterized by absence of vital organ failure, no local or systemic complications, and usually resolves within a week of presentation.
  - Moderate AP—Characterized by the development of transient organ failure/dysfunction (resolves in 48 h) or development of local or systemic complications. Local complications include development of (peri) or pancreatic fluid collections or necrosis. Recurrence of abdominal pain, fever, and worsening serum pancreatic enzyme levels could be signs indicating the development of such complications. In children, systemic complications include exacerbation of previously present co-morbid conditions of vital organs such as lung, heart, or kidneys [5].
  - Severe AP—Organ dysfunction that persists >48 h. Persistent organ failure may involve single or multiple vital organs [5].
  - In children, majority of AP include interstitial edematous pancreatitis type and necrotizing pancreatitis or infected pancreatic necrosis are rarer [6].
- **Etiology**
  - In adults, majority of AP (more than 80% of cases) are due to either biliary (gallstones) or alcohol ingestion whereas in children, the causes are diverse [5, 7]. The most common etiologies in children include biliary/obstructive, medications, and systemic inflammatory conditions (Table 43.1) [2, 5–7].

Table 43.1 Causes of pediatric acute pancreatitis [2, 5, 7]

Causes of acute pancreatitis in the pediatric population	Approximate proportion/ percentage of all cases
Biliary causes/obstruction (choledholithiasis, microlithiasis, structural causes such as choledochal cyst, pancreas divisum, and sphincter of Oddi dysfunction)	~1/3rd
Medications (some of the commonly incriminated medications for acute pancreatitis include valproic acid, azathioprine, L -asparaginase, furosemide, tacrolimus, steroids, and mesalamine)	~1/5th
"Idiopathic" (here cause cannot be determined despite extensive work up)	~1/3rd
Systemic inflammatory conditions (sepsis, hemolytic uremic syndrome, and other systemic disorders)	~1/10th
Trauma	~1/10th
Viral etiology (mumps)	~1/10th
Metabolic disorders (diabetic ketoacidosis, hypertriglyceridemia, and hypercalcemia)	~5%
Endoscopic retrograde cholangiopancreatography (ERCP)	<5%

  - In about one-fifth of patients, more than one etiology can be identified [7]
- **Clinical Presentation**
  - Abdominal pain is the most common symptom of AP. In about three-fourths of the patients, the location of pain is in the epigastric region given the location of pancreas. In some patients, the pain can be diffuse and also may radiate to the back. Nausea and vomiting can accompany the pain. In younger children and patients who are nonverbal, acute onset of feeding intolerance can be a presenting symptom.

- **Investigations**
  - In addition to serum lipase and amylase, hepatic panel, renal function panel, complete blood count, and fasting triglycerides are recommended.
  - In early stages, imaging may help us to identify the etiology of AP such as gall stones/anatomic abnormalities and in later states to evaluate complications such as fluid collections and necrosis [6].
  - Transabdominal ultrasound is the initial preferred imaging modality. Computed tomography and magnetic resonance imaging are helpful in cases of suspected pancreatic necrosis.
  - Magnetic resonance cholangio-pancreatography (MRCP) plays an important role in the diagnosis of anomalies and lesions of the biliary and pancreatic ducts. Secretin enhancement may help to further delineate the biliary and pancreatic ductal abnormalities [6].
- **Management**
  - Aggressive fluid management (both replenishment and maintenance), optimizing pain control, and early nutritional intervention are the mainstay of AP management [6]. Majority of management in children was extrapolated from literature in adults and also from retrospective pediatric studies.
  - Fluid resuscitation with intravenous (IV) hydration is a cornerstone of AP management [6]. It improves the pathogenesis of AP which is characterized by altered microcirculation of inflamed pancreatic parenchyma and formation of microthrombi [6]. Optimizing fluid status will help the progression of AP and prevention of complications such as organ failure and pancreatic necrosis. In the presence of hemodynamic compromise, fluid bolus (10–20 mL/kg body weight) should be given.
  - Crystalloids are the preferred type of IV fluids. Unlike adult literature, it is unclear if lactated Ringers's solution is superior to normal saline for fluid management in the pediatric

population [6]. In pediatric patients, 1.5–2 times the maintenance IV fluids is recommended with careful monitoring of vital signs, fluid status (input/output) in the 1–2 days after admission [4].

- For milder pain, acetaminophen or nonsteroidal anti-inflammatory drugs (NSAIDs) can be used. If NSAIDSs do not adequately control the pain or are contraindicated (e.g. acute kidney injury or bleeding diathesis), then IV opiates such as morphine should be provided.
- Children with mild AP should be started on a general (regular) oral diet and advanced as tolerated [4]. Limited evidence in chidren indicated that early initiation of oral nutrition in mild AP was associated with reduced length of hospitalization [8].
- In severe AP, enteral nutrition (oral, nasogastric, or nasojejunal depending on the tolerance) should be attempted within 72 h after fluid resuscitation and hemodynamic stabilization [4].
- No definition exists for "low-fat diet" and intake of fat need not be restricted except for patients with hypertriglyceridemia and patients with feeding intolerance [8].
- A combination of enteral nutrition and parenteral nutrition should be used in children who do not meet the caloric goals with enteral nutrition alone and have not received full calories for a week into hospitalization [4].

Acute Recurrent Pancreatitis (ARP) and Chronic Pancreatitis (CP)

- **Introduction**

  ARP leads to CP and is characterized by destruction of pancreatic parenchyma leading to irreversible inflammatory fibrosis, deformation of large pancreatic ducts, and loss of islet cell composition [7].

- **Diagnostic Criteria**

  AP—Frequent episodes of AP (requires at least two episodes of AP) plus complete resolution of symptoms between the episodes with at least one month of symptom-free interval or complete normalization of pancreatic enzymes between the episodes [9].

  CP—One of the following three criteria: abdominal pain consistent with pancreatic origin 2. evidence of exocrine pancreatic insufficiency three evidence of endocrine pancreatic insufficiency along with imaging findings suggestive consisitent with CP damage.
- **Etiology**
  - Genetic conditions (*PRSS1, CFTR, SPINK1, CTRC, CPA1, CEL, CEL-HYB*) account for nearly 50% and 70% of cases of ARP and CP, respectively [2]. Obstructive conditions and medications (similar to the medications implicated in AP) are the next common etiological causes for ARP and CP [2, 10]. Rare causes include autoimmune pancreatitis, metabolic (hypertriglyceridemia, diabetes mellitus), and toxins (alcohol/smoking) [10].
- **Clinical Presentation**
  - Patients with ARP are generally healthy between the AP episodes. Children with CP suffer from abdominal pain which may be episodic or constant [1, 10]. Patients with ARP and CP have frequent emergency department visit, hospitalizations, missed school days, and heavy economic burden [1, 2]. Family history such as *PRSS1* may be positive in genetic conditions predisposing to ARP or CP.
- **Investigations**
  - In addition to the laboratory tests noted in AP, genetic evaluation is recommended for ARP and CP cases. IgG4 can be elevated in autoimmune pancreatitis. Genetic conditions should be screened in ARP or CP.
  - Ultrasound is the most commonly used initial imaging which can utilized to assess the pancreatic size, contour, main duct diameter and its irregularity, peripancreatic fluid, and presence of calcifications [7].

- MRCP is the investigation of choice to delineate pancreatic atrophy or lipomatosis, and calcifications. It also helps to evaluate biliary stones and anatomic variants such as pancreatic divisum. Ductal anatomy can be augmented by the administration of secretin with MRCP [7, 10].
- Computer tomography is not the preferred modality in children due to radiation and poor delineation of the pancreatic duct.
- ERCP are often used in adults to evaluate CP in adults. Due to technical challenges, and invasive nature, this modality is often reserved for therapeutic interventions and not for diagnosis alone [7].

- **Management**
  - In acute presentation, management is similar to AP. Additionally, complications need to be screened and evaluated accordingly.
  - A trail of pancreatic enzyme therapy can be considered to reduce the recurrent or symptoms of ARP and CP, respectively, even though the literature surrounding this practice remains sparse [11].
  - Endoscopic or surgical or intervention radiological procedures may be needed for managing complications. For example, endoscopic retrograde cholangiopancreatography (ERCP) with biliary sphincterotomy may be needed for biliary strictures predisposing to ARP [1, 10].
  - In CP, patients with mild pain are managed with NSAIDs or neuromodulators. Patients with severe pain may need long-term opioids and this is best offered by pain specialists. In severe pain not responding to conventional pain management, patients can be referred to pancreatic centers for further management such as celiac nerve block, or aggressive surgical options such as partial or total pancreatectomy with islet cell autotransplantation can be considered [10]. Multidisciplinary team management offers the best outcome and essential team members include gastroenterologist with pancreatic expertise, pancreatic surgeon,

interventional radiologist, registered dietitian, psychologist, pain therapist, social worker, nurse coordinator, endocrinologist, and pharmacist.
- Children with CP are prone for malnutrition due to increased symptom burden, frequent hospitalizations, and increased need for interventions. Also, they are prone for exocrine pancreatic insufficiency and should have fat-soluble vitamin levels measured every 6–12 months [1, 7]. Similarly, the exocrine pancreatic insufficiency should be screening using fecal elastase or 72-h fecal fat estimation (less preferred as it is cumbersome and unpleasant) [1, 7].
- Poor bone health (osteopenia) is often associated with CP and the causes are multifactorial. Malnutrition and vitamin D deficiency are the most common reason for poor bone health followed by calcium, magnesium, phosphorus deficiencies.

Exocrine Pancreatic Insufficiency (EPI)

- **Definition**
  - Exocrine Pancreatic Insufficiency (EPI)—A reduction in pancreatic enzymes or bicarbonate or both leading to impaired digestion and absorption of macro- and micronutrients [12].
  - Even though the pancreas is involved in the digestion of various nutrients, fat and fat-soluble vitamins are predominantly affected in EPI [13]. Fat digestion is exclusively handled by pancreas and lipase is vulnerable to inactivation by gastric acid secretions. After fat, protein digestion can also be impaired in severe EPI, and carbohydrates are least affected due to compensatory digestion by the salivary amylases and other brush border disaccharidases [13].
  - Pancreas has huge functional reserve and greater than 90% of pancreatic function should be lost for clinical manifestations of EPI. Conditions causing EPI can be primary pancreatic conditions (with reduced pancreatic parenchyma as result of damage or poor development) or secondary to dis-

orders resulting in the interruption of production or function of the pancreatic enzymes (pancreatic parenchyma is not affected in secondary conditions) [12]. Table 43.2 lists the conditions with EPI.

- **Etiology**
  - Cystic fibrosis (CF) is the most common etiology for pediatric EPI. Table 43.3 details the essential aspects of the genetic conditions with EPI.
  - EPI also can also be transient during infancy, and in certain disease states such as malnutrition, post viral illness, and immediately after an episode of pancreatitis.
- **Clinical Manifestations:**
  - Patients with EPI develop symptoms related to malabsorption of nutrients and have poor quality of life.
  - In early stages, EPI can present with bloating, increased flatulence, and abdominal cramping/discomfort. These symptoms are nonspecific and may overlap with other gastrointestinal conditions such as irritable bowel syndrome (IBS), lactose intolerance, celiac disease, inflammatory bowel disease (IBD), and small intestinal bacterial overgrowth (SIBO) resulting in delay in the diagnosis of EPI [27].
  - In the later stages of EPI, steatorrhea is profound which manifests as bulky, oily/greasy, abnormally foul-smelling, and pale-colored stools [27]. Also, stools can be loose or float in the toilet and difficulty to flush. Significant weight loss despite adequate intake of calories is also a hallmark of EPI. Symptoms of fat-soluble vitamin deficiencies can also be noted in untreated patients.
  - Symptoms of the underlying conditions with steatorrhea as a feature (Tables 43.2 and 43.3) also can lead to the suspicion of EPI with subsequent confirmation.
  - In children, the disease impact can be higher than in adults due to active growth with increased nutritional demands in children. Also, the relative rarity of this condition and limited number of pediatric centers with pancreatic expertise may lead to relative difficulty in EPI diagnosis in children.

Table 43.2 Causes of exocrine pancreatic insufficiency [14]

Primary causes
Cystic fibrosis
Chronic pancreatitis
Shwachman–diamond syndrome
Other genetic causes —Johanson–blizzard syndrome, Pearson-marrow syndrome, Jeune syndrome, genetic disorders with pancreatic agenesis/aplasia, and isolated enzyme deficiencies
Pancreatectomy (either due to chronic pancreatitis or malignant conditions)
Secondary causes
Duodenitis with decreased cholecystokinin (CCK) signaling—Celiac disease and inflammatory bowel disease
Postcibal asynchrony (mismatch in mixing between meals, release of pancreatic enzymes and bile)—Bariatric surgeries and other upper gastrointestinal surgeries (e.g., short gut syndrome)
Inactivation of lipase—Zollinger Ellison syndrome, orlistat (weight loss mediation)

Table 43.3 Genetic conditions with exocrine pancreatic insufficiency [7, 15]

Name of the genetic condition	Clinical presentation
Cystic fibrosis (CF) [16]	Most common lethal genetic condition in the Caucasians. Carrier state is 1:25. Approximately 30,000 patients live in the United States. The *CFTR* gene is located on chromosome 7q codes for the CFTR protein. About 2000 mutations have been described and the most common one is F508del mutation. Approximately, 85% of CF population have EPI. Further details are separately discussed in the cystic fibrosis chapter.
Shwachman–diamond syndrome (SDS) [17]	Approximate incidence is 1 in 76, 000. The *SBDS* gene located on chromosome 7q11 codes for the SBDS protein. SBDS plays a key role in the ribosomal maturation and cellular proliferation. Pancreatic fatty infiltration is often seen and in many patients, EPI can improve spontaneously after 4 years of age. Bone marrow failure is common with tendency toward development of myelodysplasia and leukemia. Skeletal abnormalities—Short stature +/− metaphyseal involvement, and rib cage anomalies are noted as well.

(continued)

Table 43.3 (continued)

Name of the genetic condition	Clinical presentation
Johanson–blizzard syndrome (JBS) [18]	The incidence of JBS is 1 in 250,000. Mutations in the *UBR1* gene on the long arm of chromosome 15q15.2 have been noted. *UBR1* plays an important role in cell development and leucine-m-TOR signaling pathway (ubiquitin ligase). The defect in this pathway leads to dysregulated apoptosis resulting in many development anomalies such as typical facial features (nasal alar hypoplasia), scalp defects, pancreatic lipomatosis, hypothyroidism, and heart defects.
Pearson-marrow syndrome (PMS) [19]	In PMS, deletions of mitochondrial DNA lead to defective oxidative phosphorylation. Depressed bone marrow cell lines (either one cell line or more) have been described. Ringed sideroblasts and cell vacuolization in the bone marrow (Prussian blue stain) can be identified. In approximately 50% of individuals, EPI can be present, and the pancreas is fibrotic. Majority of patients die early in life secondary to severe metabolic acidosis and life-threatening infections.
Jeune syndrome [20]	Incidence—1:100,000 to 1:130,000 Small, narrow chest (asphyxiating thoracic dystrophy) leading to respiratory distress and, short-limbed dwarfism are the prominent features. Pancreatic fibrosis, abnormalities of kidneys, and liver fibrosis have been described.
Maturity-onset diabetes of the young (MODY) [21, 22]	Exocrine pancreatic dysfunction with atrophy has been noted in MODY type 5 (mutations in *HNF1B* gene) and MODY type 8 (mutations in *CEL* gene).
Hereditary fibrosing poikiloderma [23]	Patients with hereditary fibrosing poikiloderma have tendon contractures, myopathy, and pulmonary fibrosis (also referred to as by the acronym POIKTMP). Mutations in *FAM111B* have been identified. EPI and pancreatic cancers have been reported.
Pancreatic aplasia/agenesis [24]	Mutations in *PDX1 (IPF1)* locus have been identified in pancreatic agenesis

(continued)

Table 43.3 (continued)

Name of the genetic condition	Clinical presentation
Isolated enzyme deficiencies [25, 26]	Defects in *PNLIP* has been incriminated in congenital lipase deficiency and *PRSS7* mutation in congenital enterokinase deficiency.

- **Diagnosis:**
  - Pancreatic function tests can be broadly classified as direct and indirect tests [15]. Direct tests are based on the stimulation of pancreatic secretion by exogenously administered hormones such as secretin or CCK [28]. They are mostly employed as confirmatory tests and useful in early cases of EPI. They are expensive, cumbersome to perform, done in a few tertiary centers.
  - Contrarily, the indirect tests are simple, relatively cheaper, and widely used to evaluate EPI and often utilized clinically. Table 43.4 discusses the individual tests in both categories.
- **Treatment:**
  - Pancreatic enzyme replacement therapy (PERT) is the mainstay of management. Dosing recommendations are based on expert consensus and PERT dose is based either on amount of fat ingested [16]. Another easier method to calculate the dose is based on body weight and amount of food ingested (meals vs snack). In infants, 1000–2500 lipase units/kg/feed are given with breast feeding or formula. In children 1–4 years, PERT is given at a dose of 1000 lipase units/kg/meal and can be titrated to a maximum dose of 2500 lipase units/kg/meal.
  - For patients >4 years, 500 lipase units/kg/meal is provided. Dose can be titrated up to a maximum dose of 2500 units/kg/meal. Half of this dose is given for snacks. PERT is administrated just before the meal/snack. Daily maximum

Table 43.4 Pancreatic function tests for exocrine pancreatic insufficiency [3, 7, 14, 29, 30]

Direct tests
Dreiling tube test—Oroduodenal tube is used, and intravenous secretin or cholecystokinin (CCK) is used to stimulate pancreatic secretions. Obsolete in clinical practice as it is invasive and also requires fluoroscopy
Endoscopic pancreatic stimulation—Methodology very similar to Dreiling tube test [28]. Done in specialized centers only.
Secretin-enhanced magnetic resonance cholangiopancreatography—Has additional advantage of delineating the pancreatic anatomy.
Indirect tests
72-h fecal fat estimation—Gold standard method for estimating fat malabsorption. However, it is not specific for EPI as other conditions such as inflammatory bowel disease or celiac disease can also lead to fat malabsorption. Fat intake should be monitored (2 g/kg, with a maximum of 100 g daily). Co-efficient of fat absorption is calculated from (ingested fat—Excreted fat)/ingested fat. A value of at least 85% in infants <6 months and 93% in infants >6 months of age is considered normal. However, stool collection for 3 days is cumbersome and unpleasant.
Fecal elastase-1 (monoclonal test, ELISA-based)—Easy to perform, small amount of stool (5 g) is enough, a value <100 µg/g of stool is consistent with severe EPI and values 100–200 µg/g is consistent with mild to moderate EPI. False-positive values are high if the sample is watery. Only solid or semisolid stool sample should be sent. PERT can be continued and does not interfere with fecal elastase-1 estimation. Lower sensitivity in early stages of EPI.
Stool chymotrypsin test—Not used due to low sensitivity. PERT must be stopped prior to testing. Contrarily, this test is rarely utilized to evaluate adherence to treatment.
Serum immunoreactive trypsinogen (IRT)—Utilized in neonatal screening of cystic fibrosis (CF). Sweat test >60 mmol/L is diagnostic for CF.
Specific genetic tests for the diagnosis of underlying conditions
Other tests such as stool fat screening and steatocrit are often used but these are not accurate and not recommended.

dose beyond 10,000 lipase units/kg is not recommended as fibrosing colonopathy has been documented with doses exceeding this dose.

- Dose is adjusted based on improvement in symptoms. In patients with persistent symptoms, medication compliance should be evaluated. Similarly, the clinician should ensure the PERT has active enzymes by checking the appropriate storage methods and expiry date has not lapsed. A trial of acid suppression medications can also be tried.
- In children who cannot swallow, the capsule can be opened up and the microbeads/microspheres can be mixed with apple sauce or any other pureed acidic foods (with pH <4.5) and fed using a spoon [3]. Oral cavity should be checked for any left-over beads to prevent ulcerations. Similarly, in infants, the PERT can cause perianal ulcerations, and perineum should be examined for leftover enzymes.
- Diet rich in fat and high calorie diet is recommended. For example, in patients with CF, diet with 110–200% of recommended dietary allowance (RDA) is provided. In patients who don't gain weight despite maximizing oral nutritional supplements, enteral feeds (nasogastric or gastrostomy feeds) can be initiated.
- Fat-soluble vitamin supplementation is provided and regular monitoring of fat-soluble vitamin deficiencies is warranted [15].
- For CF, CFTR-directed therapies are currently available for patients with eligible mutations.
- Patients with CF are also at high risk of development of CF-related diabetes and CF-related liver disease and require periodic screening and management.
- Multidisciplinary approach is pivotal for EPI management and the team includes gastroenterologist, registered dietician, nurse coordinator, social worker, pharmacist, and other specialists (based on the underlying condition and comorbid disorders) [15].

References

1. Schwarzenberg SJ, Bellin M, Husain SZ, Ahuja M, Barth B, Davis H, et al. Pediatric chronic pancreatitis is associated with genetic risk factors and substantial disease burden. J Pediatr. 2015;166(4):890-6. e1.
2. Uc A, Husain SZ. Pancreatitis in children. Gastroenterology. 2019;156(7):1969–78.
3. Sankararaman S, Schindler T. Exocrine pancreatic insufficiency in children–challenges in management. Pediatr Health Med Ther. 2023;14:361–78.
4. Abu-El-Haija M, Uc A, Werlin SL, Freeman AJ, Georgieva M, Jojkic-Pavkov D, et al. Nutritional considerations in pediatric pancreatitis: a position paper from the NASPGHAN Pancreas Committee and ESPGHAN Cystic Fibrosis/Pancreas Working Group. J Pediatr Gastroenterol Nutr. 2018;67(1):131–43.
5. Abu-El-Haija M, Kumar S, Szabo F, Werlin S, Conwell D, Banks P, et al. Classification of acute pancreatitis in the pediatric population: clinical report from the NASPGHAN pancreas committee. J Pediatr Gastroenterol Nutr. 2017;64(6):984–90.
6. Abu-El-Haija M, Kumar S, Quiros JA, Balakrishnan K, Barth B, Bitton S, et al. Management of acute pancreatitis in the pediatric population: a clinical report from the North American Society for Pediatric Gastroenterology, Hepatology and Nutrition Pancreas Committee. J Pediatr Gastroenterol Nutr. 2018;66(1):159–76.
7. Taylor CJ, Chen K, Horvath K, Hughes D, Lowe ME, Mehta D, et al. ESPGHAN and NASPGHAN report on the assessment of exocrine pancreatic function and pancreatitis in children. J Pediatr Gastroenterol Nutr. 2015;61(1):144–53.
8. Ellery KM, Kumar S, Crandall W, Gariepy C. The benefits of early oral nutrition in mild acute pancreatitis. J Pediatr. 2017;191:164–9.
9. Morinville VD, Husain SZ, Bai H, Barth B, Alhosh R, Durie PR, et al. Definitions of pediatric pancreatitis and survey of present clinical practices. J Pediatr Gastroenterol Nutr. 2012;55(3):261–5.
10. Abu-El-Haija M, Lowe M, Barth B, Bellin MD, Fishman DS, Freedman S, et al. Pediatric chronic pancreatitis without prior acute or acute recurrent pancreatitis: a report from the INSPPIRE consortium. Pancreatology. 2020;20(4):781.
11. Freeman AJ, Ng K, Wang F, Abu-El-Haija MA, Chugh A, Cress GA, et al. Pancreatic enzyme use reduces pancreatitis frequency in children with acute recurrent or chronic pancreatitis: a report from INSPPIRE. Am J Gastroenterol. 2024;119(10):2094–102.
12. Zheng Y, Mostamand S. Nutrition in children with exocrine pancreatic insufficiency. Front Pediatr. 2023;11:943649.

13. Whitcomb DC, Duggan SN, Martindale R, Lowe M, Stallings VA, Conwell D, et al. AGA-PancreasFest joint symposium on exocrine pancreatic insufficiency. Gastro Hep Adv. 2023;2(3):395–411.
14. Capurso G, Traini M, Piciucchi M, Signoretti M, Arcidiacono PG. Exocrine pancreatic insufficiency: prevalence, diagnosis, and management. Clin Exp Gastroenterol. 2019;12:129–39.
15. Sankararaman S, Schindler T, Sferra TJ. Management of exocrine pancreatic insufficiency in children. Nutr Clin Pract. 2019;34:S27–42.
16. Freswick PN, Reid EK, Mascarenhas MR. Pancreatic enzyme replacement therapy in cystic fibrosis. Nutrients. 2022;14(7):1341.
17. Dror Y. Shwachman-diamond syndrome. Pediatr Blood Cancer. 2005;45(7):892–901.
18. Zenker M, Mayerle J, Reis A, Lerch MM. Genetic basis and pancreatic biology of Johanson-Blizzard syndrome. Endocrinol Metab Clin. 2006;35(2):243–53.
19. Pronman L, Rondinelli M, Burkardt DDC, Velayuthan S, Khalili AS, Bedoyan JK. Pearson syndrome: a rare cause of failure to thrive in infants. Clin Pediatr. 2019;58(7):819–24.
20. De Vries J, Yntema J, Van Die C, Crama N, Cornelissen E, Hamel B. Jeune syndrome: description of 13 cases and a proposal for follow-up protocol. Eur J Pediatr. 2010;169:77–88.
21. Dubois-Laforgue D, Cornu E, Saint-Martin C, Coste J, Bellanné-Chantelot C, Timsit J, et al. Diabetes, associated clinical spectrum, long-term prognosis, and genotype/phenotype correlations in 201 adult patients with hepatocyte nuclear factor 1B (HNF1B) molecular defects. Diabetes Care. 2017;40(11):1436–43.
22. Tshivhase A, Matsha T, Raghubeer S. Diagnosis and treatment of MODY: an updated mini review. Appl Sci. 2021;11(20):9436.
23. Seo A, Walsh T, Lee MK, Ho PA, Hsu EK, Sidbury R, et al. FAM111B mutation is associated with inherited exocrine pancreatic dysfunction. Pancreas. 2016;45(6):858–62.
24. Hilbrands R, Keymolen K, Michotte A, Marichal M, Cools F, Goossens A, et al. Pancreas and gallbladder agenesis in a newborn with semilobar holoprosencephaly, a case report. BMC Med Genet. 2017;18:1–5.
25. Szabó A, Xiao X, Haughney M, Spector A, Sahin-Tóth M, Lowe ME. A novel mutation in PNLIP causes pancreatic triglyceride lipase deficiency through protein misfolding. Biochim Biophys Acta (BBA) Mol Basis Dis. 2015;1852(7):1372–9.
26. Ghishan FK, Lee P, Lebenthal E, Johnson P, Bradley CA, Greene HL. Isolated congenital enterokinase deficiency: recent findings and review of the literature. Gastroenterology. 1983;85(3):727–31.
27. Berry AJ, Bilbo A. Exocrine pancreatic insufficiency and pancreatic exocrine replacement therapy in clinical practice. Nutr Clin Pract. 2024;39:S78–88.

28. Patel N, Sellers ZM, Grover A, Liu QY, Maqbool A, Morinville VD, et al. Endoscopic pancreatic function testing (ePFT) in children: a position paper from the NASPGHAN pancreas committee. J Pediatr Gastroenterol Nutr. 2021;72(1):144–50.
29. Yuzyuk TN, Nelson HA, Johnson LM. Inherited causes of exocrine pancreatic insufficiency in pediatric patients: clinical presentation and laboratory testing. CRC Crit Rev Clin Lab Sci. 2023;60(5):366–81.
30. Hopson P, Smadi Y, Mehta V, Patel S, Mehta D, Horvath K. Assessment of exocrine pancreatic function in children and adolescents with direct and indirect testing. Front Pediatr. 2022;10:908542.

Nutritional Considerations in Celiac Disease

44

Elizabeth Collyer and Rachel Goodwin

Introduction

Celiac disease is an autoimmune enteropathy occurring in genetically susceptible individuals, screening is by laboratories and confirmation by endoscopic biopsies of the small intestine demonstrating villous atrophy and intraepithelial lymphocytosis. The treatment of celiac disease is a strict, lifelong gluten-free (GF) diet. A strict GF diet is the only known treatment for celiac disease; however, a strict GF diet can present not only practical difficulties but also nutritional challenges.

Clinical Aspects of Celiac Disease

Celiac disease is an autoimmune enteropathy that occurs in genetically predisposed individuals in response to gluten ingestion. Gluten is a protein found in wheat, barley, and rye. Gluten is the

E. Collyer (✉) · R. Goodwin
Celiac Disease Specialty Clinic at Phoenix Children's Hospital, Phoenix, AZ, USA
e-mail: ecollyer@phoenixchildrens.com; rGoodwin@phoenixchildrens.com

K. Radhakrishnan (ed.), *Handbook of Clinical and Practical Pediatric Nutrition*, https://doi.org/10.1007/978-3-031-97759-6_44

protein component of wheat seed endosperm which is composed of monomers called gliadins and large polymeric structures termed glutenins. Toxicity in celiac disease is related to the gliadin fraction of the protein and its chemical structure is similar among the other cereal grains involved in celiac disease.

The strongest association of celiac disease is with the human leukocyte antigen (HLA) markers DQ2 and DQ8 which are, essentially, required for the celiac disease immune response. It is thought these markers are present on antigen-presenting cells (APCs) and allow APCS to bind gluten peptides that have been deamidated by the enzyme tissue transglutaminase (TTG). These APCS then activate CD4+ T-cells and release antibodies against gliadin and TTG as well as increase interferon (IFN)-gamma. Gliadin is also thought to directly increase other inflammatory molecules including IL-15 and IFN-Alpha [1]. Together, these inflammatory mediators then go on to damage the enterocyte directly and recruit intraepithelial lymphocytes which lead to inflammation.

Symptoms of Celiac Disease

Celiac disease can present with a host of gastrointestinal and non-gastrointestinal symptoms. Classically, celiac disease was felt to present with diarrhea, abdominal distension, muscle wasting/malnutrition, and abdominal pain. However, due to increased awareness and focus on screening, some individuals may have no symptoms, atypical symptoms, or are identified due to screening of high-risk groups. Other presentations without intestinal symptoms include short stature, iron deficiency anemia, joint pains, liver disease, and infertility (Table 44.1).

Table 44.1 Common symptoms of celiac disease

Gastrointestinal symptoms	Non-gastrointestinal symptoms
Abdominal pain	Growth failure/short stature
Diarrhea/steatorrhea	Muscle wasting
Abdominal bloating	Attention problems/"brain fog"
Constipation	Anxiety
Malnutrition/failure to thrive	Iron deficiency anemia
Nausea	Joint and/or back pains
Vomiting	Infertility
Anorexia	Acne
Liver disease	Fatigue
Oral aphthous ulcers	Irritability/irrationality
	Headache
	Hair loss
	Skin rash, multiple including dermatitis herpetiformis

Screening for and Diagnosis of Celiac Disease

It is important to note that both serologic screening and biopsy-based testing for celiac disease rely on sufficient consumption of gluten in the diet. Please see below section titled Gluten Challenge.

Indications for screening for celiac disease include those with symptoms concerning for celiac disease, as listed above. Additionally, high-risk groups for celiac disease should be screened regardless of symptoms and if symptoms develop or change. Unfortunately, there are no guidelines recommending timeframes for specific screening for every high-risk group for celiac disease. We generally screen patients at their entrance/diagnosis into a high-risk group and if symptoms change/develop.

Table 44.2 Specificity and sensitivity of various serologic tests in celiac disease

	Sensitivity	Specificity
TTG IgA	90–98	94–98
Endomysial IgA	85–98	97–100
Deamidated gliadin IgA	80–91	91–95
Deamidated gliadin IgG	88–95	86–98

Agardh 2007 [4], *Basso 2006* [5], *Hill 2005* [6], *Lewis 2010* [7]

Screening for celiac disease is performed with serum screening tests. A total serum IgA is obtained to rule out selective IgA deficiency and eliminate false negative interpretations of IgA-based celiac disease-specific serologies. The highest combined sensitivity and specificity test is IgA to tissue transglutaminase (TTG IgA). Endomysial antibody is also highly specific. In children younger than 2 years of age, endomysial IgA and TTG IgA may be less sensitive; therefore, it is recommended that deamidated gliadin IgG be obtained in children <2 years of age in addition to TTG IgA [1–3] (Table 44.2).

If screening testing is positive, or continued concern exists for celiac disease, patients should be referred to pediatric gastroenterology. It is important to continue gluten consumption in the diet until the patient is evaluated by a pediatric gastroenterologist who can discuss the risks, benefits, and alternatives of endoscopy and non-biopsy diagnosis of celiac disease with families. Additionally, it is important to remind families that testing including additional celiac disease-specific antibodies and endoscopy for evaluation of celiac disease is reliant on continued consumption of gluten in the diet. If patients are not consuming sufficient gluten, they may have false negative laboratory and endoscopy results, further complicating the diagnosis of celiac disease.

The North American Society for Pediatric Gastroenterology, Hepatology, and Nutrition (NASPGHAN) gold standard for celiac disease diagnosis is endoscopic confirmation with microscopic visualization of villus blunting, intraepithelial lymphocytosis

(>25 lymphocytes per 100 epithelial cells), and hyperplasia of the crypts [3]. Because celiac disease can be patchy, and to reduce likelihood of sampling error/increase yield of identifying celiac disease, it is recommended to obtain at least 4 biopsies from the distal duodenum and 1–2 biopsies from the duodenal bulb [3]. The scale by which the microscopic findings are evaluated was first described by Marsh in 1992 [8]. The Marsh scoring system from stage 0 (normal) to stage 3 (villus blunting) was modified by Oberhuaber et al. and is now widely used by pathologists to diagnose and stage pathologic findings in celiac disease [9]. Marsh scores of 2 and greater are considered diagnostic of celiac disease. Marsh scoring within marsh Stage 3 is subdivided on varying degrees of villus atrophy and denoted Marsh 3A, 3B, or 3C, with 3C being total villus atrophy. Severity of endoscopic findings may not correlate with symptom severity, and in many cases, children with minimal or no symptoms may have Marsh 3C findings. Visual findings are not always present on endoscopic evaluation but include scalloping or atrophy of duodenal folds, visualization of blunted areas, and nodularity of the duodenal bulb mucosa.

When pathology and serology do not agree, HLA typing can be helpful. HLA testing evaluates celiac disease susceptibility. If an individual does not carry the HLA subtypes responsible for celiac disease autoimmunity—HLADQ2 and DQ8—the likelihood of developing celiac disease approaches zero. HLA testing can be helpful in individuals who are already consuming a gluten-free (GF)diet; if no HLA Types consistent with celiac disease are present, this rules out celiac disease. About 50% of the population carries HLA DQ2 or DQ8, and therefore not everyone who is genetically susceptible to celiac disease will develop I, and therefore it is not helpful in establishing a diagnosis [10].

Non-biopsy-Based Diagnosis

Recently, the European Society for Pediatric Gastroenterology, Hepatology, and Nutrition (ESPGHAN) published and revised guidelines for non-endoscopic diagnosis of celiac disease in children [6]. By the ESPGHAN criteria, a child with an IgA TTG that is greater than 10 times the upper limit of normal and a positive endomysial antibody in a separate blood sample meets criteria for non-biopsy diagnosis. Accurate lab testing is imperative in non-biopsy diagnosis so the endomysial antibody testing must be completed from a separate blood sample to eliminate lab sample error. Previously, symptoms and HLA Testing were part of these non-biopsy-based diagnosis requirements but have since been removed in the most recent iteration of the ESPGHAN guidelines. In patients whose TTG does not meet these criteria, endoscopic biopsy is recommended [11].

The decision to undertake biopsy-based versus non-biopsy-based diagnosis for celiac disease should be a shared decision among providers and patients and their families. Important considerations include gold standard diagnostic techniques by which diagnosing physicians are bound, risk factors for anesthesia or family concern over anesthesia, importance, feasibility, and buy-in of making a significant dietary/lifestyle change without biopsy-based diagnosis, among many other factors related to the child's and family's preferences.

Gluten Challenge

In selected cases, if a gluten-free diet has previously been adopted or an individual is consuming a gluten-restricted diet, a gluten challenge becomes important for diagnostic accuracy, as intestinal healing can occur as quickly as 2 weeks after adopting a gluten-free diet. Singh et al. [12] suggested obtaining baseline serology followed by a minimum of 3–6 grams of gluten per day for over 12 weeks to optimize diagnostic accuracy for evaluation of celiac disease [12]. Increasing the dose of gluten further may improve diagnostic yield if tolerated, although in select cases a lower dose and shorter course (6–12 weeks) may be sufficient [12]. The gluten content of various foods has been estimated with 1 medium slice of bread estimated to have between 2 and 5 grams of gluten and four 2.5 inch square Graham crackers with 1.6 g gluten as examples of serving sizes [13]. In patients who are symptomatic with gluten challenge, shared decision-making should be utilized in order to discern balance between duration of gluten challenge and symptom severity.

High-Risk Groups for Celiac Disease

High-risk groups for celiac disease include a variety of diagnoses and disorders, in particular other autoimmune diseases. Both first- and second-degree relatives are at increased risk of celiac disease by approximately an eightfold and fivefold respective increased risk over the general population [14]. These groups should be evaluated with higher index of suspicion for celiac disease, and lower threshold for screening/repeated screening, and possibly endoscopy, than the general population (Table 44.3).

There are no current guidelines for ongoing screening or frequency of screening high-risk groups. However, it is recommended to screen first-degree relatives at the time of a child's diagnosis.

Table 44.3 High-Risk Groups for Celiac Disease

Autoimmune disease	Genetic disorders	Other risk groups
Type 1 diabetes mellitus	Trisomy 21	Selective IgA deficiency
Autoimmune thyroid disease (Hashimoto's and grave's disease)	Williams syndrome	First-degree relatives
Addison's disease	Turner's syndrome	Second-degree relatives
Alopecia areata		
Pernicious anemia		
Autoimmune thrombocytopenia		
Sarcoidosis		
Autoimmune hepatitis		
Primary biliary cirrhosis		

Selective IgA Deficiency

Celiac disease is found with higher prevalence in Selective IgA deficiency, making it another high-risk group for celiac disease which deserves special discussion. Serum-based testing for celiac disease relies on sufficient levels of serum IgA. In IgA-deficient patients, celiac disease screening relies on IgG-based testing. However, testing with IgG to TTG and DGP is less sensitive and specific than their IgA-based counterparts. Therefore, if concern continues to exist for celiac disease in an IgA-deficient individual, endoscopy should be undertaken [2].

With positive screening or high index of suspicion for celiac disease, referrals should be placed to pediatric gastroenterology while encouraging the patient to continue the consumption of gluten. Once that diagnosis is confirmed, referral to a registered dietitian for formal gluten-free diet education is paramount in equipping families with the management skills for success. Websites geared toward celiac disease education are a good resource for finding registered dietitians. As is noted below, gluten-free diet can be very difficult to navigate without the support and education provided by registered dietitians.

Treatment of Celiac Disease

Gluten-Free Diet-Basics

The only treatment for celiac disease remains a strict GF diet. All patients should be referred to a dietitian knowledgeable about celiac disease for thorough education on the gluten-free diet. This is particularly important in pediatrics, as both patients and families may need education and counseling tailored to the child's age and developmental level. Education can be repeated as needed, especially for children diagnosed at an early age as they become more independent. In addition to diet implementation, the overall lifestyle changes and awareness required for celiac disease are often different from those needed for patients with non-celiac gluten sensitivity. The goal of the GF diet is to achieve intestinal healing and minimize the risk of long-term complications.

Physicians and dietitians play an important role in educating and empowering patients and families to support their children in following a lifelong GF diet. At the time of diagnosis, the registered dietitian provides dietary counseling and reviews age-appropriate needs for calcium/Vitamin D and other micronutrient supplementation as needed. At follow-up visits, the dietitian assesses symptoms and diet and evaluates compliance and coping. Together, the goal is to provide care for the child and family that promotes age-appropriate growth and development while maintaining a careful GF diet.

The GF diet involves avoidance of wheat, rye, barley, and all their derivatives. While the diet avoids only three grains, these three—and wheat most commonly—are used in the production of many food and non-food items in the United States. This makes compliance with a strict GF diet more complicated (Table 44.4).

Table 44.4 Gluten-containing grains and their derivatives

Wheat	Barley	Rye
Farina	Malt[b]	Secale cereale
Tabbouleh	Malt flavoring	
Couscous	Malt extract	
Graham	Malt syrup	
Spelt	Malt vinegar	
Einkorn	Brewer's yeast	
Farro	Hordeum vulgare	
Durum		
Semolina		
Triticale		
Untested oats		
Kamut		
Udon		
Seitan		
Matzo		
Triticum		
Wheat starch[a]		

[a]Certified GF wheat starch is considered safe on a GF diet. However, eating it can feel counterintuitive and some prefer to avoid

[b]Although they contain the word "malt," the ingredients maltodextrin and maltose are considered GF [15]

Table 44.5 Naturally gluten-free alternatives

Corn	Millet	Nuts	Cassava
Rice	Teff	Seeds	Amaranth
Tapioca	Quinoa	Potatoes	Beans
Buckwheat	Wild rice	Tested GF oats	Soy

In their natural, unprocessed form, all fruits, vegetables, meats, legumes, and milk are GF. Families are encouraged to incorporate fresh fruits, vegetables, and meats into their child's diet as appropriate. Consumption of a variety of naturally GF whole grains is also encouraged. The GF diet can present a challenge to add diversity to the diet through addition of less traditional GF grains, rather than solely relying on processed GF alternatives, especially as early evidence suggests this diversity may contribute to a more robust microbiome [16] (Table 44.5).

Higher degrees of processing increase the likelihood that gluten could have been introduced. Processed and packaged foods have food labels that provide critical information about the product. Providers should be confident in educating patients and families on how to make decisions based on this information.

Gluten-Free Food Labels

The Food and Drug Administration (FDA) regulates most foods including fruits, vegetables, and packaged products. According to the FDA, GF products cannot contain wheat, rye, barley, or ingredients derived from these grains, unless they have been specially processed to remove gluten [17]. In this case, the quantity of gluten must be less than 20 parts per million, which is the equivalent of 20 milligrams per kilogram. To consume an amount of gluten that exceeds the amount considered safe, an individual would need to eat 35 servings of a food in which 1 serving contained <20 ppm gluten.

In August 2013 and August 2020, the FDA set out guidelines for the definition of GF and the labeling of products as GF [18]. Foods labeled as "gluten free," "free of gluten," "without gluten," and "no gluten" must meet these criteria. Products with statements like "made with no gluten-containing ingredients" are not required to meet the FDA GF requirements. Meat, dairy, and poultry products are regulated by the United States Department of Agriculture (USDA). The USDA does not have its own definition of GF but requires manufacturers to comply with the FDA guidelines.

Gluten-free labeling is voluntary. As a result, consumers encounter a variety of terminology which can be categorized into three groups. First are products that are "certified gluten-free," meaning they undergo third-party verification of a manufacturer's claim. Some such programs have GF cutoffs of 10 ppm gluten, which goes beyond the FDA requirements [19]. These programs may rely on analytical methods that were not available at the time of the release of the FDA regulations. Second, products may simply carry a "gluten-free" claim. These products do not necessarily have to be tested for gluten by the manufacturer but must meet the FDA definition of <20 ppm gluten. Finally, products may be GF but not labeled as such. If a product is labeled GF, whether certified or not, it is safe to consume on a strict GF diet for celiac disease (Table 44.6).

A more strategic approach is needed when making decisions on foods not labeled GF. First, patients and families should be counseled to read the ingredients list. If there are no gluten-containing ingredients or questionable gluten-containing ingredients, they consider the following 2 questions. First, does the manufacturer make other products that are labeled GF? If so, the lack of a GF claim on this product may suggest a higher risk of cross-contamination. Second, are any ingredients high risk for cross-contamination? High-risk ingredients may include ingredients made from grains, legumes, seeds, or beans, especially if milled into flours as studies have shown that naturally gluten-free

Table 44.6 Ingredients of concern if product not labeled GF

Natural flavor	Wheatgrass	Yeast extract
Modified food starch	Starch	Dextrin
Oat	Lentil	

flours are at risk for gluten contamination, especially those with higher fiber [20]. It is preferred to choose a food labeled GF if it contains a high-risk ingredient. When in doubt, patients or families can contact the manufacturer to confirm gluten content or risk.

There are two high-risk whole food ingredients that should be avoided unless a product is labeled GF: oats and lentils. Both are naturally GF but carry a high risk of cross-contact with wheat due to crop rotation, shared manufacturing equipment and other processing practices [21]. As rich sources of vitamins, minerals, fiber, and phytonutrients, the goal is to include oats and lentils in a GF diet if they have been verified to be GF. The GF diet can feel restrictive without the burden of further unnecessary eliminations.

With growing interest in fermented foods, patients and families may have questions about gluten content in products like fermented sourdough breads or miso. Fermentation and hydrolysis are not considered reliable methods to remove gluten [22]. Currently, available methods to evaluate gluten may not be accurate when testing fermented foods, including beer, yogurt, and sourdough bread. Similarly, they are not reliable when evaluating hydrolyzed products, such as those containing hydrolyzed wheat protein. It is recommended to avoid all fermented and hydrolyzed products that have gluten-containing ingredients.

Allergen Labeling

An additional complication with label reading is the fact that wheat—unlike the other gluten-containing grains—is specifically recognized by The Food Allergen Labeling and Consumer Protection Act (FALCPA) of 2004. As of 2024, this legislation requires that any of the nine major food allergens be clearly identified on a product's label. Patients and families following a GF diet should continue to avoid any product that includes wheat but should be mindful that barley and rye ingredients will never be identified with these allergen-specific labeling requirements. Put simply, "wheat free" is not the same as GF.

Moreover, there is a related type of allergen labeling called allergen advisories that may be less straightforward to interpret. The use of allergen advisory statements such as "made in a facility that processes wheat" or "may contain wheat" is voluntary. A product can have both a voluntary allergen advisory and a voluntary GF claim. If a product has both labels, the product is required to meet the definition of GF as established by the FDA and is acceptable to consume. If a product is not labeled GF and has a voluntary allergen advisory regarding wheat, it is recommended to select an alternative product. While allergen disclaimers may be useful in quickly identifying gluten-containing products, they are of limited help in determining if a product is truly GF.

Cross Contamination

Avoiding cross-contamination or cross-contact is a critical part of treatment for celiac disease. Cross contact and cross contamination are terms often used interchangeably to describe the unavoidable transfer of gluten to a GF food because of physical contact.

Patients managing celiac disease may require a higher level of lifestyle changes than those managing non-celiac gluten sensitivity. Those without celiac disease may not be concerned about low levels of gluten ingestion through cross-contamination. However, for those with celiac disease, strict avoidance of gluten even in minuscule amounts is imperative.

As gluten is a physical food particle, it is not impacted by antibacterial cleaning methods. This means that if a person is trying to clean a surface or their hands to remove gluten residue, antibacterial agents are not effective compared to more traditional cleaning methods involving soap, water, and physical scrubbing. Even with proper washing techniques certain household items are difficult to thoroughly clean. Porous surfaces or those that become scratched—like colanders, cutting boards, and well-worn nonstick pans—are likely to trap gluten particles. Consequently, patients with celiac disease should use dedicated GF versions of these items (Table 44.7).

Table 44.7 Common areas of cross-contamination

Condiments with non-squeeze tops including mayonnaise, butter, nut butters, jelly, cream cheese	Shelf with gluten foods stored above	Air fryer	Fryer/fryer basket/frying oil
Cutting board	Colander	Sifter	Grill
Griddle	Waffle iron	Toaster	Wooden utensils
Wooden rolling pin			

Some families opt to transition the entire household to adhere to GF standards. While this is an option, it involves significant time, energy, and money. Other families seek to manage gluten-containing diets alongside the dedicated GF diet for the individual with celiac disease. For example, dedicated GF items in the kitchen can be managed through color-coding and labeling to clearly identify the GF items that cannot be cross-contaminated. The exact approach should be tailored to each family. Families can be reassured that with proper precautions, a shared GF household and kitchen can still be a safe place to prepare GF foods.

Similar proactive strategies are necessary for managing meals outside the home. When a child following a GF diet attends school, families must be aware of the options available for mealtime accommodations and verify that staff members can meet the child's needs. Schools that participate in the National School Lunch Program and the School Breakfast Program are required by federal law to make necessary accommodations for a child because of disability [23]. Celiac disease is considered a disability under the Americans with Disabilities Act. However, if the child attends a private institution or any type of school that is not covered by this federal legislation, dietary accommodations may not be accommodated. Parents should be familiar with their child's rights at any type of school and seek collaborative discussion with administrators. For example, some families may benefit from requesting implementation of a Section 504 plan under the Rehabilitation Act of 1973. This is a common and federally recognized method of detailing the accommodations needed to remove barriers to learning in the school environment, such as the need for a GF diet [24].

Families may simply prefer to pack GF lunches and snacks from home. However, they must also establish plans for situations like field trips, birthdays, holiday celebrations, class parties, and other snacks. Teacher awareness and support are important as they can also discourage the sharing of food items between students. This support is crucially strengthened through the proactive engagement and communication of patient's families. Families may reach out to their managing physician for assistance completing necessary forms required by the school to make the needed accommodations.

When eating out, GF families may encounter three different types of restaurants: those that are dedicated GF, those with GF menus or items labeled GF, and those without any mention of gluten. Dedicated GF restaurants are rare, unevenly distributed geographically, and may be more costly to run because of the strict demands placed on ingredient orders. This means many families will find themselves unable to access these establishments because of distance, cost, or both.

Unable to access dedicated GF restaurants reliably. Patients with celiac disease and their families need education and support for self-advocacy when eating out, even if GF items are identified. When ordering an item identified as GF, an individual should ask targeted questions about food preparation and handling methods to help ensure that cross-contamination is avoided. Questions that relate to the preparation of a specific product may be more productive than questions on general policy, as staff familiarity with the needs of a strict GF diet can vary. For example, when ordering a GF pasta, a parent may verify that the water used to boil the pasta is fresh or used only for GF pasta and that clean or dedicated GF colanders and utensils are used to prepare it. If ordering French fries or tortilla chips labeled GF, an individual should ask what other foods are fried in the same oil.

Recently gluten detection devices have entered the market in the United States. They are marketed to individuals who want to test their foods if concerned about accidental exposure [25].

Various concerns have been raised about the use of sensors including risk for sampling error and incorrect use [26]. Currently, the American College of Gastroenterology recommends against the use of these devices as it's not clear if they provide reliable results, whether any gluten detected has clinical significance or if use improves an individual's quality of life or compliance with the diet [3].

As illustrated by the examples in this chapter, a GF diet must avoid both intentional and unintentional gluten ingestion. It is important here to highlight that gluten can also be found in products not typically thought of as food. These include medications, supplements, cosmetic products used in or around the mouth, toothpaste, lozenges, chewing gum, and more. One common non-food source of gluten in many households is pet food. It may be necessary to recognize whether family pets are consuming gluten to make strategic decisions about how patients are involved in caring for the pet. In some cases, it may be preferable to remove the source of gluten through a change in the animal's food, especially if the patient enjoys licks from their pet on their hands or face.

As they gain knowledge of the GF diet, patients and families may also have questions about gluten absorption through the skin. Physical contact with gluten to the skin does not trigger the autoimmune response in celiac disease. However, because gluten is present in certain hair products, lotions, and other cosmetics, there is a risk for accidental ingestion, and many find it easier to choose a GF version of these products. However, with these choices, it is important for families to note that the use of GF claims on cosmetic products is not regulated by the FDA.

Symptom tracking should not be used as a method of evaluating whether a certain choice was "safe". For example, if a child doesn't feel sick after eating French fries that were knowingly cross-contaminated, that does not mean choosing those French fries again is the safe choice. Some individuals with celiac disease are asymptomatic. Sometimes this may lead them to disregard concerns for cross-contamination because they do not experience immediate negative physical side effects. However, the risks of damage to the intestinal villi are the same, regardless of the degree of outwardly observable physical symptoms.

Nutritional, Financial, and Social Costs of the Gluten-Free Diet

Even as patients and their families attain understanding of the GF diet, they must also consider at least three inherent costs associated with its implementation: nutritional, financial, and social.

Nutritional Cost

Certain nutrient deficiencies may be more common in celiac disease. The explanation is twofold. First, at the time of diagnosis, the inherent intestinal damage to villi has already comprised the body's ability to absorb the nutrients consumed. Second, with the dietary elimination of gluten, there comes an attendant risk of reduction in key nutrients.

Common deficiencies at the time of diagnosis include iron, folate, Vitamin B12, Vitamin D, zinc, and magnesium [27]. Iron deficiency anemia is the most common nutritional-related deficiency associated with celiac disease [27]. However, it generally resolves with the GF diet (Table 44.8).

Deficiencies may persist despite good dietary adherence; one review found that individuals with celiac disease on the GF diet for 2 years had documented deficiencies in iron, zinc, Vitamin D, folic acid, magnesium, and calcium [28]. Wheat, rye, and barley and products made with these grains are often rich sources of B vitamins, iron, zinc, and fiber. Even refined products made of these grains may be good sources of these nutrients through the process of enrichment or fortification. Enrichment and fortification have been part of the US food industry since the 1940s when Vitamin D, iodine, B vitamins, folic acid, and iron were added to foods to address prevalent deficiencies in the population. Commonly fortified foods include flour, bread, rice, noodles, milk, plant-based milk, eggs, and salt [29].

Enriched and fortified foods continue to provide an important source of key nutrients. Fortified and enriched products were found to provide>45% of intake of vitamin B1 (thiamin) and folate and > 25% of niacin and iron in US residents >/= 2 years of

Table 44.8 Common nutrients of concern, signs of deficiency and GF food sources

Nutrient of concern [32]	Signs of deficiency	GF food sources
Calcium [33]	Fractures Osteoporosis Osteopenia Tooth decay Short stature (in children)	Yogurt Calcium-fortified orange juice Cheese Sardines Milk Fortified nondairy milk
Iron [34]	Iron deficiency anemia Fatigue/weakness Difficulty concentrating Shortness of breath Impaired cognitive function	Fortified GF breakfast cereal Oysters White beans Beef liver
Magnesium [35]	Poor appetite Fatigue/weakness Muscle tingling/cramps Abnormal heart rhythm	Pumpkin seeds Chia seeds Almonds Spinach, boiled Soy milk
Zinc [36]	Slow growth in infants Delayed puberty Hair loss Skin sores Loss of appetite Diarrhea Weight loss Slow wound healing Decreased sense of taste and smell	Oysters Beef Crab Fortified GF breakfast cereal GF oats Pumpkin seeds
Vitamin B12 [37]	Anxiety/depression (related to vitamin deficiency) Megaloblastic anemia Pernicious anemia Sore, red tongue Anorexia Low blood pressure	Beef liver Clams Oysters Nutritional yeast Salmon Tuna Ground beef Milk Yogurt

(continued)

Table 44.8 (continued)

Nutrient of concern [32]	Signs of deficiency	GF food sources
Folate/folic acid [38]	Megaloblastic anemia Anxiety/depression related to vitamin deficiency Sores on mouth/tongue Increased risk of neural tube defects (in pregnancy)	Beef liver Spinach, boiled Black-eyed peas Fortified GF breakfast cereal
Vitamin D [39]	Osteoporosis Osteomalacia Rickets	Cod liver oil Trout Salmon Mushrooms exposed to UV light

age [30]. Even with fortification, enrichment, and dietary supplementation, many individuals still consumed less than the estimated average requirement (EAR) for calcium, vitamin D, and potassium [30]. The EAR is the amount estimated to meet the needs of half of healthy individuals of a specific age. When consuming only naturally occurring sources of these nutrients a significant number of participants consumed less than the Estimated Average Requirement for age [30].

Fortification and enrichment are not mandatory in the United States, including in GF products. A study in the UK found that <30% of GF breads were fortified [31].

There are multiple ways that the risk for nutritional deficiencies can be reduced. First is compliance with the GF diet to promote intestinal healing. At the time of diagnosis, it is recommended that patients take a daily GF multivitamin that contains B vitamins (thiamin, riboflavin, B12), iron, and zinc for at least 3–6 months as the intestines heal. Patients and families should look for a supplement that is third-party verified GF and contains at least 50% of the Daily Recommended Intakes (DRI) for B vitamins based on the patient's age.

The form of vitamin preparation is important to consider when recommending a micronutrient supplement. Iron overdose was a leading cause of accidental overdose death in children 30 years ago [40]. Thankfully that statistic has improved, in part with the exclusion of iron in gummy multivitamins, which are more easily mistaken as candy. Of note, gummy vitamins may also be lower in B vitamins. Consequently, more robust supplementation can often be found in chewable tablet or liquid formulations unless the child is capable of swallowing tablets or capsules.

Inadequate calcium and Vitamin D are also concerns. Children with celiac disease may experience reduced bone mineral density. Studies have shown improved BMD in as little as 6 months with GF diet and supplementation of calcium and Vitamin D as it may not always normalize with diet alone [41]. Multivitamins do not contain calcium in sufficient quantities to make them adequate sources of calcium supplementation. If an individual does not consume sufficient calcium in their diet, a separate calcium supplement may be needed.

Calcium supplementation above recommended amounts, however, is not recommended. Calcium is best absorbed in small amounts, for children typically up to 200–300 mg per dose/instance of consumption. If more than this is needed daily, supplements should be divided [42]. Calcium carbonate or calcium citrate are the most common forms of calcium supplements available. Calcium citrate is preferred if the child is also taking any acid-suppressing medication [33]. Otherwise, families should be counseled to give the calcium supplement with meals. To facilitate these strategic decisions, dietitians can help a patient and their family assess the usual intake of calcium and then utilize calcium supplements as needed to bridge any deficits (Table 44.9).

Table 44.9 Recommended dietary allowances (RDAs) for Calcium [43]

Age	Male	Female
0–6 months	200 mg	200 mg
7–12 months	260 mg	260 mg
1–3 years	700 mg	700 mg
4–8 years	1000 mg	1000 mg
9–13 years	1300 mg	1300 mg
14–18 years	1300 mg	1300 mg

Lactase is the enzyme responsible for digestion of lactose, and its activity is often reduced when the small bowel is damaged causing secondary lactose intolerance. Foods naturally rich in calcium such as milk, yogurt, and cheese may cause GI upset in some individuals with celiac disease at the time of diagnosis. Compliance with the GF diet can reduce this intolerance over time. In the meantime, patients can opt to avoid lactose, choose lower lactose foods, or take over-the-counter lactase enzymes when consuming foods with lactose.

As Vitamin D is required for calcium to be absorbed in the GI tract, many supplements contain both calcium and Vitamin D [39]. Vitamin D is essential in bone mineralization, and vitamin D deficiency is more common in individuals with celiac disease [44]. Tailored vitamin D supplementation should be recommended based on evaluation of a child's laboratory values and age.

This evaluation—and the potential need for long-term supplementation—should be discussed with the patient's provider or dietitian and may depend on the variety of their baseline intake, reliance on processed GF alternatives, and laboratory values.

When an individual starts consuming GF alternatives, they may quickly recognize the role of gluten as both a culinary and nutritional factor in grain-based products. One of the most recognizable traits is that gluten provides elasticity and fluffiness to food [45]. A simple illustration is the difference in texture between a slice of GF bread—smaller, dense, and likely to crack and crumble—and a softer, lighter slice of gluten-containing bread. Many naturally GF starch-based staples in international cuisines are unleavened, such as crepes, injera, socca, dosa, and tortilla.

In efforts to mimic the functional role of gluten, manufacturers include alternative protein sources, fiber, hydrocolloids (gums), or emulsifiers [46]. Other ingredients may also change to improve taste and mouthfeel, with additional nutritional implications. GF products are generally higher in fat, carbohydrates, and sodium and lower in protein and fiber than their gluten-containing counterparts [47]. These differences may be of particular importance in individuals who have both celiac disease and type 1 diabetes.

Financial Cost

A patient with celiac disease has no treatment choice besides the GF diet at this time. This treatment comes at a price. A recent study found that the cost of GF products is 183% greater than the cost of their gluten-containing equivalents [48]. While some naturally GF alternatives like potatoes and corn may be affordable and accessible, many others—such as millet and teff—are not mainstream in the US and would require individuals to have strong culinary skills and knowledge to use them in ways that mimic common staples like bread, pasta, and crackers. Availability of GF alternatives also varies regionally with the highest availability on the coasts and online [48].

Some hospitals have successfully started initiatives that support patients and families in managing diet-related health conditions. For example, some have launched food pantries that include dedicated areas for GF foods so those with celiac disease have increased access [49].

The overall economic burden of the GF diet on diet adherence is not well understood currently.

Social Cost

The cultural, emotional, and psychological effects of food inherently carry a social impact for a person following a GF diet. Compliance can be difficult as the American diet relies heavily on gluten-containing products and packaged foods. Families may struggle to find grocery stores with the GF products they need or may find it difficult to afford these products given the elevated costs. Similarly, families who enjoy eating outside the home may struggle to navigate the variances in restaurant menus and practices. Added to these challenges regarding practical access to the GF diet is the problem that children feel various psychological barriers to eating differently from their peers [50, 51]. Providers need to be knowledgeable about the complex impact of the GF diet on a child's quality of life. Children and families need support to help them adapt to the lifestyle change. In fact, the adaptive or maladaptive strategies they use are associated with higher and lower quality of life [52, 53].

Children reported the highest social pressure in the school environment [54]. There is evidence that boys and girls often take different approaches in managing the GF diet. Boys often asked for more support to change their environment and did not embrace celiac disease as part of their social identity. Girls were more likely to take an active role in educating others about the diet and identified as being a "celiac" [55]. Many felt they were a burden or an outsider and that their GF diet limited daily life. Clinicians should be mindful of these differences, their social impact, and potential effect on dietary adherence when counseling in follow-up visits.

When asked about where they have the highest compliance with the GF diet, children and adolescents reported best adherence at home and school and lower compliance at social events [54]. Eating outside the home requires others responsible for food preparation to have adequate knowledge of the GF diet. When asked what could help improve adherence to the GF diet, the most common responses were improved variety and taste of GF foods, increased availability of GF foods, decreased cost of GF foods and improved education for schools and restaurants [54]. These responses highlight that supporting a patient's compliance with the GF diet requires comprehensive efforts from the medical community outside the exam room through community engagement and policy legislation (Table 44.10).

Parents play a vital role in the implementation of the GF diet, which brings its own psychological burden. For example, one study found higher levels of parenting stress among parents of children with celiac disease [56].

While a strict GF diet is the recommended treatment for celiac disease, studies have also shown that hyper-vigilance with the diet lowers quality of life [57]. Researchers highlight the need for balancing vigilance with social and emotional well-being.

With a goal of patient and family-centered care, clinicians should be aware and empathetic to the social challenges that arise

Table 44.10 A sample of quotations from survey respondents regarding positive and negative effects of a GF diet [54]

Positive effects of a GF diet	Negative effects of a gluten-free diet
"He feels so much better and is growing and looking well."	"We will not eat at restaurants because we do not want to put our child's health in the hands of a stranger."
"Our son seems to be much healthier than other kids. Sick less often. Also seems to be stronger and bigger and faster than other kids."	"Not very many items on gluten-free menus cater to children. Most often they are geared for adults."
	"Kids bully those who are different."
	"I get embarrassed because I have to eat different food at hockey tournaments and parties."
	"Religion—I am Catholic and allergic to the host." (bread or wafer consecrated in the Eucharist)

for both parents and children when embarking on a GF diet. Care teams can strive to support patients and families in the following areas that have been shown to improve dietary adherence: understanding the GF diet, feeling confident in following the diet outside the home, supporting membership in a celiac support group and resiliency in following the diet despite changes in stress or mood [50].

After Adopting the Gluten-Free Diet

Physicians should have close follow-up for their pediatric patients with celiac disease, especially following diagnosis. Celiac disease-specific antibodies are monitored every 3–6 months until normalized (Table 44.11). Ranges of 30–80% normalize at 2 years after diagnosis; however, in patients who have extremely elevated titers at diagnosis, it can take longer for normalization of these titers. The small intestine can heal fairy quickly in patients adhering strictly to a GF diet. Annually, physicians should monitor celiac disease antibodies, complete blood count, vitamin D, and thyroid screening. In patients whose titers do not normalize, he gluten-free diet should be reviewed with a registered dietitian.

Table 44.11 Recommended Laboratory Monitoring: (Adapted from NASP-GHAN Pediatric Guidelines)

Parameter	At diagnosis	Follow up (every 3–6 months until symptom resolution)	Stable patient on GF diet after titers normalize/symptom resolution
Celiac disease serology	X	X	Annual
Complete blood count	X	Optional/PRN	Optional/PRN
Hepatic panel	X	Optional/PRN	Optional/PRN
Vitamin D	X	Optional/PRN	Annual
Iron panel	X	Optional/PRN	Optional/PRN
Thyroid screening (TSH/free T4)	X	Optional/PRN	Annual
Calcium	X	Optional/PRN	Optional/PRN
B vitamins (folate, B12)	Optional/PRN	Optional/PRN	Optional/PRN
Zinc	Optional/PRN	Optional/PRN	Optional/PRN
Hgb A1C/ diabetes counseling	Optional/PRN	Optional/PRN	Optional/PRN

Optional/PRN pending dietary history, previous abnormal labs, and ongoing need

Additionally, if despite this, the patient's labs still display celiac disease autoimmunity, repeat endoscopy is recommended. In some patients, normalized titers may not indicate intestinal healing; and similarly, persistent elevation of celiac disease-specific autoantibodies may not correlate to ongoing mucosal injury [58].

The Role of Repeat Endoscopy

The role of follow-up biopsy in patients adhering to a gluten-free diet is controversial. NASPGHAN guidelines do not suggest repeat endoscopy in all celiac disease patients. However, celiac disease-specific antibody normalization may not always indicate mucosal healing. We recommended repeat intestinal biopsy in patients who have persistent symptoms or in whom celiac disease-specific serology is not normalizing as expected or is increasing despite reported adherence to gluten-free diet, or other continued concerns such as delayed growth/timing with puberty.

References

1. Wyllie R, Hyams JS, Kay M. Pediatric gastrointestinal and liver disease, Celiac disease. 5th ed; 2016. p. 395–404.
2. Hill ID, Fasano A, Guandalini S, Hoffenberg E, Levy J, Reilly N, Verma R. NASPGHAN clinical report on the diagnosis and treatment of gluten-related disorders. JPGN Rep. 2016;63(1):156.
3. Rubio-Tapia A, Hill ID, Semrad C, Kelly CP, Greer KB, Limketkai BN, Lebwohl B. American college of gastroenterology guidelines update: diagnosis and management of celiac disease. Am J Gastroenterol. 2023;118(1):59–76.
4. Agardh D. Antibodies against synthetic deamidated gliadin peptides and tissue transglutaminase for the identification of childhood celiac disease. Clin Gastroenterol Hepatol. 2007;5:1276.
5. Basso D, Guariso G, Fasolo M, et al. A new indirect chemiluminescent immunoassay to measure anti-tissue transglutaminase antibodies. J Pediatr Gastroenterol Nutr. 2006;43:613.
6. Hill ID. What are the sensitivity and specificity of serologic tests for celiac disease? Do sensitivity and specificity vary in different populations? Gastroenterology. 2005;128(4 Suppl 1):S2.
7. Lewis NR, Scott BB. Meta-analysis: deamidated gliadin peptide antibody and tissue transglutaminase antibody compared as screening tests for coeliac disease. Aliment Pharmacol Ther. 2010;31:73.
8. Marsh MN. Gluten, major histocompatibility complex, and the small intestine. A molecular and immunobiologic approach to the spectrum of gluten sensitivity ("celiac sprue"). Gastroenterology. 1992;102:330–54.
9. Oberhuber G, Granditsch G, Vogelsang H. The histopathology of coeliac disease: time for a standardized report scheme for pathologists. Eur J Gastroenterol Hepatol. 1999;11:1185–94.
10. Rostom A, Murray JA, Kagnoff MF. Medical position statement on celiac disease. Gastroenterology. 2006;131(6):1977–80.
11. Husby S, Koletzko S, Korponay-Szabó I, Kurppa K, Luisa Mearin M, Ribes-Koninckx C, Shamir R, Troncone R, Auricchio R, Castillejo G, Christensen R, Dolinsek R, Gillett P, Hróbjartsson A, Koltai T, Maki M, Mai Nielsen S, Popp A, Størdal K, Werkstetter K, Wessels M. J Pediatr Gastroenterol Nutr. 2020;70(1):141–15.

12. Singh A, Singh A, Kleinhenz J, Brill H, Fahey L, Silvester JA, Sparks B, Verma R, Lee D. A clinican's guide to gluten challenge. JPGN. 2023;77(6):698–702.
13. https://pubmed.ncbi.nlm.nih.gov/37608439/
14. Fasano A, et al. Arch of Intern Med. 2003;163:286–92.
15. FAQ [Internet]. GIG® Gluten Intolerance Group®. Available from: https://gluten.org/community/faq/
16. Lee-Sarwar KA, et al. Diversifying your diet portfolio: potential impacts of dietary diversity on the gut microbiome and human health. Am J Clin Nutr. 116(4):844–5.
17. Office of the Commissioner. "Gluten-free" now means what it says [internet]. U.S. Food and Drug Administration. 2019. Available from: https://www.fda.gov/consumers/consumer-updates/gluten-free-means-what-it-says.
18. Center for Food Safety and Applied Nutrition. Questions and answers on the gluten-free food labeling final rule [internet]. U.S. Food and Drug Administration. 2019. Available from: https://www.fda.gov/food/food-labeling-nutrition/questions-and-answers-gluten-free-food-labeling-final-rule.
19. About Us [Internet]. Gluten-Free Certification Organization. Available from: https://gfco.org/about-us/.
20. Koerner TB, Cleroux C, Poirier C, Cantin I, La Vieille S, Hayward S, et al. Gluten contamination of naturally gluten-free flours and starches used by Canadians with celiac disease. Food Addit Contam Part A. 2013;30(12):2017–21.
21. Thompson T, Lyons TB, Keller A. Lentils and gluten cross contact. Front Nutr. 2022;29:9.
22. Center for Food Safety and Applied Nutrition. Questions and answers on the gluten-free food labeling final rule [internet]. U.S. Food and Drug Administration; 2019. Available from: https://www.fda.gov/food/food-labeling-nutrition/questions-and-answers-gluten-free-food-labeling-final-rule
23. School Meals FAQs | USDA-FNS [Internet]. www.fns.usda.gov. 2019. Available from: https://www.fns.usda.gov/cn/school-meals-faqs.
24. Back-to-School and 504 Plan Guide [Internet]. Celiac Disease Foundation. Available from: https://celiac.org/about-celiac-disease/celiac-disease-in-children/504-plan/.
25. EZ Gluten—Gluten Testing—Food Testing [Internet]. ezgluten.com. Available from: https://ezgluten.com/.
26. Marić A, Scherf KA. A portable gluten sensor for celiac disease patients may not always be reliable depending on the food and the user. Front Nutr [Internet]. 2021;8:712992. [cited 2022 Jan 16]; Available from: https://pubmed.ncbi.nlm.nih.gov/34355010/
27. Caruso R, Pallone F, Stasi E, Romeo S, Monteleone G. Appropriate nutrient supplementation in celiac disease. Ann Med. 2013;45(8):522–31.

28. Rondanelli F, Gasparri P, Naso P, et al. Micronutrients dietary supplementation advices for celiac patients on long-term gluten-free diet with good compliance: a review. Medicina. 2019;55(7):337.
29. Overview of food fortification in the United States and Canada [internet]. Nih.gov. National Academies Press (US); 2015. Available from: https://www.ncbi.nlm.nih.gov/books/NBK208880/.
30. Fulgoni VL, Keast DR, Bailey RL, Dwyer J. Foods, fortificants, and supplements: where do Americans get their nutrients? J Nutr [Internet]. 2011;141(10):1847–54. Available from: https://academic.oup.com/jn/article/141/10/1847/4630521
31. Allen B, Orfila C. The availability and nutritional adequacy of gluten-free bread and pasta. Nutrients. 2018;10(10):1370.
32. Common nutritional deficiencies in people with celiac disease [internet]. wwwbidmcorg 2022. Available from: https://www.bidmc.org/centers-and-departments/digestive-disease-center/services-and-programs/celiac-center/celiacnow/nutrition-and-the-gluten-free-diet/nutritional-considerations-on-the-gluten-free-diet/common-nutritional-deficiencies-in-people-with-celiac-disease.
33. National Institutes of Health. Office of Dietary Supplements – Calcium [Internet]. Nih.gov. 2022. Available from: https://ods.od.nih.gov/factsheets/Calcium-HealthProfessional/.
34. National Institutes of Health. Office of Dietary Supplements – Iron [Internet]. NIH 2022. Available from: https://ods.od.nih.gov/factsheets/Iron-HealthProfessional.
35. National Institutes of Health. Office of dietary supplements – Magnesium [internet]. National Institutes of Health 2022. Available from: https://ods.od.nih.gov/factsheets/Magnesium-HealthProfessional/.
36. National Institutes of Health. Office of Dietary Supplements – Zinc [internet]. Nih.gov. National Institutes of Health; 2022. Available from: https://ods.od.nih.gov/factsheets/Zinc-HealthProfessional/.
37. National Institutes of Health. Office of Dietary Supplements – Vitamin B12 [internet]. Nihgov 2024. Available from: https://ods.od.nih.gov/factsheets/VitaminB12-HealthProfessional/.
38. National Institutes of Health. Office of Dietary Supplements – Folate [internet]. Nih.gov. National Institutes of Health; 2022. Available from: https://ods.od.nih.gov/factsheets/Folate-HealthProfessional/.
39. National Institutes of Health. Vitamin D [internet]. National Institutes of Health 2023. Available from: https://ods.od.nih.gov/factsheets/VitaminD-HealthProfessional/.
40. Iron Poisoning [Internet]. www.poison.org. Available from: https://www.poison.org/articles/iron-poisoning.
41. Gerenli N, Dursun F, Çeltik C, Kırmızıbekmez H. Significant improvement in bone mineral density in pediatric celiac disease: even at six months with gluten-free diet. J Pediatr Endocrinol Metab. 2020;34(3):341–8.

42. Bone Health and Osteoporosis Foundation. Calcium/vitamin D requirements, recommended foods & supplements [internet]. Bone Health & Osteoporosis Foundation 2023. Available from: https://www.bonehealthandosteoporosis.org/patients/treatment/calciumvitamin-d/.
43. Institute of Medicine (US) Committee to Review Dietary Reference Intakes for Vitamin D and Calcium; Ross AC, Taylor CL, Yaktine AL, et al. Dietary reference intakes for adequacy: calcium and vitamin D [Internet]. Nih.gov. National Academies Press (US); 2011. Available from: https://www.ncbi.nlm.nih.gov/books/NBK56056/.
44. Lungaro L, Manza F, Costanzini A, Barbalinardo M, Gentili D, Caputo F, et al. Osteoporosis and celiac disease: updates and hidden pitfalls. Nutrients. 2023;15(5):1089-9.
45. Li Y, Zheng W, Xue L, Han W, Shen J, Lin Q, et al. The role of gluten in food products and dietary restriction: exploring the potential for restoring immune tolerance. Foods [Internet]. 2023;12(22):4179-9. Available from: https://www.ncbi.nlm.nih.gov/pmc/articles/PMC10670377/
46. El Khoury D, Balfour-Ducharme S, Joye IJ. A review on the gluten-free diet: technological and nutritional challenges. Nutrients [Internet]. 2018;10(10):1410. Available from: https://www.ncbi.nlm.nih.gov/pmc/articles/PMC6213115/.
47. Fry L, Madden AM, Fallaize R. An investigation into the nutritional composition and cost of gluten-free versus regular food products in the UK. J Hum Nutr Diet. 2017;31(1):108–20.
48. Lee A, Wolf R, Lebwohl B, Ciaccio E, Green P. Persistent economic burden of the gluten free diet. Nutrients. 2019;11(2):399.
49. Boston Children's Hospital [Internet]. Childrenshospital.org. 2023 [cited 2024 Aug 30]. Available from:. https://www.childrenshospital.org/community-health/family-food-connections.
50. Leffler DA, Edwards-George J, Dennis M, Schuppan D, Cook F, Franko DL, et al. Factors that influence adherence to a gluten-free diet in adults with celiac disease. Dig Dis Sci. 2007;53(6):1573–81.
51. Macedo L, Catarino M, Festas C, Alves P. Vulnerability in children with celiac disease: findings from a scoping review. Children [Internet]. 2024;11(6):729. Available from: https://www.mdpi.com/2227-9067/11/6/729.
52. Abreu Paiva LM, Gandolfi L, Pratesi R, Harumi Uenishi R, Puppin Zandonadi R, Nakano EY, et al. Measuring quality of life in parents or caregivers of children and adolescents with celiac disease: development and content validation of the questionnaire. Nutrients [Internet]. 2019;11(10):2302. [cited 2021 Feb 10]. Available from: https://www.mdpi.com/2072-6643/11/10/2302.
53. Cadenhead JW, Wolf RL, Lebwohl B, Lee AR, Zybert P, Reilly NR, et al. Diminished quality of life among adolescents with coeliac disease using maladaptive eating behaviours to manage a gluten-free diet: a cross-sectional, mixed-methods study. J Hum Nutr Diet. 2019;32(3):311–20.

54. MacCulloch K, Rashid M. Factors affecting adherence to a gluten-free diet in children with celiac disease. J Paediatr Child Health. 2014;19(6):305–9. Available from: https://academic.oup.com/pch/article/19/6/305/2647457.
55. Rosén A, Ivarsson A, Nordyke K, Karlsson E, Carlsson A, Danielsson L, et al. Balancing health benefits and social sacrifices: a qualitative study of how screening-detected celiac disease impacts adolescents' quality of life. BMC Pediatr. 2011;11(1):32.
56. Epifanio MS, Genna V, Vitello MG, Roccella M, La Grutta S. Parenting stress and impact of illness in parents of children with coeliac disease. Pediatr Rep [Internet]. 2013;5(4) [cited 2020 Jun 20]; Available from: https://www.ncbi.nlm.nih.gov/pmc/articles/PMC3883085/.
57. Wolf RL, Lebwohl B, Lee AR, Zybert P, Reilly NR, Cadenhead J, et al. Hypervigilance to a gluten-free diet and decreased quality of life in teenagers and adults with celiac disease. Dig Dis Sci [Internet]. 2018;63(6):1438–48. Available from: https://link.springer.com/article/10.1007%2Fs10620-018-4936-4
58. Husby S, Murray J, Katzka D. AGA clinical practice update on diagnosis and monitoring of celiac disease-changing utility of serology and histologic measures: expert review. Gastroenterology. 2019;156(4):885–9.

Protein-Losing Enteropathy in Children

45

Chetan Mandelia and Donna Clement

Introduction

Protein-losing enteropathy (PLE) is a clinical syndrome characterized by excessive loss of proteins into the gastrointestinal (GI) tract, resulting in hypoproteinemia, edema, and related complications. It is not a single disease but a manifestation of various underlying conditions that disrupt the intestinal barrier or lymphatic system. Common symptoms include edema, diarrhea, ascites, malnutrition and may lead to complications such as pleural or pericardial effusion and coagulation abnormalities. The etiology often determines the clinical presentation and guides diagnosis and treatment [1, 2].

Causes and Pathophysiology

Protein-losing enteropathy (PLE) is caused by two main mechanisms—lymphatic abnormalities and mucosal injury—which result in an abnormal loss of protein into the gastrointestinal

C. Mandelia (✉) · D. Clement
Division of Pediatric Gastroenterology, Department of Pediatrics, Brody School of Medicine, East Carolina University, Greenville, NC, USA
e-mail: mandeliac20@ecu.edu; clementdo19@ecu.edu

K. Radhakrishnan (ed.), *Handbook of Clinical and Practical Pediatric Nutrition*, https://doi.org/10.1007/978-3-031-97759-6_45

lumen. Loss of protein may occur diffusely throughout the GI tract or could be limited to specific organs such as stomach or small intestine. The rate of protein loss exceeds the compensatory increase in protein synthesis and as much as 60% of the albumin pool may be lost through the GI tract daily. Proteins with longer half-lives such as albumin, immunoglobulin G, ceruloplasmin, and fibrinogen are more commonly affected compared to those with quick turnover such as pre-albumin, clotting factors, complement factors, and immunoglobulin E [1, 3] (Table 45.1).

Table 45.1 Causes of protein-losing enteropathy (PLE)

Category	Causes	Mechanism
Lymphatic abnormalities	Primary intestinal lymphangiectasia (PIL)	Lymphatic leakage of protein-rich fluid
	Secondary lymphangiectasia (e.g., Fontan-associated PLE, heart failure)	Lymphatic obstruction and leakage
	Genetic disorders (e.g., CHAPLE, Hennekam syndrome)	Congenital lymphatic defects
Mucosal injury	Inflammatory bowel disease (IBD)	Mucosal damage and increased permeability
	Infections (e.g., Salmonella, Shigella, Rotavirus)	Epithelial injury and permeability.
	Graft-versus-host disease (GVHD)	Immune-mediated mucosal injury
	Celiac disease	Villous atrophy and increased leakage
Hypertrophic gastropathy	Ménétrier's disease	Mucosal overgrowth with protein loss
Vascular disorders	Systemic lupus erythematosus (SLE)	Immune complex deposition in capillaries
	Henoch-Schönlein purpura	Vasculitis causing permeability issues
Neoplastic conditions	Lymphoma, neuroblastoma	Tumor compression causing lymphatic leakage
Cardiac conditions	Right-sided heart failure	Elevated venous pressures causing lymphatic congestion

Lymphatic Abnormalities

Lymphatic disruptions lead to leakage of protein-rich lymph into the intestine. Specific causes include:

1. **Primary Intestinal Lymphangiectasia (PIL)**:
   - Congenital malformation of intestinal lymphatic vessels. This leads to dilated lacteals in the small intestine, causing lymph leakage and subsequent protein loss [4].
   - Associated with edema, hypoproteinemia, and immune deficiencies like lymphopenia and hypogammaglobulinemia.
   - Presents in childhood but varies in severity, with some syndromic associations (e.g., Turner and Noonan syndromes).
2. **Secondary Lymphangiectasia**:
   - Results from obstructed or impaired lymphatic drainage caused by:
     – **Cardiac Diseases**: High venous pressures in conditions like congestive heart failure, constrictive pericarditis, or after Fontan procedure [3].
     – **Neoplasms**: Compression of thoracic duct by tumors such as lymphoma or neuroblastoma [2].
     – **Infections or Inflammatory Disorders**: Conditions like tuberculosis or sarcoidosis leading to localized lymphatic obstruction.

Fontan-Associated Protein-Losing Enteropathy

- Fontan-associated PLE is a severe complication of the Fontan procedure, performed for congenital heart defects that result in a single functional ventricle.
- This procedure redirects systemic venous blood directly to the pulmonary arteries, bypassing the right ventricle. Although lifesaving, it can lead to elevated systemic venous pressures and lymphatic congestion, culminating in PLE.
- Management options specific to Fontan-associated PLE include revision/fenestration of the Fontan circuit to reduce

venous pressure, lymphatic embolization or decompression and cardiac transplantation for refractory cases.
- Despite advances, Fontan-associated PLE remains a significant cause of morbidity and mortality, necessitating lifelong management and follow-up [3, 5].

Genetic Associations

- Genetic conditions like CHAPLE syndrome (*CD55* deficiency), Hennekam syndrome (*CCBE1, FAT4* gene), congenital disorders of glycosylation, disorders of triglyceride metabolism (*DGAT1* gene), yellow nail syndrome, and Klippel–Trenaunay syndrome (*PIK3CA* gene) are associated with lymphatic anomalies which result in PLE [1]. This list is vast and not limited to the causes listed above, though the ones listed above are relatively common. Genetic mutations are either from germline or somatic mutations.

Mucosal Injury

Disruption of mucosal integrity either at macroscopic or microscopic level leads to increased permeability and protein leakage. Mechanisms include:

1. **Inflammatory and Erosive Conditions**:
   - **Inflammatory Bowel Disease (IBD)**: Causes mucosal erosion and secondary lymphangiectasia, leading to significant protein loss.
   - **Infections**: Pathogens such as Salmonella, Shigella, Rotavirus, C.difficile, and Giardia lamblia cause epithelial damage, increasing permeability.
   - **Graft-Versus-Host Disease (GVHD)**: Immune-mediated injury in transplant recipients causing diffuse protein loss [3].

2. **Non-Ulcerative Conditions**:
   - **Hypertrophic Gastropathy (Ménétrier's Disease)**:
     – Characterized by excessive gastric mucosal growth, leading to loss of plasma proteins into the stomach lumen.
     – Often triggered by viral infections like cytomegalovirus in children.
   - **Eosinophilic Gastrointestinal Disorders (EGIDs)**
   - **Food Protein-Induced Enterocolitis Syndrome (FPIES)**
   - **Celiac Disease**
3. **Vascular Disorders**:
   - **Systemic lupus erythematosus (SLE) and Henoch-Schönlein purpura** cause immune complex deposition in capillaries, leading to increased permeability.

Pathophysiological Consequences

1. **Hypoalbuminemia**:
   - Albumin synthesis increases but cannot compensate for extensive losses, leading to pedal and periorbital edema, ascites, pericardial and pleural effusions.
2. **Immune Deficiencies**:
   - Loss of immunoglobulins and lymphocytes contributes to increased susceptibility to infections.
3. **Nutritional Deficiencies**:
   - Associated fat malabsorption exacerbates malnutrition and leads to fat-soluble vitamin deficiencies.
4. **Coagulation Abnormalities**
   - Loss of both pro- and anti-coagulation factors causes coagulopathy which can lead to either thrombosis or increased bleeding.

Diagnosis

The diagnosis of PLE should be suspected in the presence of edema, lymphopenia, and hypoalbuminemia (< 3.5 g/dL) after excluding other causes of low albumin such as renal or hepatic disease and protein-calorie malnutrition. Diagnosing PLE involves confirming protein loss into the GI tract and identifying the underlying cause.

1. **Stool Alpha-1-Antitrypsin (A1AT)**: Stool alpha-1-antitrypsin is a reliable marker for protein loss in the gastrointestinal tract as it is roughly the same size as albumin, resistant to enzymatic degradation (except in the stomach) and is not actively secreted or absorbed.

   Stool alpha-1-antitrypsin clearance is calculated using stool alpha-1-antitrypsin concentration, stool volume, and plasma alpha-1-antitrypsin concentration, providing a quantitative assessment of protein loss. An elevated stool A1AT clearance (>27 ml/24 hours without diarrhea or > 56 ml/24 hours with diarrhea) or spot fecal A1AT concentration (>54.0 mg/dL) can be used as a noninvasive diagnostic tool to assess disease severity and monitor treatment response (A1AT clearance is calculated by multiplying total amount of stools in milliliters in 24 hours and ratio of stool A1AT/serum A1AT) [2, 5].
2. **Endoscopy**: Identifies mucosal diseases such as IBD, Celiac disease, intestinal infections and helps visualize dilated lacteals in intestinal lymphangiectasia. Video capsule endoscopy may be useful to visualize the lesions distal to the reach of endoscopy.
3. **Lymphangiography**: Dynamic contrast-enhanced magnetic resonance lymphangiography (DCMRL) is a highly effective imaging modality for evaluating lymphatic flow disorders, including PLE. DCMRL provides detailed anatomical and functional imaging of the central lymphatic system, highlighting lymphatic vessels and potential leakage sites. It is particularly useful in detecting central lymphatic flow disorders, such as those associated with Fontan circulation, and guiding inter-

ventional therapies [6]. CT lymphangiography can also be used as an alternative if MRI is not feasible.

4. **Functional Imaging**: Scintigraphy using Tc-99 m human serum albumin and other radioisotopes has been used to localize protein loss in the gut but is not widely available.

Treatment

Management of PLE focuses on addressing the underlying cause, mitigating protein loss, and preventing complications.

Dietary Modifications: The goals are to decrease protein loss, treat clinical symptoms, and minimize nutritional consequences of PLE.

1. **Low-Fat Diet:**
   - **Purpose:** Reduce chyle production and flow, thus reducing loss of nutrients in lymphatic fluid
   - **Long Chain Triglyceride (LCT) Restriction:** Limit to 10–15% of daily calories, divided across meals to avoid chyle spikes [7].
   - **Medium Chain Triglyceride (MCT) Use:** Provides 7 kcal/g, absorbed without increasing lymph flow. Start with 0.5 g/kg/day, increasing to 1–2 g/kg/day as tolerated.
   - **Essential Fatty Acid Deficiency (EFAD):** Diets providing <10% calories from LCT can lead to EFAD, especially in growing children. Patients should be monitored closely for EFAD. Include oils high in linoleic acid (LA) and alpha-linolenic acid (ALA) to prevent EFAD. Minimum 2–4% of calories from LA is recommended to prevent EFAD [8].
   - **Duration:** While a lifetime low-fat diet may be beneficial for PLE management, adherence is difficult and extended time on a diet of 10% calories from LCT can inhibit growth and development. Frequent assessment of PLE symptoms is warranted to relax fat restrictions as feasible.

2. **High Protein Diet:**
   - **Purpose:** Though protein losses are attenuated by reabsorption of amino acids from the lumen distal to the site of lymphatic leakage, daily needs are higher than Dietary Reference Intake (DRI) for age.
   - **Recommended:** 2–3.5 g/kg in infants and children, and 1.5–3 g/kg in adolescents. If growth is faltering, prescribe the higher end of the recommended dose [8].
3. **Micronutrients:**
   - **Fat-soluble vitamins (A, D, E, K):** Deficiencies secondary to malabsorption in setting of limited formation of micelles from long-chain free fatty acids and bile salts. Additionally, losses of vitamin-D-binding protein in lymphatic chyle can worsen the vitamin D deficiency. Children with PLE have increased risk of low bone mineral density [7].
   - **Supplementation:** Prescribe water-miscible fat-soluble vitamins while dietary fat is limited to 10–15% of total calories.
   - **Trace minerals:** Monitor serum iron, zinc, and copper.
4. **Oral Supplements, Enteral Formulas**
   - **Fat-modified formulas** are available for infants, children, and adolescents with high MCT:LCT ratio. Less palatable than standard oral supplements. Monitor for EFAD when using a low LCT formula long-term.
   - **Protein:** Moderate- and high-protein oral supplements and formulas are available. Commercial protein powders can be added to low-LCT formulas and to foods and beverages.

Pharmacological Interventions

- **Steroids** such as budesonide have been used for treatment of Fontan-associated PLE with some success.
- **Octreotide**: Reduces splanchnic blood flow and enteric protein loss.
- **Sirolimus and Everolimus** (mTOR inhibitors) have also been tried for selected situations involving abdominal lymphatic disorders.
- **Albumin infusion** can be used only as a short-term measure for patients with severe low albumin and severe edema to

increase plasma oncotic pressure and concomitant diuretics can be utilized.

Surgical and Interventional Approaches:

- **Fontan Revision**: Addresses Fontan-associated PLE
- **Lymphatic Embolization and Microsurgery**: Emerging therapy for focal lymphatic leaks [3].
- **Surgical resection of intestine** can be planned for localized bowel involvement with primary intestinal lymphangiectasia.

Conclusion

Protein-losing enteropathy in children is a complex condition requiring a multidisciplinary approach. Early recognition, accurate diagnosis, and targeted treatment are essential to improving outcomes and quality of life. Future advancements in genetic testing and interventional techniques hold promise for better management of this challenging syndrome.

References

1. Brownell JN, Piccoli DA. Protein-losing enteropathy. Wyllie and Hyams' Pediatric Gastrointestinal and Liver Disease; 2021.
2. Braamskamp MJAM, Dolman KM, Tabbers MM. Protein-losing enteropathy in children. Eur J Pediatr. 2010;169:1179–85.
3. Ozen A, Lenardo MJ. Protein-losing enteropathy. N Engl J Med. 2023;389:733–48.
4. Waldmann TA, et al. Primary intestinal lymphangiectasia. N Engl J Med. 1961;265:431–8.
5. Alsaied T, et al. Protein losing enteropathy after the Fontan operation. Int J Cardiol Congenit Heart Dis. 2022;7:100338.
6. Ramirez-Suarez KI, Tierradentro-Garcia LO, Smith CL, et al. Dynamic contrast-enhanced magnetic resonance lymphangiography. Pediatr Radiol. 2022;52:285–94.
7. Savoca ML, Brownell JN. Comprehensive nutrition guidelines and management strategies for enteropathy in children. Semin Pediatr Surg. 2024;33:151425.
8. Mogensen KM. Essential fatty acid deficiency. nutritional issues in gastroenterology, Series #164. Practical gastroenterology. June 2017.

Nutrition Requirements in Neurological Disorders

46

Amanda Abou-Fadel and Catherine Wills

Approach of Nutrition in Children with Neuromuscular Disorders

Pediatric neuromuscular disorders (NMD) are a group of disorders that are acquired or inherited, leading to muscle weakness, decreased muscle mass, and impaired motility and function. These patients are at an increased risk for a range of nutrition and feeding complications related to their neuromuscular state. Common complications include inadequate or excessive weight gain, swallowing difficulties, constipation, diarrhea, and gastroesophageal reflux disease (GERD). They are prone to malnutrition (whether it's failure to thrive or overweight/obese).

Previous studies have reported a 50% prevalence of obesity at 10 years of age in boys with Duchenne muscular dystrophy (DMD), which is more than double the general population. Exact prevalence rates can vary by study, but generally 30% to 50% of children with DMD experience undernutrition or are at risk of it as the disease progresses. Mehta et al. revealed prevalence of

A. Abou-Fadel (✉) · C. Wills
Pediatric Gastroenterology, Hepatology and Nutrition, Akron Children's Hospital, Akron, OH, USA
e-mail: AAbou-Fadel@akronchildrens.org; cwills@akronchildrens.org

K. Radhakrishnan (ed.), *Handbook of Clinical and Practical Pediatric Nutrition*, https://doi.org/10.1007/978-3-031-97759-6_46

severe malnutrition increased from 2 to 17% after a period of 3 years in patients aged 2–12 years old but with SMA (not DMD).

Nutrition is very important and can be challenging to optimize in this patient population. Malnutrition affects their overall development and quality of life and is associated with worse overall outcomes such as increased mortality and prolonged hospital stay.

A multidisciplinary approach is critical for a comprehensive nutritional management and should include a dietician, a gastroenterologist, speech therapist, physiotherapist, occupational-therapist, behavioral psychologist, registered nurse, and social worker (Fig. 46.1) [1]

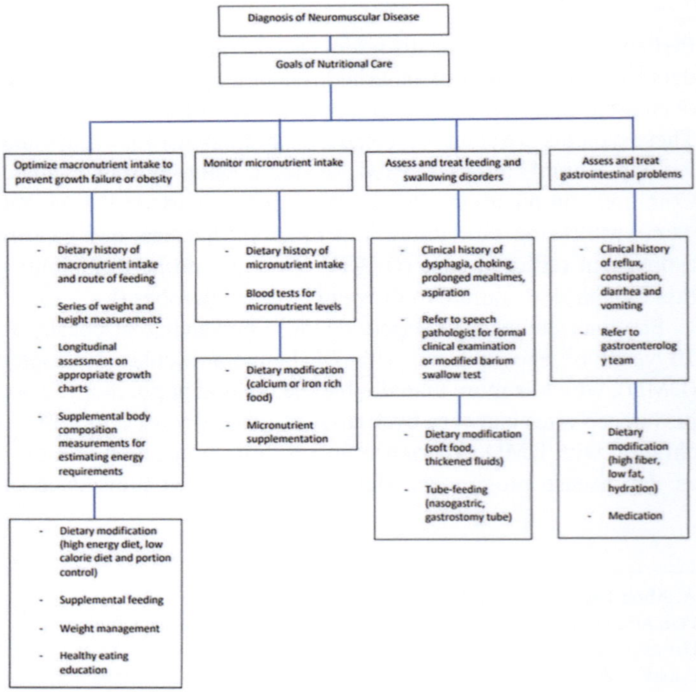

Fig. 46.1 Summary of recommended dietetic approach for children with neuromuscular disorders [1]

Nutritional assessment should include weight, height, and body mass index (BMI), though height measurements can be challenging (contractures, unable to stand, scoliosis). Segmental measures can be used.

Knee height is superior to ulnar length and arm span in estimating standing height in ambulatory patients and supine length in nonambulatory patients.

Ulnar length is preferred for children with significant lower limb contractures.

Expected height for age and weight for age are generally lower than those of reference population.

Child may also have an underlying genetic condition that impacts growth potential [1].

BMI has a moderate correlation with body fat percentage in ambulatory children with CP. Thus, body composition is important (including dynamics of fat, lean tissue mass, and water content).

Patients with neurological disability usually have increased total body water, depleted fat stores, and decreased bone density.

DEXA scan can be used to assess body composition [2].

– But not always easy to perform.
– Needs specialized center and equipment.
– Costly.

Skin fold thickness (SFT) (triceps and subscapular SFT measurements) are sensitivity and specific predictors of malnutrition [2].

Triceps SFT is recommended in patients with CP [2].

Risk of Osteopenia

- Predictors of low bone mineral density include significant immobilization, stunted growth, previous fractures, and use of anticonvulsants.

Dual-energy X-ray absorptiometry scan evaluation is the standard for evaluating BMD in children.

Assess feeding ability, nutritional status, if GERD or aspiration risks are present.

- Child may or may not be able to communicate hunger or thirst leaving it to the caregiver to decide how much the child should have.
- Impaired oral motor dysfunction.
  Inadequate lip closure, drooling, persistent tongue thrust, poor bolus formation.
  Difficulty swallowing can increase the risk of aspiration.
- Assess if feeds can be oral or enteral.
- Oral feeds should always be preferred.
- Enteral tube feeds should be considered if weight gain continues to be inadequate despite oral nutritional supplementation.
- Follow-up should be every 1–3 months initially when on oral nutrition, assessing nutritional status.
- Infants or children with poor nutritional status might need to be seen more frequently.
- Older children should be seen at least annually.

As NMD progresses, energy requirements can change, and patients might have lower energy needs after loss of ambulation.

Nutritional issues do impact energy regulation. Wide range of clinical features and mobility complicate ability to estimate energy needs.

Fat-free mass is a greater predictor of energy requirement than ambulatory status.

Predictive equations using height/length may not be as accurate as measurements are difficult to obtain and each patient needs careful assessment.

Important to individualize goals, monitor, and adjust.

Additional energy can be required during periods of growth, illness, pre- or post-surgery, so it's important to plan for nutritional optimization if needed or have sick days plan in place.

Enteral Tube Feeds

- For patients who are unable to meet their nutritional requirements by mouth [3].
- Undernourished despite optimized oral nutrition.
- Feeding and swallowing dysfunction
  - Dysphagia, Risk of aspiration, prolonged mealtime >30 min

  Different types of enteral feeding tubes vary per indication [2].

- NG
  - Short-term, less invasive, can be used prior to G-tube placement for nutrition optimization and ensuring tolerance of enteral feeds.
  - Not for long term, can be easily dislodged.
- PEG/G-tube
  - Most clinicians consider a minimum weight limit as 2.3 kg for placement [2].
  - Increased risk of GERD, so evaluate for it prior to placement.
- Nissen's fundoplication (if indicated)
- Post-pyloric feeds (NJ-tube, GJ-tube, J-tube) for patients with severe GERD, persistent vomiting, severe gastroparesis, growth failure, and increased risk of aspiration
  - But has higher frequency of complications and challenges in tube replacement

Formula selection

Formula selection should be based on age of child, energy requirements, and mode of access.

Commercially available formula

Precise amounts of micro and macronutrients.

Polymeric, semi-elemental, elemental, and disease-specific formulations available.

Whey-based formulas may be beneficial in patient with severe NI and GERD, or gagging/retching.

Blenderized foods

Home blenderized foods can be labor intensive and increase risk for bacterial contamination if strict hygienic precautionary measures are not followed.

Commercial products are available (Fig. 46.2 and Table 46.1).

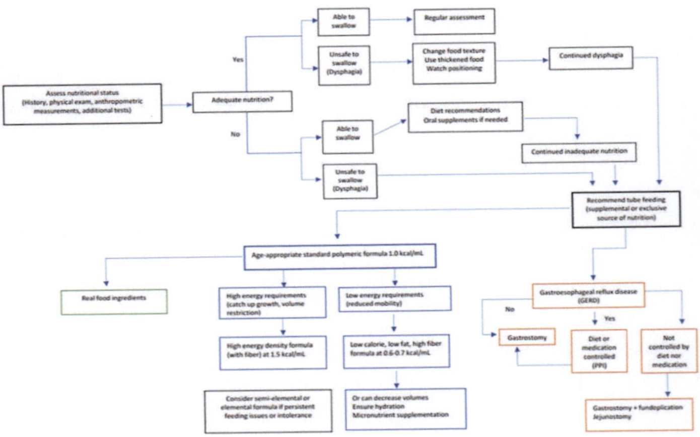

Fig. 46.2 Nutritional management of children with neurological impairment [3].

Table 46.1 Nutritional issues and recommended diet interventions for patients with neuromuscular disorders [1].

Issue	Dietetic intervention
Swallowing difficulties/aspiration	Modify food consistency (thicken fluids, semisolid diet) Adjust feeding position and seating, devices to ensure good support for self-feeding and safe swallowing. Refer to speech pathologist and occupational therapist for swallowing assessment Consider supplementation if insufficient oral intake, aspiration, prolonged mealtimes or poor weight gain

(continued)

Table 46.1 (continued)

Issue	Dietetic intervention
Poor caloric/nutrient intake	Review food preferences, eating habits Increase calories and proteins in the diet Provide education regarding mealtime routines and also include plans for sick days
Gastrointestinal issues	Constipation: Increase fiber intake, hydration, bowel regimen Refer to gastroenterologist for management of acid reflux and delayed gastric emptying
Corticosteroid side effects (DMD)	Education for parents about potential for increased appetite Monitor for weight gain especially if family history of obesity. Refer to endocrinology if growth plateaus or side effects of steroids are intolerable

Disease States

Cerebral Palsy

Nutrition Concerns/Intervention Assess swallow function, drooling, dentition, postural difficulties (pain, spasticity, hip luxation), GERD, esophageal motility, vomiting, aerophagia, delayed gastric emptying, constipation, bone health.

Children have a different body composition.

Assess for malnutrition (ESPGHAN) weight > 2 standard deviations below mean.

Triceps skin fold or MUAC below 10%ilie.

Obtain height—segmental measurements.

Bone mineral density + labs for micronutrients.

Enteral feeding if unable to meet nutritional requirements orally, are undernourished despite supplementation, or are at risk of aspiration secondary to swallow dysfunction [4].

Bone growth: children with CP have deficient bone growth and increased risk for nontraumatic fractures.

Supplement calcium and Vitamin D
Vitamin D: 800-1000 IU/day

Growth specific growth curves are available and defined by gross motor function classification system (ESPGHN)).

Energy Needs [5]

Dietary reference intake (DRI) (please see Chap. 2)
Specific to the individual and depends on severity of motor function and disease, mobility, and degree of altered metabolism.
Nonambulatory in wheelchair may need 60–70% of calories compared to healthy age-matched peers.
Severe malnutrition: additional 15–20% increase in calories +2gm protein/kg/day to support catch-up growth.
Orally fed patients who are undernourished.
Add extra calories utilizing high-fat spreads, avocado, fortify milk with cream, milk powders, flavorings, commercially available modulars (carbohydrate polymers, protein powders, combined carbohydrate, and fat supplements)
Add extra protein using diced or pureed meats, dairy products, eggs, lentils, and legumes.
High energy-dense formulas are available for oral or enteral supplementation.
Add fiber depending on needs of child (fiber goals are same as for average developing child ((age + 5 in children 2 years of age)

Important to ensure that intake of nutrients does not exceed recommended upper limits.

Fluid Goals

May have fluid loss through drooling of saliva, sweating, respiratory distress and may be unable to communicate thirst or be unable to consume adequate fluids.
Use Holiday Segar equation and actual body weight.
Feasible goal may be 90% of estimated need.

Duchenne Muscular Dystrophy

Disease State Progressive muscle degeneration and the loss of the ability to walk independently. Estimated 4% loss of muscle mass/year.

Milder forms intermediate muscular dystrophy and Becker muscular dystrophy which can result in loss of walking ability by ages 13–16 and over 16.

Nutritional Concerns/Intervention

First line of treatment is Glucocorticoids to maintain muscle strength and functionality [6].

Monitor serum calcium and 25-hydroxyvitamin D levels yearly.
Consider vitamin D and mineral supplementation.

Optimize macronutrient intake to avoid growth failure or obesity [7].

Reduced calorie requirements secondary to decreased energy expenditure attributed to decreased physical activity and decreased REE.

Steroids increase appetite.

Later stages of disease patient may be malnourished and underweight secondary to muscle weakness, which contributes to dysphagia, constipation, delayed emptying, prolonged mealtimes, and dependent food intake. Respiratory failure at this stage can increase calorie requirements.

Manage feeding and swallowing issues [6].

Progression of the disease leads to difficulty chewing/swallowing [6].

- Consider tube feeding [6].
  - Polymeric formula or blended diet [6]

Treat GI symptoms [6]

GERD.

Treat with H2Blockers or PPI

Constipation

Polyethylene glycol after gastrostomy placement is recommended.

To prevent aspiration with high volume of intake

Increase fiber or blended diets can help with constipation.

Monitor micronutrient intakes such as Vitamin D and calcium [6].

Growth Specific growth curves are available

Not always accepted in clinical practice, as they represent how children typically grow and not how they should grow.

Energy Needs Based on DRI (Chap. 2)

Gene therapies that have been approved recently may have an impact of clinical course and therefore nutritional needs. Clinical judgment will need to exercised in these settings to ensure that the nutritional recommendations are optimal.

Spinal Muscular Atrophy

Disease state: neurodegenerative disease. Defects in survival motor neuron 1 (SMN1) cause selective destruction of alpha motor neurons in anterior horn cells of spinal cord and brainstem. There are four subtypes [6].

Type 1: Very weak infant unable to sit unsupported with onset <6 months.

Type 2: Non-ambulant patients able to sit independently with onset between 6–18 months.

Type 3: Ambulant patients with onset between 18 months and 18 years.

Type 4: Adult onset.

Nutrition concerns: goals differ for each subtype.

Weight control, dysphagia management, manage GI dysfunction.
Type 1 and Type 2:
Gastrostomy placement in first few months of life to avoid risk of malnutrition.
Polymeric formula or blended feeds
Type 1 obtain VFSS after diagnosis and if clinical indications such as weak suck, fatigue, wet voice, pneumonia.
Type 1: increased risk of malnutrition caused by respiratory issues, dysphagia, weak masticatory muscles, and tachypnea.
Reduce risk of respiratory infections.
"Non-sitter" patients need to have evaluation to ensure they have safe swallowing and no bulbar dysfunction that can lead to aspiration and lung infections.
"Sitter" patients have a higher risk of overweight as result of decrease physical activity, altered body composition.
"Walkers"—swallowing disorders and feeding problems are rare in this subtype.
Main nutrition concern is obesity due to impaired mobility and increased risk of comorbidities such as metabolic syndrome, hypertension, and diabetes [6]

Growth: use standardized growth curves and monitor growth trends [6]

Assess body composition using dual-energy X-ray absorptiometry and bioelectrical impedance analysis.

Energy needs: use DRI's (Chap. 2) [6]

Multiple gene therapy options and disease-modifying medications have been approved recently, and they can have an impact of clinical course and therefore nutritional needs. Clinical judgment will need to be exercise in these settings to ensure that the nutritional recommendations are optimal.

Congenital Myopathies

Disease state: includes a group of inherited diseases of the skeletal muscle, which cause static or progressive muscle weakness or developmental delays.

Nutrition Concerns

Feeding and swallowing difficulty [8].

Attributed to weakening of bulbar muscles as part of disease process.
Increased risk of aspiration [8].
Recommended to have VFSS.

GERD

Delayed gastric emptying.
Constipation.

Growth
- No specific data or growth charts.

Many patients with neuromuscular disorders have short stature and growth trajectory that is below age.
Patients with NMD often have an increased fat to muscle ratio which may result in a lower healthy weight.
Important to monitor serial growth data and avoid over feeding.

Nutrition
- Typical childhood problem is malnutrition.

Nutrition assessment should consider.

Length of meals
Frequency of meals
Frequency of lung infections
Difficulty chewing

Changes to texture of food

Stress in family or enjoyment of meals for the child and parents

Ability to eat independently.

In the event of feeding problems, optimize treatment strategies.

Patient most often require a feeding tube- preferably gastrostomy feeds.

Energy Needs: No specific data on energy and protein needs

Monitoring growth and other nutritional parameters are important to avoid under, as well excess feeding and weight gain.

Charcot-Marie Tooth Disease

Disease state: A collection of inherited genetic disorders that affect the peripheral nerves [3, 1]. Progressive distal-proximal muscular weakness and sensory loss.

Nutrition Concerns

- Limited literature on specific nutritional issues [8].

Nutrition approach must be evaluated individually based on clinical assessments [6].

References

1. Chou E, Lindeback R, Sampaio H, Farrar MA. Nutritional practices in pediatric patients with neuromuscular disorders. Nutr Rev. 2020;78(10):857–65. https://doi.org/10.1093/nutrit/nuz109.
2. Prasad D, Bhriguvanshi A. Nutritional issues and Management in Children with Cerebral Palsy. Published online April 30, 2022. https://www.researchgate.net/publication/361950340_Nutritional_Issues_and_Management_in_Children_with_Cerebral_Palsy.
3. Nutritional Management of Cerebral Palsy in Children. EMJ 20205429–38. Published online October 2, 2020. https://www.emjreviews.com/wp-content/uploads/2020/12/Nutritional-Management-of-Cerebral-Palsy-in-Children.pdf.
4. Rebelo F, Mansur IR, Miglioli TC, Meio MDB, Junior SCG. Dietary and nutritional interventions in children with cerebral palsy: A sys-

tematic literature review. Grammatikopoulou MG, ed. Plos One. 2022;17(7):e0271993. https://doi.org/10.1371/journal.pone.0271993.
5. Corkins MR, Balint J, Bobo E, Plogsted S, Yaworski JA. The A.S.P.E.N. Pediatric Nutrition Support Core Curriculum. 2nd ed. Silver Spring, MD: American Society for Enteral and Parenteral Nutrition; 2015.
6. Dipasquale V, Morello R, Romano C. Gastrointestinal and nutritional care in pediatric neuromuscular disorders. World J Clin Pediatr. 2023;12(4):197–204. https://doi.org/10.5409/wjcp.v12.i4.197.
7. Salera S, Menni F, Moggio M, Guez S, Sciacco M, Esposito S. Nutritional challenges in Duchenne muscular dystrophy. Nutrients. 2017;9(6):594. https://doi.org/10.3390/nu9060594.
8. Chou E, Lindeback R, D'Silva AM, Sampaio H, Neville K, Farrar MA. Growth and nutrition in pediatric neuromuscular disorders. Clin Nutr. 2021;40(6):4341–8. https://doi.org/10.1016/j.clnu.2021.01.013.

Neonatal Nutrition and Prematurity

47

Taylor Rice, Audrey Ruthenberg, and Subhash Puthuraya

Neonatal Gastrointestinal Tract

Development of GI Tract [1, 2, 3]

- The alimentary canal begins as a primitive gut tube by the lateral folding of endoderm and splanchnic mesoderm at about 3–4 weeks of gestation.

T. Rice
Pediatric Nutrition Support, Division of Pediatric Gastroenterology, Hepatology, and Nutrition, Cleveland Clinic Children's Hospital, Cleveland, OH, USA
e-mail: ricet3@ccf.org

A. Ruthenberg
Pediatric Gastroenterology, Hepatology, and Nutrition, Pediatric Nutrition Support, Cleveland Clinic, Cleveland, OH, USA

Cleveland Clinic Children's Hospital, Cleveland, OH, USA
e-mail: ruthena@ccf.org

S. Puthuraya (✉)
Neonatology, Cleveland Clinic Lerner College of Medicine of Case Western Reserve University, Cleveland, OH, USA

Cleveland Clinic Children's Hospital, Cleveland, OH, USA
e-mail: puthurs@ccf.org

K. Radhakrishnan (ed.), *Handbook of Clinical and Practical Pediatric Nutrition*, https://doi.org/10.1007/978-3-031-97759-6_47

- During the formation of the head fold, the cranial part of the yolk sac becomes enclosed within the embryo forming the foregut.
- The caudal part of the enclosed yolk sac becomes the hindgut.
- The midgut, formed between the foregut and the hindgut remains in communication with the yolk sac, until it is closed at about the 10th week.
- The cranial oropharyngeal membrane starts breaking down at the 4th week followed by the caudal cloacal membrane at about 6 weeks.

Esophagus [1, 2, 3]

- During the 4th week, the tracheoesophageal septum divides the foregut with the posterior part forming the esophagus.
- The esophagus elongates as the body grows cranially by the 7th week.
- Muscular layers of the esophagus develop from the 6th to 9th week of gestation, and the lumen of the esophagus is present by the 10th week.
- Initially, the epithelium of the esophagus, derived from endoderm, is ciliated. However, it is replaced by stratified, non-keratinizing squamous epithelium by the 9th month of gestation.
- Earliest uncoordinated swallowing is present at 16 weeks gestation, and coordinated swallowing and sucking is present by about 34–36 weeks gestation.

Stomach [1, 2, 3]

- The caudal part of the foregut shows a fusiform dilation forming the stomach at the end of the 4th week.
- During the 6–10 weeks, the stomach rotates in two planes growing differentially along the margins leading to its shape and position.
- There is a 90-degree counterclockwise rotation along the longitudinal axis, which makes the dorsal aspect come on to the left and the ventral aspect to the right.

- The mesentery from this rotation forms the lesser omentum and gastrosplenic ligaments. A second clockwise rotation along the anteroposterior axis and rapid growth of the caudal part of the dorsal mesentery form the greater omentum.
- The mucus-secreting cuboidal epithelium with gastric pits is seen from the 6th to 9th week of gestation. Parietal and chief cells, found in the fundus and body of the stomach appear by the tenth and 12th week of gestation.
- The enteroendocrine cells appear around the 8th to 9th week.
- The mucosa of the stomach is mature in appearance by the 20th week of gestation.
- The gastric secretory function starts at 12 weeks with the detection of gastrin, hydrochloric acid, pepsin, and intrinsic factor.

Small Intestine, Pancreas, and Biliary System [1, 2, 3]

- During the 6th to 12 weeks of gestation, the gut herniates out and the duodenum undergoes a 270-degree rotation around the superior mesenteric artery (SMA) axis to bring it under the SMA leading to its retroperitoneal position.
- The duodenal epithelium proliferates to form a solid tube, and a recanalization process subsequently makes it become hollow again.
- The duodenum is supplied both by the celiac axis and superior mesentery artery, with the transition defining the junction of the foregut and midgut.
- The intestine returns to the enlarged abdominal cavity by the 11th week.
- The small intestine doubles its length from 26 weeks (100–125 cm) to 38 weeks to measure about 200–300 cm at birth.
- The circular and longitudinal muscles of the small intestine appear at 6 and 8 weeks of gestation. Neuroblasts are seen at 7 weeks, and myenteric and sub-myenteric plexus appear by the 9th to 13 weeks of gestation.
- Mature villi are present throughout the intestine by the 14th week of gestation.

- By 20 weeks of gestation, endocrine cells proliferate and secrete peptide hormones and neurotransmitters.
- Enteric ganglion cells, derived from neural crest cells start from the esophagus at 5 weeks and migrate downwards to the anal canal in the craniocaudal direction until the 12th week of gestation. The submucous plexus formed by neuroblasts also progresses in a craniocaudal direction during the 12th to 16th weeks of gestation.
- The liver and biliary system develops from a hepatic diverticulum on the ventral aspect of mesentery.
- The rotations of the stomach and intestines lead to the final location of the liver in the right upper quadrant.
- The ventral and dorsal pancreatic buds also fuse during the rotation to become a single organ of pancreas.
- The biliary and pancreatic drainage systems fuse during development, so that the common bile duct and main pancreatic ducts drain at the ampulla of vater.

Colon, Rectum, and Anus [1, 2, 3]

- From 10th to 12 weeks, the colon undergoes a 270-degree rotation which brings the cecum into the right lower quadrant, the ascending colon in the right gutter, the transverse colon from hepatic flexure to the splenic flexure and the descending colon in the left gutter.
- Further along the sigmoid colon connects to the rectum.
- During development, the ascending and descending colon become retroperitoneal structures, and the transverse and sigmoid colon become attached to the mesentery.
- The colon is supplied by the superior and inferior mesenteric artery with the junction being the mid-transverse colon to splenic flexure. This represents the transition of the midgut and hindgut.
- The cloacal membrane is formed during the third week of gestation.

- From the 4th to 6 weeks, this membrane gets partitioned by the urogenital septum anteriorly to the urogenital sinus and posteriorly to the anorectum.
- The ectoderm around this region forms the anal pit which forms the distal third of the anal canal. The proximal two-thirds are derived from the mesoderm.
- The anal membrane breaks down during the 8th week forming the pectinate line.
- In addition to neural crest-derived ganglion cells, the anorectum receives parasympathetic innervation from spinal nerves at sacral levels 2, 3, and 4.

Fetal Accretion and Preterm Neonatal Digestion of Nutrients

Carbohydrate [4, 5]

- Glucose is the major source of energy metabolism in the fetus with lactate and amino acids accounting for the rest.
- Both glycogenolysis and gluconeogenesis are minimal in the fetus, and fetal glucose uptake is closely regulated by maternal plasma glucose level.
- There is a steady increase in hepatic glycogen stores with a rapid increase around 36 weeks gestation.
- At the time of birth, the epinephrine, norepinephrine, and glucagon levels increase, and insulin levels decrease leading to mobilization of glycogen and fatty acids.
- This, along with initiation of gluconeogenesis, helps to maintain the glucose homeostasis after birth.
- Overall, the neonate demonstrates adequate carbohydrate absorption.
- Pancreatic amylase is present by 22 weeks of gestation.
- Intestinal disaccharidases and lactase reach adult levels at about 28 weeks and 36 weeks gestation, respectively.
- Premature newborns have less efficient glucose transport across their intestinal wall. In preterm infants, the colonic salvage pathway formed by colonic bacterial fermentation also

helps in efficient absorption of lactose breakdown products-short chain fatty acids.

Protein [5]

- Due to rapid growth and energy needs, the fetus receives quantitatively large amounts of amino acids.
- The amino acids are actively transported across the placenta leading to higher fetal circulation levels than maternal levels.
- Preterm infants also have a higher protein turnover on a body weight basis when compared to adults.
- A high protein intake by low-birth-weight neonates results in higher rates of weight gain and nitrogen accretion.
- Amino acid transport capacity is well-developed in neonates.
- Secretion of dipeptidase is well-developed early in life.
- Preterm infants have higher gastric pH and increased buffering ability of stomach contents.
- Both chymotrypsin and trypsin are decreased in preterm infants.

Fat [5]

- Rapid weight gain of the fetus during the 26–40 weeks gestation is due to an increase in water, fat, and nonfat components.
- However, beyond 30 weeks, the fat component accumulation is far greater than the nonfat component.
- Lipids are also essential constituents of the brain and form the main component of the myelin sheath.
- Essential fatty acids are important during the structural expansion of the brain in the last trimester.
- Preterm infants have decreased bile acid secretion with adult values reached at 2 months of age.
- Pancreatic lipase has reduced activity in preterm infants, and they rely on lingual, gastric, and lipases in breast milk for triglyceride breakdown.
- Absorption of fat in preterm is similar to term infants, and it increases during the first month of life.

Nutritional Care and Growth Parameters of the Preterm Infant

Anthropometric Assessment [6, 7, 8]

The assessment of growth using appropriate anthropometrics in the preterm population is critical to providing insight on the nutritional status and goals of the neonate.

- Anthropometrics obtained at birth are used to determine infant maturity and intrauterine growth, which will then guide clinical care needs, while growth trends post birth will inform nutritional interventions long-term.
- Additionally, growth trends can provide insight on potentially serious underlying chronic illnesses such as metabolic disorders and congenital syndromes; therefore, they should be obtained by a trained professional in a consistent manner using the below outlined tools to be considered reliable.
- Refer to Table 47.1 for anthropometric tools and frequency. Measurements most commonly used to assess growth include weight, length, and head circumference, which are then plotted on a preterm growth chart at birth and on a weekly basis to determine trends.
- The Fenton and Olsen Growth Chart are common tools utilized on neonates to inform preterm growth trends, with a transition

Table 47.1 Anthropometric Assessment of Neonate [6, 8]

Anthropometric	Tools to measure	Frequency	Goals
Weight	Calibrated gram scale	Daily	15–20 g/kg/day[a]
Length	Length board[b]	Weekly	0.9–1 cm/week
Head circumference	Tape measure	Weekly[c]	0.9–1 cm/week

[a]Dependent on patient growth trajectory and should not include postnatal weight loss, which is expected to be between 5–14%, with the nadir reached by day of life 5 [6]

[b]Should be done by 2 people, one to hold the infant's head and one to guide the footboard and lengthen legs [6]

[c]May need to be monitored more frequently if concern for micro or macrocephaly [6]

Table 47.2 Birth weight and size for age [6]

Birth weight	Categorization
≥2500 grams	Normal birth weight
<2500–1500 grams	Low birth weight
<1500 grams-1000 grams	Very low birth weight
<1000 grams	Extremely low birth weight
Weight percentile at birth	Size for age
<10th%ile	Small for gestation (SGA)
10-90th%ile	Appropriate for gestation (AGA)
>90th%ile	Large for gestation (LGA)

to the WHO Growth Chart at 40 weeks corrected age, all of which can be plugged into publicly accessible electronic calculators on Peditools in order to obtain reliable percentile and z-score datapoints. The Fenton and Olsen Growth Charts are both endorsed by the American Academy of Pediatrics and the Academy of Nutrition and Dietetics to assess preterm growth (any infant born <37 weeks gestational age).

- Infants are classified at birth as either Small for Gestational Age (SGA), Appropriate for Gestational Age (AGA), or Large for Gestational Age (LGA), based on their birth weight.
- Table 47.2 outlines the definitions for birth weight categorization and size for age. A patient's size for age helps practitioners anticipate potential clinical needs and complications, as each of the SGA and LGA categories holds a set of risks associated with it, such as hypoglycemia, respiratory failure, temperature instability, and feeding issues.
- It is important that birth anthropometrics are obtained in the most accurate and reliable manner in order to help guide the patient's care plan.

Enteral Nutrition [6, 8, 9]

- The nutritional goals of preterm infants aim to support growth, which imitates normal intrauterine growth patterns, while supporting overall development.
- Preterm nutrition is linked with outcomes such as infection risk, necrotizing enterocolitis (NEC), bronchopulmonary dys-

Table 47.3 Micro and macronutrient needs[6, 9]

	<1000 g	1000–1500 g	1500–2000 g	2000–2500 g
Macronutrients				
Energy (cal/kg/day)	110–130	110–130	110–130	105–125
Protein (gm/kg/day)	3.5–4.5	3.5–4.5	3.0–4.0	2.5–3.5
Fat (gm/100 kcal)	4.1–7.4			
Micronutrients				
Calcium (mg/kg/day)	120–220			
Phosphorus (mg/kg/day)	70–120			
Iron (mg/kg/day)	2–3			
Vitamin D (IU/day)	400–700; Max 1000			
Sodium (mEq/kg/day)	3–5			
Zinc (mg/kg/day)	2–3			

plasia, and retinopathy of prematurity; therefore, special attention needs to be made to the nutrients provided to this population.
- Preterm infants cannot be considered a homogenous group due to a host of medical conditions they may encounter, decreased nutrient stores, altered gastrointestinal absorption, and rapid growth goals.
- Furthermore, nutritional care should be individualized based on the extent of prematurity, body weight, growth trends, feeding tolerance, and disease conditions.
- Nutrients in which special attention should be paid in the preterm population are energy, protein, calcium, phosphorus, iron, vitamin D, sodium, and zinc (Table 47.3).

Feeding Protocols [8, 10]

Feeding guidelines vary across NICUs.

- There is currently no consensus on the optimal protocol for feeding advancement in the neonate; however, there's evidence supporting that when units have a standardized feeding protocol it improves outcomes, such as central line days, parenteral

Table 47.4 Feeding protocol elements to consider [8, 10]

Trophic feeds	When to initiate and duration	Usually considered trophic if <20 ml/kg/day is provided. Given for 3 days or less
Feeding advancement schedule	Volume and frequency of advancement	Rate of advancement should balance the risk of prolonged use of central venous lines, potential feeding intolerances and the benefits of achieving full feeds
Feeding type	Maternal breast milk Donor breast milk Preterm formula	Maternal breast milk is preferred, when available
Fortification plan	When to advance calories beyond 20 calorie/ounce	Early fortification has been observed in the literature as promoting improved growth without adverse consequences. Once feeds reach 50–80 ml/kg/day, it should be considered

nutrition use, time to reach full enteral feeds and time to regain birth weight, all without increasing the risk of NEC and central line-associated bloodstream infection.

- Additionally, evidence is in favor of early enteral nutrition (EN) initiation versus maintaining a period of NPO in order to prevent atrophy of the gut, so a consistent standard of EN care should be established when determining feeds for the preterm infant (Table 47.4).

Human Milk and Donor Milk [11]

- Human milk is the preferred feeding choice for all infants due to the vast amount of research exhibiting its benefits, specifically in the preterm population; however, maternal breast milk is not always available as soon as an infant is born.
- Breast milk production typically picks up between day of life 3 and 5, so there are times other options must be available to meet the nutritional needs of the neonate, while still helping stimulate and protect gut development. (Table 47.5).

Table 47.5 Maternal and donor breast milk uses and contraindications [6, 11]

Breast milk	Indications for use	Benefits of use	Contraindications for use	Composition
Maternal	All infants Considered the gold standard feed	Improved developmental outcomes, decreased NEC risk, decreased incidence of late-onset sepsis, decreased incidence of retinopathy of prematurity and decreased time to reach full enteral feeds; economical and social benefits for mother and child	Infants with galactosemia Mothers infected with HIV Mothers infected with human T-cell lymphotropic virus, type I or II Mothers with active illicit drug use[a]	Carbohydrate: Lactose Protein: Whey-predominant Fat: Long-chain triglycerides
Donor	Infants born <1500 grams Gastro-intesinal anomalies Intrauterine growth restriction Secondary choice when mother's milk is not available or there's insufficient quantity	May reduce NEC risk vs formula	Infants with galactosemia Infants with poor growth	

[a]If enrolled in a supervised methadone treatment program, breast milk can be provided

Human Milk Fortification and Premature Formula, Transition Formulas [6, 8, 11]

- Human milk, although the gold standard for all infants, is insufficient in energy, protein, and minerals, which are needed to promote growth and healthy bone development in preterm infants.
- Unfortified breast milk can lead to nutritional inadequacy, growth failure, and poor outcomes for preterm infants; therefore, the use of multicomponent fortifiers is recommended.

Human Milk Fortifiers (HMF) [6, 8, 11]

A. Available as a sterile liquid.
B. Protein source options: bovine or human.
C. Human milk-based fortifiers are produced from pasteurized donor milk, whereas bovine fortifiers are produced from cow's milk.
   (a) Protein structure options: intact or hydrolyzed
   (b) Designed to be mixed with human milk
   (c) Standard versus targeted fortification
      (i) Standard fortification assumes an average composition of breast milk and provides nutrients in a fixed dose through the use of HMF.
      (ii) Targeted fortification utilizes human milk analysis to determine specific macronutrient needs, which may be added individually.
         1. Only practical when there is a human milk analyzer available and there are properly trained individuals to run it.

Preterm Formulas [6]

A. Designed to be used on preterm infants when mother's milk is not available and/or donor breast milk is no longer recommended.
   (a) Similar nutrient composition as breast milk mixed with HMF
   (b) Available as sterile, ready-to-feed formulas in varied calorie concentrations

Transitional Formulas [6, 12]

A. Designed for late preterm infants (>/= 34 weeks) when mother's milk is not available and/or donor breast milk is no longer recommended or as a home-going formula for all preterm infants.
B. Available as sterile ready-to-feed formula as well as powder.
C. Can be added to breast milk as a powdered calorie enhancer or provided straight as an exclusive formula.
D. Higher in calories, protein, calcium and phosphorus versus standard term formula.

Parenteral Nutrition (PN) [6, 8, 13, 14]

Due to the immature gastro-intestinal tract of premature infants, most preterm infants will require PN with a slow advancement of enteral feeds.

- PN should be started once line access is obtained, especially for those <1500 grams at birth. Initiation of PN after birth has been found to decrease length of time to regain birth weight and improve short-term growth.
- Starter PN is initiated first, and typically contains carbohydrates and protein to prevent excessive catabolism and calcium to prevent hypocalcemia.
- Once diuresis has occurred, typically after 24 h of life, electrolytes can be added to the TPN.
- Advancement of PN to meet the needs for preterm infants should occur over the first week of life; however, it may be delayed if the patient is unable to tolerate advancement in glucose concentration.

Macronutrients

Carbohydrates [6, 8]

- Glucose is the main energy source for preterm infants.
- Preterm infants, especially those <1500 grams, are at high risk for hyperglycemia (Blood glucose levels >150 mg/dL) as glucose tolerance and insulin sensitivity are reduced.
- Dextrose should be introduced and advanced in a stepwise manner (Table 47.6) to reduce risk for hyperglycemia.
- Glucose levels should be monitored with initiation and advancement of GIR(Glucose infusion rate).
- For those infants with peripheral lines, dextrose concentration should not be increased beyond 12.5%.

Protein [6, 8, 13, 14]

Adequate protein intake is essential to promote optimal growth, body composition, and neurodevelopment in premature infants.

- Protein should be initiated at a dose <3 gm/kg/d and advanced to a maximum of 3.5 gm/kg/d. Pediatric Amino Acid (AA) solutions are used for preterm infants to provide both essential and non-essential Amino Acids in a ratio to produce plasma amino acid concentrations similar to term breast-fed infants.
- These solutions also have a lower pH, which allows for higher calcium and phosphorus delivery.
- Cysteine, a conditionally essential amino acid, is added to PN solutions at a usual dose of 40 mg/g of amino acid.
- Starting AA soon after birth improves glucose stability, promotes nitrogen balance, and prevents catabolism.

Table 47.6 Parenteral nutrition macronutrient recommendations [15]

	Initial	Advance by	Goal
Dextrose (mg/kg/min)	6–8	1–2	10–14 (max 14–18)
Protein (gm/kg/d)	1–3	–	3–3.5
Fat (gm/kg/d)	0.5–1	0.5–1	3

Intravenous Fat Emulsion [6, 8, 16]

- Preterm infants are at high risk of developing Essential Fatty Acid Deficiency (EFAD); therefore, Intravenous Fat Emulsions (IVFE) should be started by DOL 1–2.
- In addition to Essential Fatty Acids, IVFE provide a significant source of calories. To prevent EFAD, a dose of 0.25 gm/kg/d of linoleic acid is required [8]. The type of lipid emulsion used determines the minimum IVFE required.
- Several fat emulsions are available, each with specific infusion rates. See Parenteral Nutrition Chap. 6 for specifics.
- Preterm infants are at high risk for hypertriglyceridemia. Monitoring of plasma triglycerides levels may be beneficial in SGA infants, those with hyperglycemia, evidence of lipemia in blood samples or those suffering from a systemic infection.

Micronutrients

Electrolytes [6, 8, 14, 17]

Electrolytes are added to PN once postnatal diuresis occurs and urine output is adequate. See Table 47.7 for estimated requirements.

- Sodium and potassium are added to PN in the form of acetate, chloride, or phosphate (less likely potassium phosphate).
- As diuresis occurs, additives should be adjusted to maintain acid-base balance.

Table 47.7 Estimated parenteral electrolyte requirements [15]

Electrolyte	
Calcium	0.5–4 meq/kg/d
Magnesium	0.3–0.5 meq/kg/d
Phosphorus	0.5–2 mmol/kg/d
Sodium	2–5 meq/kg/d
Potassium	2–4 meq/kg/d
Chloride	As needed to maintain acid-base balance
Acetate	As needed to maintain acid-base balance

- Limiting chloride in the first week of life is recommended to prevent hyperchloremic acidosis.
- Frequent monitoring of labs should occur during the first week of life with initiation and advancement of PN as fluid status changes.
- The addition of calcium and phosphorus to PN is essential to optimize bone mineralization and prevent metabolic bone disease.
- Calcium is typically added to PN as calcium gluconate. Phosphorus can be added as potassium phosphate or sodium phosphate.
- Not only is the dose of calcium and phosphorus important for bone mineralization, but also the ratio. Calcium and phosphorus should be initiated at a molar ratio of 0.8:1 with advancement to goal of 1.3:1 (molar ratio).
- The requirements for calcium and phosphorus are higher in preterm infants compared to term infants due to the limited stores at birth in preterm infants.
- Unfortunately, it is often difficult to provide adequate calcium and phosphorus because of precipitation that occurs with higher doses.
- The addition of cysteine to the PN of preterm infants aids by lowering the pH of the solution and increasing solubility, allowing for higher intakes of calcium and phosphorus.

Vitamins [6, 14, 15]

Both water-soluble and fat-soluble vitamins are added to the PN as a compounded solution. Vitamin content of the compounded solutions is listed in Parenteral Nutrition Chap. 6.

- The multivitamin solution is added at 2 ml/kg/d up to 5 ml. Infants less than 2.5 kg will not receive the full 5 ml dose and therefore, additional supplementation may be needed pending diagnosis.

Minerals [6, 8, 18]

Trace elements are added to PN individually, as trace element packages do not meet the needs for preterm infants. Zinc, chromium, selenium, copper, and occasionally manganese should be

Table 47.8 Estimated parenteral nutrition trace element requirements [6]

Trace element	
Zinc	400 mcg/kg
Copper	20 mcg/kg
Chromium	0.05–0.3 mcg/kg
Selenium	2 mcg/kg/d
Manganese	1 mcg/kg/d

added to neonatal PN. Recommended doses are listed in Table 47.8. Dosing may be affected by multiple factors.

Special Considerations

- Zinc—Zinc requirements may be elevated in elevated in those infants with excessive GI losses due to diarrhea or ostomy output, rapid growth, or for skin healing.
- Copper—Those infants with increased GI losses may have increased copper needs. The reduction or elimination of copper form PN solutions may result in copper deficiency.
- Chromium and Manganese—Both trace elements are contaminants in many PN additives, and therefore intake may be adequate without additional supplementation. In infants with chronic renal failure, chromium requirements may be reduced.
- Iron is not routinely added to PN solutions due to risk of iron overload. The enteral route is preferred if iron is needed; however, if parenteral iron is needed, iron should be supplemented at a dose of 200–250 mcg/kg/day.

Refeeding Syndrome [8, 19]

- Preterm infants are at risk for refeeding syndrome (RS) due to the poor nutrient stores present at birth, followed by the immediate supply of dextrose and AA via starter PN with limited or no phosphate.
- Those at highest risk for RS are those infants whose pregnancies were complicated by placental insufficiency, causing fetal growth restriction leading to chronic and prolonged malnutrition.

- RS typically occurs within 2–6 days after initiation of PN.
- RS in the neonatal population may be characterized by hypophosphatemia, hypokalemia, hypercalcemia, hypomagnesemia, and/or hyperglycemia.
- Close monitoring of serum electrolytes should begin within 24 hours of initiation of PN.
- Specific recommendations on protein, dextrose, and lipids to prevent refeeding syndrome are currently not available; however, some suggest lower doses of AA to prevent hypophosphatemia.
- Phosphorus should be added to PN as early as can be provided.

Intrauterine Growth Restriction (IUGR)[20–22]

- Refers to a fetus who has not achieved expected in-utero growth. IUGR is a result of placental insufficiency and insufficient nutrient transfer across the placenta. Infants can be defined as having symmetrical growth restriction or asymmetric growth restriction.
  - Symmetric growth restriction: weight, length, and head circumference are all proportionally affected. Typically occurs early in gestation.
  - Asymmetric growth restriction: Head circumference is preserved while weight and length velocity are compromised. Typically occurs late in the second trimester or the third trimester.
- Nutritional risks associated with IUGR:
  - Hypoglycemia/hyperglycemia.
  - Hypocalcemia.
  - Feeding intolerance/increased risk for Necrotizing Enterocolitis.
  - Electrolyte abnormalities.
  - Acidemia.
-

References

1. Schoenwolf GC, Bleyl SB, Brauer PR, Francis-West PH. Development of the gastrointestinal tract. Larsen's Human Embryology. 14:335–67.
2. Fanaroff MD. Development of the neonatal gastrointestinal tract. Martin's Neonatal-Perinatal Medicine. 85:1598–604.
3. Bolender DL. Basic embryology. Fetal and Neonatal Physiology. 3:23–38.
4. Garg M, Sherin U, Fanaroff D. Disorders of carbohydrate metabolism in the neonate. Martin's Neonatal-Perinatal Medicine. 90:1672–96.
5. de la Cruz D, Fetal JN. Digestive-absorptive functions in fetuses, infants, and children. Neonatal Physiology. 86:881–888.e2.
6. Hodges B. Pediatric nutrition practice, group P. Academy of Nutrition and Dietetics Pocket Guide to Neonatal Nutrition; 2022.
7. Chou JH, Roumiantsev S, Singh R. PediTools electronic growth chart calculators: applications in clinical care, research, and quality improvement. , Journal of Medical Internet Research [Internet] 2020 Jan 30 [cited 2020 Oct 16];22(1):e16204. Available from: https://pubmed.ncbi.nlm.nih.gov/32012066/
8. Koletzko B, Cheah FC, Domellöf M, Poindexter BB, Vain N, van Goudoever JB. Nutritional Care of Preterm Infants. Karger Medical and Scientific Publishers; 2021.
9. Barbieri J, Petrea CM. Select micronutrients for the preterm neonate. Nutr Clin Pract. 2023;38:S66–83.
10. Lagerquist E, al-Haddad B JS, Irvine J, Muskthel L, Rios A, Upadhyay K. Feeding volume advancement in preterm neonates: a level 4 neonatal intensive care unit quality improvement initiative. Nutr Clin Pract. 2023 Oct;38:1175–80.
11. Adamkin DH. Use of human milk and fortification in the NICU. J Perinatol. 2022;43:551–9.
12. Groh-Wargo S, Thompson M. Managing the human-Milk-fed, preterm, VLBW, infant at NICU discharge: the sprinkles dilemma. Infant, child and adolescent. Nutrition. 2014;XX(X):1–8.
13. Robinson D, Calkins K, Chen Y, Petrea Cober M, Falciglia G, Church D, Mey J, McKeever L, Sentongo T. Guidelines for Parenteral Nutrition in Preterm Infants: The American Society for Parenteral and Enteral Nutrition. 2023;47:830–58.
14. Goday PS, Walia CS. Pediatric nutrition for dietitians. Boca Raton: CRC Press; 2022.
15. ASPEN recommendations on appropriate parenteral nutrition dosing for neonatal and pediatric patients. [Internet]. 2020 [cited 2024 June 28]. Available from https://www.nutritioncare.org/uploadedFiles/Documents/GuidelinesandClinicalResources/PN Dosing 1-Sheet-Nov 2020-Final.pdf.

16. Tsang C, Uauy R, Koletzko B, Zlotkin S. Nutrition of the preterm infant: scientific basis and practical guidelines. 2nd ed; 2005.
17. Mihatsch W, Fewtrell M, Goulet O, Molgaard C, Picaud J, Senterre T. The ESPGHAN/ESPEN/ESPR/CSPEN working group on pediatric parenteral nutrition. ESPGHAN/ESPEN/ESPR/CSPEN guidelines on pediatric parenteral nutrition: calcium, phosphorus and magnesium. Clin Nutr. 2018;37:2360–5.
18. Domellof M, Szitanyi P, Simchowitz V, Franz A, Mimouni F. The ESPGHAN/ESPEN/ESPR/CSPEN working group on pediatric parenteral nutrition. ESPGHAN/ESPEN/ESPR/CSPEN guidelines on pediatric parenteral nutrition: iron and trace minerals. Clin Nutr. 2018;38:2354–9.
19. Cormack B, Jiang Y, Harding J, Crother C, Bloomfield F, ProVIDe Trial Group. Neonatal refeeding syndrome and clinical outcome in extremely low-birth-weight babies: secondary cohort analysis from the ProVIDe trial. J Parenter Enter Nutr. 2020;0(0):1–14.
20. Bozzetti V, Tagliabue PE. Enteral feeding of intrauterine growth restriction preterm infants: theoretical risks and practical implications. Pediatr Med Chir. 2017;39(2)
21. Bozzetti V, Tagliabue PE, Visser GHA, van Bel F, Gazzolo D. Feeding issues in IUGR preterm infants. Early Hum Dev. 2013;89:S21–3.
22. Mandy, GT. UpToDate [Internet]. Uptodate.com. 2024 [cited 2024 Nov 6]. Available from: https://www.uptodate.com/contents/fetal-growth-restriction-fgr-and-small-for-gestational-age-sga-newborns?search=IUGR%20feeding%20&source=search_result&selectedTitle=1%7E150&usage_type=default&display_rank=1.

Pediatric Pulmonary Disorders and Nutritional Concerns

48

Parevi Majmudar, Sara Bewley, Kristina Pytlak, and Diana Schnee

Children are in a constant state of growth and development, which means they need more air, water, and food to maintain an anabolic state. This results in increased caloric needs to support their growth [1].

Sufficient nutrition and supplementation have been associated with better outcomes in children with lung diseases, including cystic fibrosis, chronic lung disease of prematurity, chronic mechanical ventilation, and acute respiratory failure [2].

P. Majmudar (✉)
Pediatric Nutrition Support, Division of Pediatric Gastroenterology, Hepatology, and Nutrition, Cleveland Clinic Children's Hospital, Cleveland, OH, USA

Center for Pediatric Pulmonology Diseases, Cleveland Clinic Children's Hospital, Cleveland, OH, USA
e-mail: MAJMUDP@ccf.org

S. Bewley · K. Pytlak · D. Schnee
Pediatric Nutrition Support, Division of Pediatric Gastroenterology, Hepatology, and Nutrition, Cleveland Clinic Children's Hospital, Cleveland, OH, USA
e-mail: BEWLEYS@ccf.org; pyllakk@ccf.org; SCHNEED2@ccf.org

K. Radhakrishnan (ed.), *Handbook of Clinical and Practical Pediatric Nutrition*, https://doi.org/10.1007/978-3-031-97759-6_48

Cystic Fibrosis

- Malnutrition and undernutrition from cystic fibrosis (CF) result from an imbalance between energy demand and energy intake.
- Energy needs of children with CF are estimated to be 1.5–2 times the needs of those without CF.
- A high-calorie, high-fat diet is generally recommended [3].
- Those with CF have higher energy expenditure due to pancreatic insufficiency and lung disease unique to CF [4].

Lung disease in CF increases energy demand through several mechanisms:

- Continuous cycle of chronic inflammation, bacterial colonization, recurrent infections causing a systemic hypermetabolic state with elaboration of proinflammatory cytokines.
- Increasing airflow obstruction and hyperinflation, all of which increase the cost of ventilation.
- Maintenance of normal weight and stature for age in children is associated with lung function and survival.
- A 2003 study in children between 3 and 6 years of age found that children with weight for age less than the fifth percentile at 3 years of age had significantly lower pulmonary function at 6 years of age compared with those with a weight for age greater than the 75th percentile at 3 years.
- The CF Foundation Patient Registry data consistently shows that children with higher body mass index (BMI) percentile have better lung function [2].
- Nutrition in CF should take into account pancreatic enzyme replacement, fat-soluble vitamin, and micronutrient supplementation.

Nutritional Management of the Cystic Fibrosis Patient

Estimating Needs

- Consensus statements and guidelines recommend that people with CF require anywhere from 110 to 200% of the RDA. The Estimated Energy Requirements (EER) formulated from the Recommended Daily Allowances (RDA) are commonly used to determine energy needs in the pediatric CF population [5].
- This is due to increased energy needs due to: pancreatic insufficiency and secondary malabsorption, infections, increased work of breathing, and/or higher metabolic rate.
- When estimating needs, keep in mind the goals of sustained weight gain and growth in infants and children.
- A high-calorie, high-fat diet (35–40% of total calories) is recommended to meet increased needs.
- Infants who are newly diagnosed with cystic fibrosis typically need their feedings adjusted to promote adequate weight gains.
- Typically plan on increasing caloric density of feedings for the cystic fibrosis patient proactively. Most infants will need feedings concentrated to 24–27 calorie/ounce.
- To note, CF Foundation recommends all infants to be plotted on the CDC growth chart rather than the WHO growth chart to establish optimal growth trends early in life [5].

Lab Monitoring [5]

- Vitamins A, D 25-OH, prothrombin time (PT) (or PIVKA-II) and E levels should be checked annually, fasting levels of A are preferable.
- PIVKA-II or DCP level recommended as more sensitive measures of vitamin K status (vs PT).
- Vitamins A and D are acute phase reactants; level should not be measured if patient is acutely ill.
- Possible vitamin A deficiency if night blindness/difficulty seeing at night.
- Unclear if individuals with pancreatic sufficiency require annual fat-soluble vitamin levels.

Enzyme Therapy

- Pancreatic enzyme replacements contain lipase, amylase, and protease.
- Goal of 1000–2500 units/lipase/kg/meal.
- Please refer to chapter on pancreatic disorders for more details.

Vitamin/Mineral Supplementation [5]

- Those individuals with CF with pancreatic insufficiency have an increased need for fat-soluble vitamins.
- There are options for water-miscible CF-specific multivitamin preparations that contain fat-soluble vitamins in an amount greater than in a non-CF-specific multivitamin.
- Vitamins are available in liquid, chewable, or soft gel.

Salt

- A high salt diet is recommended for all CF patients secondary to losses.

  Dosing Guidelines

  – Infants from birth to 6 months require 1/8 teaspoon salt daily.
  – Infants >6 months–12 months require 1/4 teaspoon salt daily.
    May add to formula or in applesauce when giving PERT.
  – Children 12 months and older liberal salt diet.
- Consider recommending salt supplementation of 1/4 teaspoon daily be continued past first birthday and until child is consuming a full diet with added salt.

Iron

- Iron deficiency can occur in individuals with CF; more often in adults and those with severe lung disease.
- CF-specific vitamins do not contain iron.
- Monitor for anemia with an annual hemoglobin and hematocrit.

Modulators

- New modulator therapies show promising results regarding improved weight gain.
- Individualizing counseling regarding the high-calorie diet, as needed to adjust for patients on gene modulators [5].
- Excessive weight gain can be a complication.
- The clinical incidence and relevance of this in CF is currently unknown and warrants closer monitoring.

Bronchopulmonary Dysplasia

- Bronchopulmonary dysplasia (BPD) is an inflammatory lung disease found in infants born before 32 weeks of gestation who require ongoing respiratory support at 36 weeks postmenstrual age.
- Often, these infants have minimal energy reserves and limited stores of essential nutrients.
- Achieving optimal nutrition in infants with BPD is complicated as estimating total energy needs is difficult.
- This can lead to inadequate nutrition in at-risk infants, which in turn compromises lung development and function characterized by delayed somatic growth, delayed alveolar development, and abnormal lung healing [6].

- As such, children with BPD require more total energy than age-matched controls without BPD, due to increased work of breathing and increased metabolic demands [6].
- Factors that can contribute to nutritional deficiency in infants with BPD include:
  - Frequent discontinuation of feedings during periods of instability or acute hospitalization.
  - Systemic steroids are often used in the management of BPD. Corticosteroids are known to have a negative impact on linear growth and cause slower weight gain velocity, independent of energy expenditure and intake.

  - Diuretics are commonly used in BPD to manage pulmonary edema. Prolonged use can result in electrolyte derangements with negative effects on bone mineralization.
  - Rapid and frequent changes in respiratory support may lead to increased levels of stress, work of breathing, and energy expenditure.
- Children with BPD who demonstrate catch-up weight gain or above-average weight gain have greater improvement in their lung function testing over time compared to children with BPD who have average or below average weight gain [6].

Acute and Chronic Respiratory Distress in the Pediatric Patient

Introduction

Acute Respiratory Distress Syndrome (ARDS) occurs when fluid builds up in the alveoli in the lungs, thus preventing them from filling up with air [7]. To improve oxygen levels in the body, patients with ARDS often require mechanical ventilation or oxygen therapy [7]. Mechanical ventilation can become a chronic need if a child cannot be weaned from support.

Types of mechanical ventilation [8]:

1. Noninvasive ventilation: oxygen delivery via a mask over the patient's nose and/or mouth.
   (a) Continuous Positive Airway Pressure (CPAP) provides a constant positive pressure for air delivery into the lungs.
   (b) Bilevel Positive Airway Pressure (BiPAP) provides a higher pressure at the time of inhalation and lower pressure at the time of exhalation.
   (c) High Flow Nasal Canula (HFNC) provides oxygen flow rate of up to 60 liters per minute.
2. Invasive ventilation: use of an endotracheal tube placed directly into the trachea and connected to the ventilator. Air is delivered directly to the lungs.

Nutrition considerations with noninvasive ventilation[8]:

1. Oral or nasal feeding tubes can often prevent the tight seal that is needed with noninvasive ventilation for optimal air delivery.
2. Sometimes the air being delivered by the CPAP or BiPAP machine does not only deliver air to the lungs, but can be unintentionally delivered to the stomach causing abdominal distention, which can increase vomiting or feeding intolerance.
   (a) Post-pyloric tubes can help overcome this problem to prevent aspiration.

Nutrition considerations with invasive ventilation [8, 9]:

1. Patients who are intubated are often fluid restricted and on diuretics, which can lead to inadequate energy intake and electrolyte disturbances.
2. Patients with limited mobility along with chronic ventilator support may have higher or lower nutrient and fluid needs depending on their underlying diagnosis.

Growth Assessment

Children with need for pulmonary support have increased risk for malnutrition due to the inability to consume nutrition orally.

Enteral nutrition (EN) support should be initiated within 24 hours of admission in critically ill children, unless contraindicated [10]. EN, even in small amounts, can improve gastrointestinal mucosal integrity [10]. The goal is to provide at least 2/3 of energy expenditure in invasively ventilated children within the first week [10]. Initiate parenteral nutrition (PN) support if unable to initiate EN support.

In those with chronic ventilatory support outside of the hospital, issues with both under- and overweight status maybe observed. These issues are exacerbated by limited mobility, infections, and altered metabolism associated with underlying diagnoses.

Estimating Needs

During acute illness, patients are often in a catabolic state due to the production of acute phase proteins, repair of tissues, and the production of immune proteins; thus, their protein requirements are increased [7]. A prolongation of this catabolic state can result in decreased cardiopulmonary function in the setting of the breakdown of cardiac and respiratory muscle mass [7]. See Table 48.1 for estimating protein requirements.

For chronic care, the DRI for protein intake should be sufficient provided the patient does not have any other issues, such as pressure wounds which would increase protein needs.

Sufficient energy from carbohydrates, fat, and protein should be provided to preserve lean muscle mass in acutely ill and chronic patients [7]. Excessive carbohydrate intake may prolong mechanical ventilation as excess carbohydrates are converted into fat, which generates carbon dioxide [7]. Indirect calorimetry is the gold standard for estimating energy needs in the critically ill patient; however, predictive equations are often used with indirect calorimetry is not available [7]. Children who are ventilated may have lower energy requirements; however, adjustments should be made to ensure adequate protein, and vitamin and mineral intake while preventing excessive weight gain [10].

Table 48.1 ASPEN critical care guidelines [9]

Age	gm/kg/day
0–2 years	2–3
2–13 years	1.5–2
13–18 years	1.5

Asthma Patients

Asthma is an inflammatory condition of the lower airways. It is the most common chronic disease of childhood in the United States. If asthma is poorly controlled, children may require repeated courses of systemic corticosteroids to manage acute asthma exacerbations. Systemic corticosteroids can cause, among other side effects, increased appetite and excessive weight gain.

If the ability to exercise is limited by inadequate asthma control, this will also contribute to worsening weight gain.

Asthma in patients with obesity is more difficult to control, for various reasons:

- Increased mass in the abdomen by adipose tissue decreases the functional residual capacity of the lungs, and this in turn can increase airway reactivity.
- Adipose tissue releases proinflammatory mediators, which are associated with poor asthma control. These markers are elevated in patients with asthma and obesity.
- High saturated fatty acids can acutely increase airway inflammation and decrease lung function.
- Altered adaptive and innate immune cell function, contributing to airway inflammation in obesity.

Patients with asthma and metabolic syndrome have blunted responses to common asthma medications, and it is worthwhile to refer these patients for dietary counseling.

Nutritional Needs in Patients with Asthma

Children with asthma can be at risk for overnutrition and malnutrition. They often require steroids, which can result in growth failure, but are also susceptible to sodium and fluid retention, glucose intolerance, and increased appetite, which can lead to excessive weight gain [11]. Obesity is associated with greater asthma morbidity and while the relationship has not been clearly described, excess body weight may contribute to inflammation of the lung or steroid resistance [12]. Additionally, children with asthma may have limited exercise tolerance due to asthmatic flares thereby perpetuating the cycle of obesity and asthma. In some cases, malnutrition may be present because of increased energy expenditure with work of breathing or due to repeated post-tussive emesis during flares.

Working toward normalized growth trends is an important aspect of treatment. Lifestyle changes to help achieve a healthful body weight and reduce inflammation in pediatric patients include:

- Reduction/elimination of refined carbohydrates and added sugars.
- Focus on minimally processed, whole foods.
- Minimize food consumed that is prepared outside of the home.
- Increase in consumption of lean proteins, produce, legumes, whole grains, and healthy fats.
- Increase in physical activity (as tolerated) and reduce sedentary behavior.
- Limit consumption of red meat.
- If underweight, oral dietary supplements may be warranted.

Reduction in dairy products with the goal to reduce mucous production is not effective and can put children at risk for poor intake of calcium, phosphorus, and vitamin D [13]. However, if a family opts to remove dairy from their child's diet, appropriate alternatives should be. In the case of chronic oral steroid use, calcium and vitamin D intake should also be optimized to protect bone growth.

Implementation of specific diets for asthma is likely not founded; however, dietary practices, such as the Mediterranean diet, adopt the themes mentioned above. When warranted, weight loss can lead to an improvement in asthma symptoms [14].

References

1. Marostica PJC, Stein RT. Kendig & Chernick's disorders of the respiratory tract in children. 2012.
2. Knebusch N, et al. Macronutrient and micronutrient intake in children with lung disease. Nutrients. 2023;15(19):4142.
3. Stallings VA, et al. Evidence-based practice recommendations for nutrition-related management of children and adults with cystic fibrosis and pancreatic insufficiency: results of a systematic review. J Am Diet Assoc. 2008;108(5):832–9.
4. Solomon M, Bozic M, Mascarenhas MR. Nutritional issues in cystic fibrosis. Clin Chest Med. 2016;37(1):97–107.
5. Leonard A, Schindler T, Padula L, Altman K, Vavrina K. In: Chin M, editor. Cystic fibrosis nutrition 101: getting started. 9th ed; 2022.
6. Miller AN, Curtiss J, Kielt MJ. Nutritional needs of the infant with bronchopulmonary dysplasia. NeoReviews. 2024;25(1):e12–24.
7. Wilson B, Typpo K. Nutrition: a primary therapy in pediatric acute respiratory distress syndrome. Front in Pediat. 2016; 4. Praveen Goday, Mehta N. Pediatric critical care nutrition. Chapter 15: Respiratory failure. McGraw Hill Professional; 2014.
8. Kratochvíl M, Klučka J, Klabusayová E, Musilová T, Vafek V, Skříšovská T, et al. Nutrition in pediatric intensive care: a narrative review. Children. 2022;9(7):1031.
9. American Dietetic Association. Ventilator Issues [Internet]. Pediatric nutrition care manual. American Dietetic Association; [cited 2024 Oct 10]. Available from: https://www.nutritioncaremanual.org/topic.cfm?ncm_category_id=13&lv1=144632&lv2=144777&ncm_toc_id=144777&ncm_heading=Nutrition%20Care%20home%20page.
10. Mehta NM, Compher C. A.S.P.E.N. Clinical Guidelines: Nutrition Support of the Critically Ill Child. Journal of Parenteral and Enteral Nutrition [Internet]. 2009 [cited 2024 Oct 10];33:260–76. Available from: https://doi.org/10.1177/0148607109333114.
11. A.S.P.E.N. Clinical Guidelines: Nutrition Support of the Critically Ill Child Mehta NM, Compher C; A.S.P.E.N. Board of Directors. A.S.P.E.N. Clinical guidelines: nutrition support of the critically ill child. JPEN J Parenter Enteral Nutr 2009;33(3):260–276.
12. Soczewka M, Kędzia A, Skowrońska B, Niechciał E. Importance of diet in children and adolescents with obesity and asthma. Pediat Endocrinol Diabetes Metabol. 2024;30(2):91–6.
13. Wüthrich B, Schmid A, Walther B, Sieber R. Milk consumption does not lead to mucus production or occurrence of asthma. J Am Coll Nutr. 2005;24(6 Suppl):547S–55S.
14. Calcaterra V, Verduci E, Ghezzi M, Cena H, Pascuzzi MC, Regalbuto C, et al. Pediatric obesity-related asthma: the role of nutrition and nutrients in prevention and treatment. Nutrients. 2021;13(11):3708.

Nutritional Considerations in Kidney Disease

49

Raed Bou Matar and Merideth Miller

Acute Kidney Injury

Acute kidney injury (AKI) is defined as the sudden loss of kidney function that lasts days to weeks. The Kidney Disease Improving Global Outcomes classify AKI into three stages as detailed in Table 49.1. Possible nutrition-related concerns related to AKI are addressed in Table 49.2.

R. B. Matar (✉) · M. Miller
Center for Pediatric Nephrology, Cleveland Clinic Children's Hospital, Cleveland, OH, USA
e-mail: BOUMATR@ccf.org; MILLERM5@ccf.org

K. Radhakrishnan (ed.), *Handbook of Clinical and Practical Pediatric Nutrition*, https://doi.org/10.1007/978-3-031-97759-6_49

Table 49.1 Stages of AKI based on the 2012 Kidney Disease Improving Global Outcomes (KDIGO) clinical practice guidelines [1]

AKI stage	Definition
Stage 1	Increase in serum creatinine by 0.3 mg/dL within 48 hours Or Increase in serum creatinine to 1.5–1.9 × baseline within 7 days Or Urine output <0.5 mL/kg/h for 6–12 h
Stage 2	Increase in serum creatinine to 2.0–2.9 × baseline within 7 days Or Urine output <0.5 mL/kg/h for more than 12 h
Stage 3	Increase in serum creatinine to 3.0 × baseline within 7 days. Or Increase in serum creatinine to 4.0 mg/dL Or Initiation of kidney replacement therapy Or Urine output <0.3 mL/kg/h for 24 h Or Anuria for 12 h Or In patients <18 y of age, decrease in eGFR to <35 ml/min per 1.73 m^2

Table 49.2 Nutrition considerations and recommendations in AKI

Concerns	Considerations/recommendations[a]
Hyponatremia	Target rate of correction should not exceed 10 mEq/L/day Dilution due to fluid retention and/or hypotonic fluids—free water restriction, adjust free water content in IVF Dehydration—fluid resuscitation with isotonic fluids. Hyperglycemia—correct glucose level [2]
Hypernatremia	Target rate of correction should not exceed 10 mEq/L/day Dehydration—fluid resuscitation with isotonic or hypotonic fluids. Excessive sodium in IV fluids—adjust fluids [2]

Table 49.2 (continued)

Concerns	Considerations/recommendations[a]
Hyperkalemia	Remove potassium from IVF and/or TPN [3] Low potassium diet (2000 mg in older children, examples of high potassium foods: bananas, potatoes, tomatoes, dairy products[a])
Hyperphosphatemia	Low phosphorus diet (800–1000 mg in older children, examples of high phosphorus foods: dairy products, whole wheat, hot dogs[a]) [4]
Hypoalbuminemia	Dilutional due to fluid retention (mild) Nutritional (most common) Proteinuria Treat by optimizing dietary protein intake (nuts, seeds, legumes, chicken)
Hypertension and fluid retention	Loop diuretics and/or sodium restriction [5]: Ages 1–3 years: < 1200 mg sodium/day Ages 4–8 years: < 1500 mg sodium/day Ages 9–13 years: < 1800 mg sodium/day Ages 14–18 years: < 2300 mg sodium/day [6] (Foods high in sodium include soups, frozen meals, pizza, hot sauce, ketchup[a])
Anorexia	Offer nutritional supplements and/or modulars Meal planning and increasing calories with high-calorie additives such as butter, vegetable oil, sour cream, avocado Tube (enteral) feeding or parenteral nutrition may be required [7]

[a]See nutrient-specific section for additional foods

Nutrition Recommendations/Considerations

- Critically ill patients are at an increased risk for malnutrition. AKI increases this risk due to impaired metabolism of fats and carbohydrates, electrolytes, and fluid imbalances.
- Continuous Kidney Replacement Therapy (CKRT) is commonly administered in patients with severe AKI who are unable to maintain homeostasis.
- Nutrients such as proteins, glucose, trace elements, and water-soluble vitamins are removed during CKRT. This highlights

Table 49.3 Macronutrient needs during CKRT [8, 9]

Nutrient	Recommendation
Calories/ energy[a]	Limit to 20–30% above basal needs to avoid overfeeding Indirect calorimetry is gold standard for calculating Resting Energy Expenditure (REE) Ensure all calories are accounted for: medications, glucose-containing fluids added to the CKRT
Carbohydrates	20–25% of total calories Citrate may induce insulin resistance
Protein[a]	Goal is a positive nitrogen balance: 40–50% of total calories Protein losses in CKRT are significant Start with the American Society of Parenteral and Enteral Nutrition (ASPEN) protein needs for Critically ill: 0–2 years: 2–3 g pro/kg 2–13 years: 1.5–2 g pro/kg 13–18 years: 1.5 g pro/kg An additional 10–20% in protein may be needed to account for CKRT losses
Fat[a]	30–40% of total calories Limit infants to 3–4 g/kg/d Limit children to 2–3 g/kg/d Supplement with L-carnitine, which is essential for fatty acid movement into the mitochondria and is cleared by CKRT [10]. Monitor for hypertriglyceridemia and hypocholesterolemia (common on CKRT)
Fluids	CKRT facilitates controlled fluid removal, allowing for provision of adequate nutrition

[a]Use established dry weight for calculation

the importance of optimizing nutrition early in patients on CKRT [7]. See Tables 49.3 and 49.4 for macro- and micronutrient recommendations for nutrition support.

- Enteral nutrition should be started within the first 24–48 hours. If unable to provide nutrition enterally, parenteral nutrition is a viable alternative.
- Citrate is often used for regional anticoagulation of the CKRT circuit. However, citrate is commonly associated with metabolic alkalosis and may induce insulin resistance.

Table 49.4 Micronutrient needs during CKRT [8, 9]

Nutrient	Recommendation
Electrolytes	
Sodium	Adjust CKRT fluids and/or parenteral nutrition
Potassium	Adjust CKRT fluids and/or parenteral nutrition
Phosphorus	Adjust CKRT fluids and/or parenteral nutrition
Calcium	Adjust CKRT fluids and/or parenteral nutrition Patients on citrate anticoagulation are at risk for both hypocalcemia and hypercalcemia. Calcium drip and citrate rates are adjusted based on blood and circuit calcium levels, respectively.
Magnesium	Adjust CKRT fluids and/or parenteral nutrition
Vitamins monitor frequently while on CKRT	
Thiamine	Check within the first week of CKRT initiation Supplementation based on age: < 12 months = 0.3 mg/d 1–3 years = 0.5 mg/d > 3 years = up to 1.2 mg/d Alternatively, 83 mcg/L added to CKRT fluid
Vitamin B6	Check within the first week of CKRT initiation High dose B6 recommended to be guided by serum levels
Folic Acid	Check within the first week of CKRT initiation Supplementation based on age: < 1 year = 48 mcg/d 1–3 years = 90 mcg/d > 4 years = 240 mcg/d Alternatively, 4.4 mcg/L added to CKRT fluid
Vitamin C	Check within the first 2 weeks of CKRT initiation Supplementation based on age: < 1 year = 50 mg/d 1–3 years = 15 mg/d > 3 years = 90 mg/d Alternatively, 1.9 mg/L added to CKRT fluid
Fat-soluble vitamins (ADEK)	Not seen to be removed in effluent

(continued)

Table 49.4 (continued)

Nutrient	Recommendation
Trace elements—monitor frequently while on CKRT	
Selenium	May need extra dose once weekly based on clearance Optimal dose not established in children
Copper	Monitor levels, low levels not consistently seen Optimal dose not established in children
Zinc	Monitor levels, low levels not consistently seen Optimal dose not established in children
Manganese	Monitor levels, may be elevated Adjust/remove from parenteral nutrition

Chronic Kidney Disease

Chronic kidney disease (CKD) is defined as abnormalities of kidney structure or function present for at least 3 months. It is often characterized by progressive gradual decline in kidney function over time. CKD is classified into various stages based on estimated GFR (see Table 49.5 for classifications of CKD) and degree of albuminuria [11] (see Table 49.6 for classification of albuminemia).

- Patients with early stages of chronic kidney disease (CKD) should maintain a healthy diet based on the general Dietary Guidelines for Americans.
- As CKD progresses, more specific recommendations and restrictions may be necessary to achieve appropriate homeostasis.
- Children with CKD may develop insufficient growth and poor weight gain due to inadequate energy and/or protein intake. CKD may progress quickly during periods of rapid growth.
- Growth hormone (GH) may be indicated for impaired GH utilization in CKD patients. GH is generally started if height or height velocity z-score for age remains < -2 and/or a height/length for age remains <fifth percentile after delivery of adequate calories and correction of metabolic bone parameters.

Table 49.5 Stages of CKD

Stage	Description	GFR (mL/min/1.73 m^2)
G1	Normal or high	>90
G2	Mildly decreased	60–89
G3a	Mildly to moderately decreased	45–59
G3b	Moderately to severely decreased	30–44
G4	Severely decreased	15–29
G5	Kidney failure	<15

Table 49.6 Stages of albuminemia

Stage	Description	Urine albumin to creatinine ratio (mg/g)
A1	Normal to mildly increased	< 30
A2	Moderately increased	30–300
A3	Severely increased	> 300

- Oral intake may be limited in infants and young children with CKD with increased caloric needs. Therefore, oral supplementation or enteral tube feedings is often needed to achieve adequate nutrition and growth.

Nutrient deficiencies are common in patients with CKD due to dietary restrictions and poor appetite. Table 49.7 addresses nutrition considerations for patients with CKD and recommendations to address each.

Table 49.7 Nutrition considerations and recommendations for CKD

Nutrient	Recommendation	Nutrition considerations
Calories	Based on Dietary Reference Intake (DRI) equations (Chap. 2) for age adjusting for activity level and growth needs [12]	Monitor overall growth trends Use estimated dry weight to calculate needs Infants have particularly high energy needs to achieve adequate growth
Protein	CKD stage 3: 100–140% DRI for age[a] CKD stage 4–5: 100–120% DRI for age[a] Peritoneal dialysis: 100% DRI[a] + 0.15–0.3 g pro/kg/day Hemodialysis: 100% DRI[a] + 0.1 g pro/kg/day [12]	Use protein modulars and supplements to maintain growth and serum albumin levels Limit protein intake in patients >18 y of age [13] Infants on peritoneal dialysis may need up to 3 g pro/kg/day due to dialysis losses
Potassium	Restriction: 2000 mg/day [14][a]	Foods high in potassium include bananas, potatoes, tomatoes, dairy products Potassium binding medications (e.g., kayexalate) to decant formula or orally
Phosphorus	Restriction: 800–1000 mg/day [14][c]	Foods high in phosphorus include dairy products, whole wheat, hot dogs. Phos is often added as a preservative to various highly processed foods. Start phosphorus binding medication (e.g., sevelamer) as needed
Fluid	Based on urine output and/or fluid retention Fluid restriction as needed Additional fluid may be necessary in infants and young children with polyuria	Evaluate sodium intake Provide suggestions to help with thirst: hard candy, gum, ice, frozen grapes, decrease sodium intake Monitor serum sodium levels and adjust fluids as needed

Table 49.7 (continued)

Nutrient	Recommendation	Nutrition considerations
Sodium	Loop diuretics and/or sodium restriction [5]: Ages 1–3 years: <1200 mg sodium/day Ages 4–8 years: <1500 mg sodium/day Ages 9–13 years: <1800 mg sodium/day Ages 14–18 years: <2300 mg sodium/day [6] Infants/young children with kidney salt wasting may need sodium supplements	Sodium restriction is based on fluid retention and blood pressure In children with salt wasting, monitor serum levels and supplement as needed (low levels may impair growth)
B Vitamins	Start kidney specific multivitamin at CKD stage 4–5	B vitamins are removed during dialysis and are limited in diet due to restrictions. Kidney-specific multivitamin provides higher B vitamins
Vitamin D3	Supplement based on serum levels, see chapter on vitamin D for repletion recommendations	Vitamin D absorption is impaired in patients with CKD Vitamin D activation in the kidney is limited. Vitamin D3 is generally preferred due to more reliable absorption [15]
Vitamin A	Vitamin A can accumulate in patients with CKD Limit vitamin A intake in supplements and formulas	High vitamin A levels can cause toxicity

[a]See chapter on protein for DRI
[b]See chapter on estimated energy needs for appropriate equations
[c]Nutrient recommendations may need to be adjusted based on lab values and patient size

Nephrotic Syndrome

Nephrotic syndrome is defined by a triad of high-grade proteinuria, hypoalbuminemia, and edema.

See Table 49.8 for common nutrition considerations and recommendations for patients with nephrotic syndrome based on their lab values and symptoms.

Table 49.8 Nutrition recommendations and considerations in nephrotic syndrome

Nutrient of concern	Recommendation	Consideration
Protein	Ensure adequate protein intake for growth	Excessive animal protein intake may exacerbate hyperfiltration glomerular injury and dietary acid load.
Sodium	Loop diuretics and/or sodium restriction: Ages 1–3 years: <1200 mg sodium/day Ages 4–8 years: <1500 mg sodium/day Ages 9–13 years: <1800 mg sodium/day Ages 14–18 years: <2300 mg sodium/day [6]	Restriction in all children, with greater benefit in those with significant edema and/or hypertension
Cholesterol and triglycerides	Monitor cholesterol panel Dietary restriction is often insufficient to control dyslipidemia in nephrotic patients, and antilipidemic agents may be considered if severe [7].	Nephrotic syndrome causes elevated cholesterol and triglyceride levels
Potassium	Monitor labs, consider 2000 mg/day restriction based on blood levels[a] [7]	- Restrict only as needed
Phosphorus	Monitor labs, consider 800–1000 mg/day[a] restriction based on blood levels	- Restrict only as needed

[a]Nutrient recommendations may need to be adjusted based on lab values and patient age

Renal Tubulopathies

- Selective deficiencies in kidney tubular function may result in impaired acid-base balance and various electrolyte disturbances.
- Impaired tubular acid excretion usually results in renal tubular acidosis (RTA).
- On the contrary, rare genetic disorders such Bartter's syndrome and Gitelman syndrome are associated with impaired tubular salt and chloride reabsorption leading to metabolic alkalosis and hypokalemia.
- Nutritional management generally centers on the correction of the underlying deficits with enteral or intravenous supplements [16]. Table 49.9 presents information regarding different renal tubulopathies and nutrition considerations based on the diagnosis.

Table 49.9 Tubular disorders and Nutrition Considerations

Tubular disorder	Underlying tubular defect	Nutritional consideration(s)
Fanconi syndrome (Includes Type II RTA) [16]	Global dysfunction of the proximal tubules resulting in impaired reclamation of bicarbonate, phosphorus, amino acids, and glucose	Supplement with sodium citrate (young children) or sodium bicarbonate (teenagers and adults) to correct the metabolic acidosis Supplement with phosphorus as needed to correct hypophosphatemia Glucose and amino acid losses are usually inconsequential and do not require specific therapy
Isolated proximal RTA (Type II RTA, rare) [16]	Impaired reclamation of filtered bicarbonate	Supplement with sodium citrate (young children) or sodium bicarbonate (teenagers and adults) to correct metabolic acidosis

(continued)

Table 49.9 (continued)

Tubular disorder	Underlying tubular defect	Nutritional consideration(s)
Distal RTA (Type I RTA) [16]	Impaired secretion of H+ in the distal convoluted tubules Calcium reabsorption is also often impaired resulting in hypercalciuria and nephrocalcinosis or kidney stones	Supplement with sodium citrate (young children) or sodium bicarbonate (teenagers and adults) to correct metabolic acidosis If hypercalciuria present, manage with proper hydration and citrate supplements
Type IV RTA (Aldosterone deficiency or Aldosterone resistance) [16]	Impaired aldosterone function results in urinary sodium wasting and impaired potassium excretion in the cortical collecting ducts	Restrict dietary potassium. High salt diet.
Bartter's syndrome [17]	Severely impaired reabsorption of sodium, potassium, calcium, and chloride in the thick ascending loop of Henle	Salt craving is common, and generous salt intake should be encouraged Supplement with sodium chloride and potassium chloride as needed Adequate hydration to help prevent kidney stones
Gitelman's syndrome [17]	Mildly impaired reabsorption of sodium, potassium, magnesium, and chloride in the distal convoluted tubules	Salt craving is common, and generous salt intake should be encouraged Supplement with sodium chloride, potassium chloride, and magnesium salts as needed

References

1. Kellum JA, Lameire N, Aspelin P, et al. Kidney disease: Improving global outcomes (KDIGO) acute kidney injury work group. KDIGO clinical practice guideline for acute kidney injury. Kidney Int Suppl. 2012;2(1):1–138. https://doi.org/10.1038/kisup.2012.1.
2. Sterns RH, Nigwekar SU, Hix JK. The treatment of hyponatremia. Semin Nephrol. 2009;29(3):282–99. https://doi.org/10.1016/j.semnephrol.2009.03.002.

3. Rodan AR. Potassium: friend or foe? Pediatr Nephrol Berl Ger. 2017;32(7):1109–21. https://doi.org/10.1007/s00467-016-3411-8.
4. Leaf DE, Christov M. Dysregulated Mineral Metabolism in AKI. Semin Nephrol. 2019;39(1):41–56. https://doi.org/10.1016/j.semnephrol.2018.10.004.
5. Brater DC. Diuretic therapy. N Engl J Med. 1998;339(6):387–95. https://doi.org/10.1056/NEJM199808063390607.
6. Dietary Guidelines for Americans | health.gov. Accessed 19 Sep 2024. https://health.gov/our-work/nutrition-physical-activity/dietary-guidelines.
7. Sethi SK, Maxvold N, Bunchman T, Jha P, Kher V, Raina R. Nutritional management in the critically ill child with acute kidney injury: a review. Pediatr Nephrol Berl Ger. 2017;32(4):589–601. https://doi.org/10.1007/s00467-016-3402-9.
8. Fishman G, Singer P. Metabolic and nutritional aspects in continuous renal replacement therapy. J Intensive Med. 2023;3(3):228–38. https://doi.org/10.1016/j.jointm.2022.11.001.
9. Jonckheer J, Vergaelen K, Spapen H, Malbrain MLNG, De Waele E. Modification of Nutrition Therapy During Continuous Renal Replacement Therapy in Critically Ill Pediatric Patients: A Narrative Review and Recommendations. Nutr Clin Pract Off Publ Am Soc Parenter Enter Nutr. 2019;34(1):37–47. https://doi.org/10.1002/ncp.10231.
10. Sgambat K, Moudgil A. Carnitine deficiency in children receiving continuous renal replacement therapy. Hemodial Int Int Symp Home Hemodial. 2016;20(1):63–7. https://doi.org/10.1111/hdi.12341.
11. Disease K. Improving Global Outcomes (KDIGO) CKD Work Group. KDIGO 2024 Clinical Practice Guideline for the Evaluation and Management of Chronic Kidney Disease. Kidney Int. 2024;105(4S):S117–314. https://doi.org/10.1016/j.kint.2023.10.018.
12. Shaw V, Polderman N, Renken-Terhaerdt J, et al. Energy and protein requirements for children with CKD stages 2-5 and on dialysis-clinical practice recommendations from the Pediatric Renal Nutrition Taskforce. Pediatr Nephrol Berl Ger. 2020;35(3):519–31. https://doi.org/10.1007/s00467-019-04426-0.
13. KDOQI Clinical Practice Guideline for Nutrition in CKD. 2020. Update - PubMed. Accessed 15 Sep 2024. https://pubmed.ncbi.nlm.nih.gov/32829751/
14. Nutrition for Children with Chronic Kidney Disease – NIDDK. National Institute of Diabetes and Digestive and Kidney Diseases. Accessed September 15, 2024. https://www.niddk.nih.gov/health-information/kidney-disease/children/helping-child-adapt-life-chronic-kidney-disease/nutrition-chronic-kidney-disease
15. Tripkovic L, Lambert H, Hart K, et al. Comparison of vitamin D2 and vitamin D3 supplementation in raising serum 25-hydroxyvitamin D sta-

tus: a systematic review and meta-analysis. Am J Clin Nutr. 2012;95(6):1357–64. https://doi.org/10.3945/ajcn.111.031070.
16. Rodríguez SJ. Renal tubular acidosis: the clinical entity. J Am Soc Nephrol JASN. 2002;13(8):2160–70. https://doi.org/10.1097/01.asn.0000023430.92674.e5.
17. Kleta R, Bockenhauer D. Salt-Losing Tubulopathies in Children: What's New, What's Controversial? J Am Soc Nephrol JASN. 2018;29(3):727–39. https://doi.org/10.1681/ASN.2017060600.

Nutrition in Malignancy and Stem Cell Transplant

50

Rachel N. Zeno, Seth Rotz, Sara Bewley, and Alexis Payton

Weight loss and poor appetite are common presenting symptoms for patients with malignancy due to the energy utilized in rapid malignant cell proliferation. This is further exacerbated by many side effects of commonly used chemotherapeutic agents, including:

- Taste changes.
- Nausea.
- Vomiting.
- Mucositis (inflammation and enterocyte damage causing pain with enteral intake and poor intestinal absorption).

Radiation therapy can induce similar side effects. For these reasons, all patients should have a pre-therapy nutritional assessment and be reassessed periodically throughout therapy by a registered dietitian (RD)[1]. Some types of cancer and their associated therapies put patients at higher risk for nutritional deficiencies than others:

R. N. Zeno (✉) · S. Rotz · S. Bewley · A. Payton
Division of Pediatric Hematology, Oncology, and BMT, Cleveland Clinic Children's Hospital, Cleveland, OH, USA
e-mail: ZENOR2@ccf.org; ROTZS@ccf.org; BEWLEYS@ccf.org; PAYTONA4@ccf.org

K. Radhakrishnan (ed.), *Handbook of Clinical and Practical Pediatric Nutrition*, https://doi.org/10.1007/978-3-031-97759-6_50

- Highly emetogenic chemotherapy
  - Cisplatin (solid tumors, brain tumors)
  - Stem cell transplant conditioning
- Head and neck radiation (head and neck tumors)

Good nutrition is essential in aiding recovery from the systemic impacts of chemotherapy.

- Many patients undergoing chemotherapy experience severe neutropenia (suppression of neutrophil counts to less than 500 cells/uL).
- Due to the risk of infection with decreased leukocytes and impaired mucosal barrier integrity, many have historically suggested that patients with neutropenia maintain highly restricted diets that avoid "high microbial risk" foods to decrease infectious risk.
- However, recent studies have demonstrated no reduction in foodborne illnesses in those on a highly restrictive "neutropenic diet" when compared to focusing on safe food handling, a diet which emphasizes:
  - Cleaning hands and food
  - Safely preserving food between consumption
- Highly restrictive diets have been found to negatively impact quality of life and reduce consumption of calories, protein, fiber, and vitamin C by a population often already in a nutritional deficit. With this new knowledge, recent clinical practice has shifted away from restrictive diets and toward safe food handling [2–5] (Fig. 50.1).

Micronutrient deficiencies are common among children with cancer, especially those with solid tumors, and studies have suggested that micronutrient deficiencies are associated with worse outcomes [6].

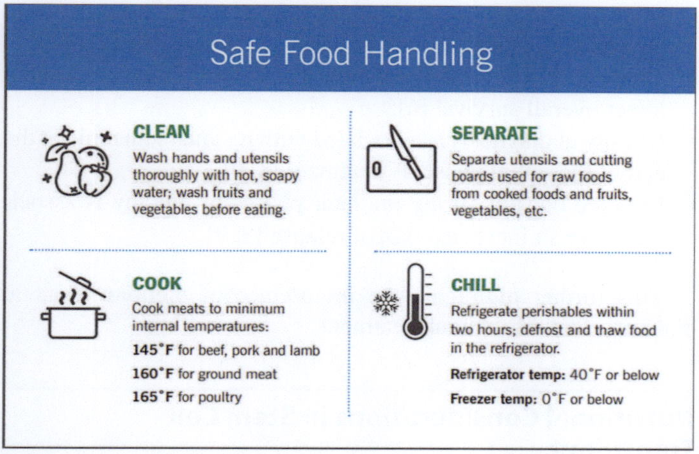

Fig. 50.1 Recommended processes for safe food handling. Published with permission from the Cleveland Clinic

- Zinc—inferior survival in patients with solid tumors.
- Selenium—inferior survival in patients with hematologic malignancies.
- Vitamin B-12 – inferior survival in patients with solid tumors.
- Multiple micronutrients—inferior survival across all malignancies.
- Folate—conflicting evidence regarding role of deficiency in promoting vs lowering cancer risk.
  - Avoid supplements containing folate in patients receiving antifolate chemo.

Among children with acute lymphoblastic leukemia, the most common pediatric cancer diagnosis, weight at either extreme of the spectrum (obesity and underweight) is associated with an increased risk of relapse.

- Patients who are underweight at diagnosis are more likely to relapse than those who were normal or overweight [7].
- Those with a decrease in weight early during treatment had a lower overall survival [6].
- Obesity at diagnosis is associated with residual leukemia at the end of the initial phase of treatment [8, 9]
- Extreme obesity during the later phases of therapy is associated with an increased risk of relapse [8, 9].

This further highlights the importance of dietitian input at diagnosis and throughout treatment.

Nutritional Considerations in Stem Cell Transplant

Hematopoietic stem cell transplant (HSCT), also known as bone marrow transplant (BMT), is the process of replacing one's bone marrow with either donated stem cells (allogenic) or one's own stem cells (autologous). Prior to receiving a HSCT, the patient must undergo preparative conditioning with high-dose chemotherapy and/or total body irradiation (TBI). The intensity of chemotherapy and/or TBI result in more extreme versions of previously mentioned side effects along with additional toxicities such as hepatic veno-occlusive disease (VOD)/sinusoidal obstruction syndrome (SOS) and graft versus host disease (GVHD)[3].

- VOD/SOS is chemotherapy-induced hepatocyte damage causing hepatic venule occlusion.
- VOD/SOS presents with weight gain and elevated bilirubin and transaminases, followed by oliguria, ascites, hepatic failure, and encephalopathy [10].
- Fluid overload is a strong predictor of the development of VOD/SOS, which is why fluid status requires careful monitoring with frequent weight and volume assessments [11].

GVHD occurs when donor graft cells attack host antigens.

- GVHD is classified as acute (<100 days post-) or chronic (>100 days posttransplant) and may present in the skin, gastrointestinal (GI) tract, liver, or chronically across a multitude of tissues.
- Hyperglycemia and obesity have both been shown to increase the risk of GVHD development [3, 11].
- Acute GVHD of the GI tract presents with diarrhea, which may be associated with nausea, vomiting, melena, hematochezia, and abdominal pain, and can progress to ileus or intestinal perforation.
- The severity of lower GI GVHD is quantified by the volume of stool output:
- Stage I = 10–19.9 ml/kg/day.
- Stage II = 20–30 ml/kg/day.
- Stage III (severe) > 30 ml/kg/day.

Severe diarrhea management (timeline is patient-dependent):

Step 1: Make patient NPO and initiate total parenteral nutrition (TPN) until stool volume decreases.

Step 2: Gradual re-introduction of oral intake can begin with low-residue and low-lactose liquid nutrition.

Step 3: Low-residue, lactose, and fat solid foods can be gradually re-introduced starting with smaller, frequent meals before progressing back to a normal diet [13].

Chronic GVHD can present with –

- Dysphagia, odynophagia, anorexia, nausea, diarrhea, weight loss, and cachexia.
- The mainstay of treatment is a prolonged course of systemic steroids followed by a prolonged taper, although newer steroid-sparing treatments are being used more frequently [14].
- All patients should have their nutritional status evaluated prior to HSCT due to the high risk of protein-calorie malnutrition and vitamin deficiencies.

- Many patients who undergo HSCT have an underlying malignancy for which they have already received prior treatment.
- Significant weight loss during the treatment period between diagnosis and HSCT is associated with inferior survival outcomes.
- Pretransplant vitamin testing is important to assess for deficiencies.
- Studies have shown that large doses of vitamin D prior to transplant, termed "Stoss dosing," reduce the incidence of GVHD [15].
- Vitamin C and E also help reduce oxidative stress through anti-inflammatory properties, which can contribute to a reduced incidence of GVHD, and there are ongoing studies investigating whether these vitamins can prevent or treat acute GVHD [12].
- Increased enteral nutrition (EN) posttransplant is associated with shorter time to engraftment, fewer infections, more stable glucose levels, and decreased GVHD (especially grade III and IV) when compared to parenteral nutrition (PN), especially compared to total parenteral nutrition (TPN)[11].
- When considering initiating tube feeds, consider the cancer types and associated treatments that increase the risk of nutritional deficiencies:
- Higher-risk cancers typically have tolerance issues and need more gradual feed advancement.
- Assessing patient's current symptom patterns when devising a feeding schedule.
- When choosing a formula:
  - Standard formulas: good starting point unless suspecting tolerance issues.
  - High-calorie formulas: helpful if volume intolerance is a concern (due to chemotherapy or tumor burden).
  - Hydrolyzed formulas: often needed in those at risk of absorption intolerance.
  - Free amino acid formulas: considered if hydrolyzed formulas are still not tolerated.

Despite this, many patients end up requiring some amount of PN.

- Mucositis is often a driver of poor oral intake and can make patients intolerant of oral intake.
- PN is generally considered when a patient is:
  - Is unable to consistently meet at least 60–70% of their calorie needs.
- Lose >5% of their body weight.

PN guidelines emphasize a focus on meeting nutritional needs while balancing the risk of VOD/SOS:

- PN should not be initiated before day +1 of transplant (the day following cell infusion)[14.]
- Advance dextrose slowly to watch for hyperglycemia.
- Too much sodium can increase risk for VOD secondary fluid overload versus worsening ascites and requires daily lab monitoring[10.]
- Lipids should not be provided for at least 2 weeks after TPN initiation.
- May need higher magnesium doses in the setting of certain immunosuppressive medications.

Long-Term Impacts of Cancer and Its Treatment

It is important to recognize the long-term impacts of various cancer treatments on later metabolism and nutrition as more children are surviving their pediatric malignancies as cancer therapies continue to improve.

- Glucocorticoids, used in many leukemia and lymphoma treatment regimens as well as GVHD, increase the risk of osteoporosis, so emphasizing the importance of calcium and vitamin D intake during and after therapy along with physical activity and exercise may help offset this risk.
  - Some patients may also benefit from bisphosphonate therapy.

- Metabolic syndrome is more common in survivors of ALL and HSCT, particularly those who received cranial radiation as part of treatment, when compared to the general population [7].
  - Important to follow patients in survivorship clinic with height, weight, BMI.
  - Screen for each element of metabolic syndrome.
    Refer to endocrinology if concern for secondary causes of obesity.
- Dietary interventions during therapy including diet education and modification can help offset these long-term effects [1, 3].

Future Directions

Similar to other areas of medicine, there is an increasing emphasis on individualizing patient care. Within nutrition in pediatric malignancy and HSCT, there too is an increasing drive to focus on individual needs to improve outcomes.

References

1. Fabozzi F, Trovato CM, Diamanti A, Mastronuzzi A, Zecca M, Tripodi SI, et al. Management of Nutritional Needs in Pediatric Oncology: A Consensus Statement. Cancer. 2022;14(14):3378.
2. Morris A, O' Connor G, Renshaw G. A Cross-sectional Survey to Review Food Safety Practices Within Pediatric Oncology and Stem Cell Transplant Centers in the United Kingdom. J Pediatr Hematol Oncol. 2023;45(4):e471–8.
3. Casirati A, Salcedo I, Cereda E, Chabannon C, Ruggeri A, Kuball J, et al. The European Society for Blood and Marrow Transplantation (EBMT) roadmap and perspectives to improve nutritional care in patients undergoing hematopoietic stem cell transplantation on behalf of the Cellular Therapy and Immunobiology Working Party (CTIWP) and the Nurses Group (NG) of the EBMT. Bone Marrow Transplant. 2023;58(9):965–72.
4. Fox N, Freifeld AG. The neutropenic diet reviewed: moving toward a safe food handling approach. PubMed. 2012;26(6):572–5, 580, 582 passim.

5. Is Your Food Safe? | Leukemia and Lymphoma Society [Internet]. Lls.org. 2024 [cited 2024 Jun 17]. Available from: https://www.lls.org/article/your-food-safe.
6. Ganguly S, Srivastava R, Agarwala S, Dwivedi S, Bansal PG, Gonmei Z, et al. Prevalence of micronutrient deficiency and its impact on the outcome of childhood cancer: A prospective cohort study. Clin Nutr. 2022;41(7):1501–11.
7. MAH d H, Pluijm SMF, de Groot-Kruseman HA, te Winkel ML, Fiocco M, ELT v d A, et al. The negative impact of being underweight and weight loss on survival of children with acute lymphoblastic leukemia. Haematologica. 2015;100(1):62–9.
8. Gibson TM, Ehrhardt MJ, Ness KK. Obesity and Metabolic Syndrome Among Adult Survivors of Childhood Leukemia. Current Treatment Options. Oncology. 2016;17(4)
9. Orgel E, Tucci J, Alhushki W, Malvar J, Sposto R, Fu CH, et al. Obesity is associated with residual leukemia following induction therapy for childhood B-precursor acute lymphoblastic leukemia. Blood. 2014;124(26):3932–8.
10. Dalle JH, Giralt SA. Hepatic Veno-Occlusive Disease after Hematopoietic Stem Cell Transplantation: Risk Factors and Stratification, Prophylaxis, and Treatment. Biol Blood Marrow Transplant. 2016;22(3):400–9.
11. Mahadeo KM, McArthur J, Adams RH, Radhi M, Angelo JP, Jeyapalan AS, et al. Consensus Report by the Pediatric Acute Lung Injury and Sepsis Investigators and Pediatric Blood and Marrow Transplant Consortium Joint Working Committees on Supportive Care Guidelines for Management of Veno-Occlusive Disease in Children and Adolescents: Part 2—Focus on Ascites. Fluid Electrolytes Renal Trans Issues. 2017;23(12):2023–33.
12. Martin-Salces M, de Paz R, Canales MA, Mesejo A, Hernandez-Navarro F. Nutritional recommendations in hematopoietic stem cell transplantation. Nutrition. 2008;24(7–8):769–75.
13. Koç N, Mehmet Gündüz M, Azık F, Tavil B, Gürlek-Gökçebay D, Özaydın E, et al. Stepwise diet management in pediatric gastrointestinal graft versus host disease. Turk J Pediatr. 2016;58(2):145–55.
14. Zeiser R. Novel approaches to the treatment of chronic graft-versus-host disease. J Clin Oncol. 2003;41(10):1820–4.
15. Bodea J, Beebe K, Campbell C, Salzberg D, Miller H, Adams R, et al. Stoss therapy is safe for treatment of vitamin D deficiency in pediatric patients undergoing HSCT. Bone Marrow Transplant. 2021;56(9):2137–43.

Eating Disorders in the Child and Adolescent 51

Ellen S. Rome, Veronica E. Issac, Jennifer Hyland, and Hanna Leikin

Eating disorders represent a set of life-threatening, biopsychosocial illnesses. They impact children, adolescents, young adults, and adults of all shapes and sizes. Early recognition and prompt intervention decrease morbidity and mortality.

Eating disorders recognized in DSM-5 are found in Table 51.1 below.

E. S. Rome (✉) · V. E. Issac
Center for Adolescent Medicine, Cleveland Clinic Children's Hospital, Cleveland, OH, USA

Cleveland Clinic Lerner College of Medicine, Cleveland, OH, USA
e-mail: Romee@ccf.org; issacv@ccf.org

J. Hyland
Pediatric Nutrition Support, Division of Pediatric Gastroenterology, Hepatology & Nutrition, Cleveland Clinic Children's Hospital, Cleveland, OH, USA
e-mail: hylandj2@ccf.org

H. Leikin
Cleveland Clinic, Cleveland, OH, USA

Cleveland Clinic Children's Hospital, Cleveland, OH, USA
e-mail: leikinh@ccf.org

K. Radhakrishnan (ed.), *Handbook of Clinical and Practical Pediatric Nutrition*, https://doi.org/10.1007/978-3-031-97759-6_51

Table 51.1 Diagnostic criteria for eating disorders, adapted from DSM-5

Anorexia nervosa	Restriction of energy intake relative to requirements leading to a significantly low body weight in the context of age, sex, developmental trajectory, and physical health Intense fear of gaining weight or becoming fat or persistent behavior that interferes with weight gain, even though already being at a significantly low weight Disturbance in the way in which one's body weight or shape is experienced, undue influence of body weight or shape on self-evaluation, or persistent lack of recognition of the seriousness of the current low body weight	**Subtypes:** **Restricting type:** predominantly restricts; during the last 3 months, the person has not engaged in recurrent episodes of binge eating or purging behavior (i.e., self-induced vomiting or the misuse of laxatives, diuretics, or enemas) **Binge-eating/purging type**: during the last 3 months, the person has engaged in recurrent episodes of binge eating or purging behavior (i.e., self-induced vomiting or the misuse of laxatives, diuretics, or enemas)
Bulimia nervosa	Recurrent episodes of binge eating, characterized by both eating, in a discrete period of time (e.g., within any 2-hour period), an amount of food larger than most people would eat during a similar period of time and under similar circumstances, and a sense of lack of control over eating during the episode Recurrent inappropriate compensatory behavior to prevent weight gain, such as self-induced vomiting; misuse of laxatives, diuretics, or other medications; fasting; or excessive exercise The binge eating and inappropriate compensatory behaviors both occur, on average, at least once a week for 3 months Self-evaluation is unduly influenced by body shape and weight The disturbance does not occur exclusively during episodes of anorexia nervosa	Bulimia nervosa is defined by the BINGES with compensatory behavior (vomiting, hyperexercising, laxatives, etc.)

Avoidant/restrictive food intake disorder (ARFID)	Eating or feeding disturbance (including but not limited to apparent lack of interest in eating or food; avoidance due to sensory characteristics of food; or concern about aversive consequences of eating) as manifested by persistent failure to meet appropriate nutritional and/or energy needs associated with one or more of the following: Significant weight loss (or failure to gain weight or faltering growth in children) Significant nutritional deficiency Dependence on enteral feeding Marked interference with psychosocial functioning No evidence of lack of available food or an associated culturally sanctioned practice	
Binge eating disorder (BED)	Recurrent episodes of binge eating are characterized by: Eating, in a discrete period of time, an amount of food larger than what most individuals would eat in a similar period of time under similar circumstances A sense of lack of control overeating during the episode Occurs 1 time/week over at least 3 months Eating behaviors associated with the binges (≥ 3 of the following): Eating much more rapidly than normal Eating until feeling uncomfortably full Eating large amounts of food when not feeling physically hungry Eating alone because of feeling embarrassed by how much is eaten Feeling disgusted with oneself, depressed, or very guilty afterward Marked distress regarding binge eating No compensatory behaviors	

(continued)

Table 51.1 (continued)

Other specified feeding and eating disorders (OSFED)	**Atypical anorexia nervosa (AAN)**: All of the criteria for AN except that despite significant weight loss, the individual's weight is within or above the normal range **Subthreshold bulimia nervosa of low frequency and/or limited duration** All of the criteria for BN except that the binge eating and inappropriate compensatory behaviors occur, on average, less than once a week and/or for less than 3 months **Binge eating disorder of low frequency and/or limited duration** All of the criteria for BED except that the binges occur, on average, < once a week and/or < 3 months **Purging disorder:** Recurrent purging behavior to influence shape or weight (e.g. self-induced vomiting, misuse of laxatives, diet pills or diuretics) in the absence of binge eating **Night eating syndrome:** Recurrent episodes of night eating, as manifested by eating after awakening from sleep or by excessive food consumption after the evening meal. There is awareness and recall of the eating. The night eating causes significant distress and/or impairment in functioning	Layman's terms: AAN sounds like AN, but they have not yet lost so much that they are underweight Layman's terms: Subthreshold BN sounds like BN, but not happening as often or as consistently Layman's terms: as above; same symptoms but not happening as often or as consistently

Other Forms of Disordered Eating

Grazing, non-compulsive subtype refers to those with non-compulsive eating but without the sense of loss of control. This subtype involves "mindless" eating, eating in a distracted way, and eating whatever is available on the spur of the moment.

Grazing, compulsive subtype refers to those individuals trying to resist but going back and eating small or modest amounts of food, perhaps eating what is most tempting in the moment, and responding to cravings for food.

Relative Energy Deficiency in Sport (RED-S) replaced the term Female Athlete Triad in 2014, when the International Olympic Committee consensus group coined the phrase to be more inclusive of males and other subgroups. This phrase captures descriptively those whose low energy intake disrupts their overall physiologic function. In layman's terms, their energy expenditure is greater than their energy intake. This term does not appear in DSM-5.

Essential aspects of the history can be seen in Table 51.2, with elements of the physical examination in Table 51.3. For all clinicians, attention to the growth chart remains a first-line screen for eating disorders. Children and adolescents tend to follow a consistent growth trajectory; crossing 1 Z score standard deviation in weight and/or BMI and/or lowed linear growth in the presence of malnutrition should alert the clinician to investigate for abnormal eating attitudes and behaviors, while simultaneously assessing for thyroid disease, inflammatory bowel disease, onset of celiac disease, or other disease processes. The more precipitous the drop in weight, the more urgent the evaluation should be. Brief screening tools such as the SCOFF (Table 51.4) may aid in early assessment; a score of 2 or more "yes" responses indicates likelihood an eating disorder, deserving of further referral for evaluation in order to initiate earlier treatment [1].

Laboratory evaluation and Differential Diagnosis can be found in Table 51.5.

Table 51.2 Useful questions on history

How much of your day is spent on food/body thoughts?
Are there body areas that truly distress you or that you check repeatedly? Which areas?
What is the most you've ever weighed? How tall were you then? When was that?
What is the least you've ever weighed? How tall were you then? When was that?
What do you think you ought to weigh?
Are there weights that feel too high? Too low?
Do you ever make yourself vomit? If yes, how often? When did you start?
Have you ever used laxatives, diet pills, diuretics,other methods to manipulate weight? If yes, which kinds, how many and how often?
Has anyone ever bullied or teased you? If yes, at school? At home? Where?
Do you count calories or fat grams? If so, how much do you allow?
What do you do for exercise? How much, how often? **How stressed are you if you miss a workout?**
How old were you for your first period? (for girls or individuals with a uterus)
When was your last period? What weight were you then? On or off OCs/ hormones?
Are your periods regular? How long do they last? Cramps?
HEADS questions—asked confidentially
Who lives at **H**ome? What happens when there is an argument at home?
Education: what grade are you in? How are your grades this year? Last year?
Activities: how do you spend your time?
Drugs (cigs/vape, marijuana and other drugs, alcohol, OTC drugs),
Depression (including passive and active suicidal ideation, and self-harm)
Sex: do you see yourself as male, female, nonbinary, other? Are you attracted to men/guys, women/girls, both, neither, other? Have you had sex ever (oral, vaginal, anal)? Has anyone ever done anything to you sexually that made you uncomfortable.
Other mental health questions:
Anxiety? With or without panic attacks?
Obsessive compulsive thoughts or behaviors? (having to do things a certain way, rituals that gets stuck on, extra time on tasks to get them exactly so, etc.).
Full review of systems, including cold intolerance, weakness/fatigue, dizziness, syncope and near-syncope, headaches, GI symptoms including bloating, abdominal pain, early satiety, nausea, vomiting, reflux/heartburn, diarrhea and constipation. Also acrocyanosis, easy bruising, carotonemia (orange skin), amenorrhea or irregular periods, muscle cramps, history of fractures.

Table 51.3 Relevant aspects of the physical examination

General: marked weight loss/gain, lanugo, hypothermia, flat or anxious affect, pallor
HEENT: perimolysis (dental erosions on lingual and occlusal surfaces), dental caries; parotid gland enlargement; cheilosis (dry cracked skin at the corners of the mouth)
Cardiac: bradycardia, orthostatic increase in HR (>20 beats/min) or decrease in diastolic BP (>10 mm HG) when going from lying to standing, low blood pressure, cardiac murmur (1/3 pts. with AN with mitral valve prolapse)
Abd: scaphoid, hepatomegaly, palpable loops of stool, epigastric tenderness
Breasts: atrophic
Neuro: psychomotor retardation (slow speech and thought), loss of muscle mass, slow DTRs, sciatica/nerve compression from lack of padding
Skin: dry skin, acrocyanosis, edema from third spacing;cuts/burns or other evidence of self harm, carotonemia, angular stomatitis, Russell sign (callous over knuckles from self-induced emesis), bruising over spine or other areas; acanthosis nigricans and straie in pts. with obesity
Physical examination may be entirely normal!

Table 51.4 The SCOFF questionnaire adapted from the American Psychiatric Association

Do you make yourself Sick because you feel uncomfortably full?
Do you worry you have lost Control over how much you eat?
Have you recently lost >14 lbs. (one Stone) in 3 months?
Do you believe yourself to be Fat when others say you are too thin?
Would you say that Food dominates your life?

Table 51.5 Appropriate laboratory evaluation

Complete blood count	Pts with disordered eating can have pancytopenia, with leukopenia first, anemia second, thrombocytopenia last
Complete metabolic panel including magnesium and phosphorus	Hypokalemia in pts. who purge or restrict for a prolonged time; Hypoglycemia (from restricting); Hyponatremia (with water loading and/or laxatives) Hypochloremia (with laxative abuse or vomiting); Abnormal bicarbonate (elevated with volume contraction from restricting and/or purging; decreased with laxative abuse); Creatinine (elevated with dehydration and renal dysfunction, lowered with decreased muscle mass) Phosphorus (decreased in refeeding syndrome and with malnutrition) Magnesium (decreased with malnutrition and with laxative abuse) Calcium (slight decrease with malnutrition and impact on bone) AST and ALT: elevated with passive congestion of liver with the early heart failure of refeeding syndrome Total protein/albumin (increased in early malnutrition with loss of muscle mass or misuse of milk of magnesia; decreased with chronic malnutrition) Alkaline phosphatase (lowered with malnutrition, also with magnesium deficiency, zinc deficiency, celiac disease, hypothyroidism and other illnesses.
Thyroid hormone testing	TSH: decreased or normal T4: decreased or normal (euthyroid sick syndrome) T3: may be decreased if below metabolically normal weight

(continued)

Table 51.5 (continued)

FSH and LH Estradiol and testosterone Prolactin	Low FSH, LH, estradiol (bio females), testosterone (bio males) consistent with starvation LH:FSH 3:1 consistent with polycystic ovary syndrome FSH, LH elevated (r/o ovarian failure) Prolactin >20 (r/o prolactinoma)
Erythrocyte sedimentation rate	Low [1–3] with starvation; elevated >15 warrants evaluation for inflammatory or infectious process in face of starvation
Celiac diagnostic panel	Useful to r/o celiac disease in children and adolescents who have fallen off growth curve
Vitamin D, thiamine	Low with starvation and inadequate intake of either

Nutrition Assessment

A full malnutrition assessment should be completed for all patients based on malnutrition criteria in chapter on Nutrition Theory—Chap. 2.

Features which may be concerning for nutrition insufficiency include:

- Sudden change in growth trajectory (weight and/or height) when plotted on growth chart.
- A decrease in BMI/age percentiles and Z-scores.
- A decrease in weight/age Z-score of −1 or greater.
- Physical findings including pallor or dry skim, thinning hair and/or lanugo.

Do not just look for weight loss. Absence of weight gain, or cessation of linear growth velocity can be an indicator of malnutrition and disordered eating patterns [1].

Nutrition Intervention

Patients with weight loss and malnutrition may be initially hypometabolic and then experience rapid hypermetabolism as refeeding begins.

- Typically recommend 120–150% of predicted energy needs using standard equations.
- Patients can safely start refeeding usually at 2250–2500 kcal per day, and will often need between 3000–4000 kcal/day during medical and nutritional repletion [2, 7–9].
- Avoid excessive protein intake; therefore, fat and carbohydrate needs are higher than typical.
- Patients without malnutrition can be prescribed similar energy and protein needs of children and adolescents without eating disorders.

Inpatient (IP) Nutritional Insufficiency Protocol [7, 9]

- Patient is initiated on a 2250-calorie diet with maintenance fluids unless otherwise directed by MD.
- Calories are advanced by 250 kcals daily until bradycardia resolves.
- Patient is required to drink an evening shake that is approximately 600–700 kcals to improve vitals, as a means of more expedient correction of bradycardia due to malnutrition.
- The RD is responsible for meal planning with the family to ensure balanced intake from protein, carbohydrates, and fats to meet their caloric demand.
- If patient is <18 years of age, the RD meal plans alone with parents. This follows the family-based therapy model and recommendations for treatment of eating disorders.
- Patients' likes and dislikes are taken into account, with a priority on safe foods, expanded choices to foods that were safe before onset of the eating disorder, and usually not initially inclusive of foods the patient never liked.
- If patient is >18 years of age, the patient may be a part of meal planning.

IP supplement requirements (1.5 kcal/mL supplements)

- 50–90% of meal consumed, need to drink 8 ounces of supplement.
- <50% of meal consumed, need to drink 16 ounces of supplement.
- If <100% of snack consumed, need to drink 8 ounces of supplement.
- *If patient refuses supplement PO, nasogastric tube will be placed to administer.

Criteria for admission can be found in Table 51.6 [7–9].

Prevention of Refeeding Syndrome

- Refeeding syndrome occurs when a patient goes from starvation, with total body phosphorus depletion, to a sudden increase in cellular influx of phosphorus that occurs with refeeding.
- The high glucose load that occurs after a rapid increase in caloric intake stimulates secretion of insulin, which further increases cellular uptake of glucose, phosphorus, potassium, and magnesium.
- As the body makes ATP from ADP, within 12 to 72 hours, there is little to no available phosphate in the face of chronic starvation, causing each cell's mitochondrial pump to fail.

Table 51.6 Medical criteria for hospitalization for acute medical stabilization

Bradycardia (heart rate < 50 beats per minute)
Other cardiac arrhythmia (prolonged QTc defined as >450 for <18yo, >460 for >18yo)
Orthostatic hypotension
Hypothermia
Precipitous weight loss
Hypokalemia, hypglycemia, other electrolyte imbalance
High risk for refeeding syndrome
Failure of outpatient management

- This leads to congestive heart failure, elevated liver enzymes from passive congestion, and peripheral/dependent edema.
- Refeeding syndrome can be prevented with proactive use of a phosphorus supplement for the first 5 days of acute refeeding; we use Nutra-Phos (Willen Drug Co., Teva Pharmaceutical Industries, Ltd., Baltimore, MD), a mixture of 250 mg phosphorus, 164 mg sodium phosphate, and 278 mg potassium phosphate.
- Caloric intake can be safely started for most adolescents at 2200–2500 calories per day, as well as the administration of Nutra-Phos or other similar supplement twice a day for 5 days (packet mixed with 8 oz. juice or other fluid) [9].
- A complete metabolic panel (CMP) along with magnesium and phosphorus can be followed upon admission or initially, then the morning after admission, then every other morning unless laboratory abnormalities suggest closer monitoring. With a CMP, both liver and renal function can be followed.
- Strict counting of intake and output (Is and Os) can help identify risk for fluid overload, ongoing dehydration, isosthenuria, and other concerns.

Vitamin/Mineral Deficiencies

Vitamin and mineral labs are routinely drawn on eating disorder patients.

- Initial screening labs include CMP, CBC + Diff, ferritin, and vitamin D.
- Additional labs may be ordered depending on their degree of malnutrition and dietary restrictions (i.e., vegan, avoiding dairy, etc.).
- Studies have shown that patients with anorexia nervosa are at risk for deficiencies in selenium [3], B9, and zinc [3, 4] (Table 51.7).

Table 51.7 Treatment for the vitamin and mineral deficiencies common with eating disorders [5]

Vitamin/mineral deficiencies	Treatment
Vitamin D	2000 international units (IU) per day vitamin D3 OR 50,000 IU per week vitamin D2 for 6–12 weeks followed by maintenance dosing 600–1000 IU per day vitamin D3
Calcium	Calcium carbonate total of 1500 mg/day divided into 500 mg doses
Iron	Children <12 years: 3–6 mg/kg/d ferrous sulfate Adolescents: Standard recommended dosing in adolescents and adults varies widely, ranging from 60 to 300 mg elemental iron per day administered once or divided in three doses

Outpatient Nutrition Counseling

- There is no gold standard for nutrition therapy for outpatient interventions.
- Ensuring adequate energy intake for medical stabilization is the goal.
- It is recommended that children under 18 years of age participate in family-based therapy and nutrition therapy. This is a proven effective method for recovery.

Basics of Any Meal Plan

- Three meals per day.
- Two to three snacks per day.
- Establishing regular meal and snack patterns.
- Adequate fluid intake.
- Patients with severe malnutrition with brain starvation typically benefit from nutritional supplementation to help optimize nutrient intake and promote weight gain.
- In severe cases, placement of nasogastric tube is indicated.
- The above recommendations should be applied to all patients with eating disorders, including anorexia nervosa, bulimia nervosa, binge eating disorder, and avoidant restrictive food intake disorder (Table 51.8).

Table 51.8 Common meal plan patterns

Exchange system	The US food exchange lists divides foods into six groups: grains, proteins, fruits, vegetables, dairy, fat (lipids) Patient is given a meal plan with an exchange list. The exchange list gives portion sizes for one exchange Foods within each category can be substituted or "exchanged" for another food Challenge is that nutritional value of exchanges can vary, and patients may choose exchanges lower in calories Most often used in residential treatment when patients are monitored Ex: a meal should contain 3 grains +3 proteins +2 fats +1 fruit
Macronutrient focus	Recommend each meal contains protein, carbohydrates, and fat sources. Review adequate portion sizes with patient/parent Provide education on the role of each nutrient. Highlight need for increased carbohydrates and fat sources during periods of growth and development Ensure adequate calcium intake Ensure fruit/vegetable intake, but these do not count as carbohydrate options at a meal Snacks should each contain two food groups (vegetables do not count)
MyPlate	MyPlate model is based off of the USDA guidelines ¼ plate protein, ¼ plate grains, ½ plate fruits and vegetables + dairy This meal pattern is often used for younger children and patients with ARFID It does not review the adequacy of fat needed for an adolescent, so would need to provide additional education on needs
Plate by plate method	A visual approach to plating meals, that was designed to aid in treatment of eating disorders, across all diagnoses, without measuring, counting or numbers. The approach can be used alongside family-based treatment, as well as other treatment modalities [6]

Monitoring and Growth Expectations

- Initial expected growth goals include inpatient weight gain of 0.2 kg/day to stabilize physiology.
- Caloric intake is increased daily to sustain that rate of gain, while monitoring for refeeding syndrome.
- Outpatient weight gain goals are slower, aiming for 0.2–1 kg (½ lb. to 2 lbs) a week for those who need to gain.
- Outpatient weight goals are individualized, as based on previous BMI trends; considering linear growth velocity potential and stage of pubertal development.
- Weight ranges should change as each person tracks along an expected growth curve with age and with expected pubertal milestones achieved.
- Use caution when stating a weight goal to a family, as they may not be thinking through the expected changes of age and pubertal stage.
- As for height expectations, after menarche, girls can be expected to grow 1–4 inches.
- Boys may continue growing through high school and into college years.

Prognosis

- The prognosis for youth with eating disorders can be explained in terms of the rule of thirds; a third of children and adolescents will recover fully, a third will recover but when stressed will click into abnormal eating attitudes and behaviors, and a third will have a chronic and relapsing course, with up to 25% of this bottom third at risk for dying prematurely due to the complications of their illness.
- Fertility can be expected to be preserved for those in recovery; in the midst of an eating disorder, one cannot assume that ovulation will be consistently suppressed. Thus, contraceptive options may need to be discussed for those who are sexually active.

When counseling patients and families, prevention of relapse can include the following:

- Decrease weight and body talk in the home and elsewhere. That includes self-deprecating body disparagements as well as weight teasing of the child or adolescent.
- Provide a supportive food environment, including family dinners as frequently as possible.
- Help children build self-esteem beyond looks and physical appearance.
- Encourage healthy coping skills and appropriate expression of feelings.
- Educate parents on the signs and symptoms of eating disorders, and when to seek help.
- Validate the parents' struggles, and help engage them in their own self-care in order to better care for their child.

References

1. Goday PS, Walia CS. Chapter 22 Adolescent Medicine. In: Pediatric nutrition for dietitians. Boca Raton: CRC Press; 2022. p. 323–35.
2. American Dietetic Association. Pediatric Nutrition Care Manual®. Adolescent Medicine. https://www.nutritioncaremanual.org/. Accessed 26 Aug 2024.
3. Achamrah N, Coëffier M, Rimbert A, Charles J, Folope V, Petit A, et al. Micronutrient Status in 153 Patients with Anorexia Nervosa. Nutrients [Internet]. 2017 Mar 2 [cited 2020 May 26];9(3). Available from: https://www.ncbi.nlm.nih.gov/pmc/articles/PMC5372888/.
4. Katz RL, Keen CL, Litt IF, Hurley LS, Kellams-Harrison KM, Glader LJ. Zinc deficiency in anorexia nervosa. J Adoles Health Care [Internet] 1987 [cited 2020 May 28];8(5):400–406. Available from: https://www.sciencedirect.com/science/article/abs/pii/0197007087902270.
5. National Institutes of Health. Vitamin and mineral supplement fact sheets [Internet]. Nih.gov. 2017. Available from: https://ods.od.nih.gov/factsheets/list-VitaminsMinerals/.
6. Sterling W, et al. The Use of the Plate-by-Plate Approach for Adolescents Undergoing Family-Based Treatment. J Acad Nutr Diet. 119(7):1075–84.
7. Golden NH, Katzman DK, Rome ES, Gaete V, Nagata JM, Ornstein RM, Garber AK, Starr T, Kohn M, Sawyer SM. Medical Management

of Restrictive Eating Disorders in Adolescents and Young Adults: Position Statement of the Society for Adolescent Health and Medicine. J Adolesc Health. 2022;71:648–54.
8. Hornberger LL, Lane MA. Committee on adolescence. Identification and management of eating disorders in children and adolescents. Pediatrics. 2021;147(1):e2020040279. https://doi.org/10.1532/peds.2020-040279.
9. Strandjord SE, Sieke EH, Richmond M, Khadlikar A, Rome ES. Medical stabilization of adolescents with nutritional insufficiency: a clinical care path. Eat Weight Disorders 2016 21(3):403–410, epub 2015 Nov 23. https://doi.org/10.1007/s40519-015-0245-5. PMID 26597679.

Nutrition in Disorders of Gut-Brain Interaction and Motility

52

Sujithra Velayuthan, Ben Freiberg, Diana Schnee, and Maria Haught

Disorders of Gut-Brain Interaction

- Disorders of Gut-Brain Interaction (DGBI) are a group of disorders classified by gastrointestinal symptoms. They are diagnosed using Rome IV criteria.
- Irritable bowel syndrome (IBS), functional dyspepsia (FD), and functional constipation (FC) are among the frequently studied DGBI. FD is common in children with a community prevalence of 5–10% in developed countries [1]. The prevalence

S. Velayuthan (✉)
Division of Pediatric Gastroenterology, Hepatology and Nutrition, Cleveland Clinic Children's Hospital, Cleveland, OH, USA
e-mail: VELAYUS@ccf.org

B. Freiberg
Division of Pediatric Gastroenterology, Hepatology, and Nutrition, Cleveland Clinic Children's Hospital, Cleveland, OH, USA
e-mail: FREIBEB@ccf.org

D. Schnee · M. Haught
Pediatric Nutrition Support, Division of Pediatric Gastroenterology, Hepatology, and Nutrition, Cleveland Clinic Children's Hospital, Cleveland, OH, USA
e-mail: SCHNEED2@ccf.org; HAUGHTM4@ccf.org

K. Radhakrishnan (ed.), *Handbook of Clinical and Practical Pediatric Nutrition*, https://doi.org/10.1007/978-3-031-97759-6_52

of IBS varies from 1.2 to 5.4 depending on where they live [2]. The pooled prevalence of FC in children is 9.5% [3].

- Rome IV criteria define IBS as having all the following criteria: 1. Abdominal pain occurring more than 4 days per month and related to defecation, change in frequency or form of stools, 2. Pain not resolved with resolution of constipation in children with constipation and 3. Not fully explained by another medical condition after appropriate evaluation [2].
- FD is characterized by one or more of the following symptoms for at least 4 days a week: early satiety, post prandial fullness, epigastric pain/ burning and not explained by other medical conditions after appropriate evaluation [2].
- According to Rome IV criteria, functional constipation should meet at least 2 of the following criteria: 1. Two or fewer defecations in toilet per week, 2. At least one episode of fecal incontinence per week, 3. History of retentive posturing or excessive voluntary stool retention, 4. History of painful or hard bowel movements, 5. Presence of a large fecal mass in rectum and 6. History of large diameter stools that can obstruct the toilet [2].
- Although the pathophysiology of DGBI is not completely understood, it is found to be due to a complex interplay between various factors such as altered gastrointestinal motility, visceral hypersensitivity, mucosal barrier, microbiota, and its interaction with the mucosal immune function and central nervous system processing [4].
- It is better understood using a biopsychosocial model which takes into account the psychological and social domains, in addition to the biomedical aspect of the symptoms [4].

Nutritional Impact

- While the burden of symptoms can lead to reduced food intake resulting in malnutrition, various dietary modifications are utilized to improve symptoms of DGBI which in turn improves nutrition.

- Out of all the pediatric DGBI, the association of food with FD and IBS is well studied.
- Symptoms of FD are found to be associated with the amount of retained food in the stomach rather than impaired accommodation of the stomach [5]. Fat and acid also cause symptoms in FD patients due to hypersensitivity of the duodenum [6].
- Children with IBS suffer from frequent abdominal pain and bloating associated with bowel movements. Dietary factors that aggravate the symptoms of IBS are lactose, fructose, and sweeteners [7]. Fermentable oligosaccharides, disaccharides, monosaccharides, and polyols (FODMAP) are short-chain carbohydrates that are not easily digested in the small intestine and can be fermented by bacteria in colon. This results in increased gases and short-chain fatty acids which in turn draw water into colonic lumen increasing motility. The resulting increased gas and water in the lumen causes abdominal distension and pain in susceptible individuals [8].

Management

- Given the association of delayed gastric emptying and symptoms of FD, reduced fat meals and small frequent meals are recommended despite no solid evidence [5]. Avoiding spicy and acidic foods as well as caffeinated beverages is also recommended [9].
- Diets with FODMAPs show increased gastric pressure in both IBS and control patients but worsened symptoms only in patients with IBS. Diets low in FODMAPs are shown to reduce symptoms in children with IBS. Multiple adult and pediatric studies also show improvement of abdominal symptoms in IBS on low FODMAP diet [8]. Common foods with high and low FODMAP are noted in Table 52.1.

Table 52.1 Common foods with high and low FODMAPs [43–45]

	High FODMAP foods	Low FODMAP foods
Grains	Wheat, rye, barley in large quantities, semolina, bulgur, spelt	Brown rice, white rice, oats, oat bran, quinoa, gluten-free bread, cereals, pastas, crackers without honey, polenta, tapioca, buckwheat, corn tortillas, corn chips, plain rice cakes
Vegetables	Brussell sprouts, broccoli, cauliflower, asparagus, garlic, onions, mushrooms, peas, artichokes, cabbage	Carrots, cucumbers, celery, bell peppers, lettuce/spinach/arugula, green onions/chives, ginger, potatoes/root vegetables, squash (Eggplant, zucchini)
Fruit	Dried fruits, apples, pears, stone fruit (peaches, plums, apricots, avocado, nectarines), watermelon, mango, juice of these fruits	Honeydew, cantaloupe, citrus fruit, kiwi, pineapple
Legumes	Most legumes and legume-based foods	Small portions of chickpeas, lentils, green peas, edamame
Meats and high-protein foods	Meats breaded with wheat ingredients or marinated in high FODMAPS (i.e., garlic, onion, honey, buttermilk) or in a cream sauce	Firm tofu, can season or marinate with lemon/ lime juice, vinegar (except apple cider vinegar), olive oil, herbs.
Dairy	Products made from cow's milk: ice cream, milk, evaporate milk/ sweetened condensed milk, yogurt, soft cheese	Hard cheese/low lactose cheese (parmesan, cheddar, provolone, Colby, etc.), almond milk, rice milk, lactose-free milk, lactose-free yogurt

(continued)

Table 52.1 (continued)

	High FODMAP foods	Low FODMAP foods
Nuts and seeds	Cashews, pistachios, soy nuts; more than 2 tablespoons of almonds	10–15 or 1–2 Tbsp of almonds. No more than 1/4 cup of macadamia nuts, pecans, pine nuts, walnuts, pumpkin seeds, sesame seeds, sunflower seeds; peanuts
Sweeteners	Honey, agave, high fructose corn syrup, Sugar alcohols (sorbitol, mannitol, xylitol, maltitol) fructose	Sugar (sucrose), glucose, pure maple syrup, aspartame, corn syrup solids, brown sugar, sucralose, stevia
Additives	Inulin, FOS (fructo-oligo-saccharides), chicory root	
Miscellaneous	Onion powder, garlic powder, dehydrated onion, whey protein concentrate (unless lactose-free), molasses	Baker's yeast, baking powder, coconut water (8 oz.), whey protein isolate, chocolate, guar gum, jam/jelly (1 1/2 Tbsp.—avoid those made with high fructose corn syrup), vinegar (except apple cider), maltodextrin, pectin, coffee (1 cup per day), tea (1 cup), sucrose-sweetened soft drink, salt, pepper, soy sauce

- In children with lactose intolerance, administration of lactase (beta galactosidase) tablets has demonstrated improvement in abdominal pain, diarrhea, bloating, and flatulence [10].
- Normal fluid and fiber intake and a healthy diet are recommended for all children. Addition of fiber to the diet has shown improvement in bowel habits and abdominal pain in patients with IBS [11, 12].
- In patients with FC, drinking additional fluids has not been shown to improve stool frequency [13]. However, increased intake of water while taking osmotic laxative does increase

stool frequency [14]. Although soluble fibers bulk up the stools and help with constipation, taking fiber supplements has not been shown to improve symptoms of pediatric constipation in contrast to adult studies [5].

Small Intestinal Bacterial Overgrowth (SIBO)

- The gut microbiota performs multiple beneficial effects on the host such as prevention of colonization by pathogenic bacteria, maintenance of integrity of the intestinal epithelium, and development of gut lymphoid tissue. In addition, they also contribute nutritionally by synthesizing vitamin K, folic acid, and short-chain fatty acids.
- An intact ileocecal valve maintains the gradient of bacterial colonization (abundance on the colonic side) across it. Additionally, the migrating motor complex (MMC) in the small intestines and the gastric acid in stomach also help to keep the bacterial count low in the small intestine.
- Previously called blind loop syndrome, SIBO is defined as an excessive growth of bacteria in the small intestine with a predominance of colonic-type bacteria. This results in symptoms such as bloating, diarrhea, constipation, nausea, abdominal pain, flatulence, and malabsorption [15]. These symptoms overlap with other conditions and high degree of suspicion in susceptible children is recommended for proper diagnosis.
- SIBO is seen in association with conditions causing intestinal stasis (dysmotility), altered anatomy of the gastrointestinal tract bypassing the ileocecal valve, failure of the gastric acid secretion and pancreatic enzyme defense, and immunodeficiency. Children with chronic diseases such as celiac

disease, cystic fibrosis, and IBS have high risk of developing SIBO [15].

- Although culture of the jejunal aspirate is the gold standard, due to the invasiveness of the procedure and complexity of culturing process, hydrogen and methane breath testing are now widely used to diagnose SIBO. DNA sequencing of the duodenal aspirate can also be done.

Nutritional Impact

- SIBO causes host intestinal epithelial injury resulting in diarrhea and steatorrhea. The absorption of all macronutrients (carbohydrate, protein, and lipid) is impaired [16].
- Bacterial deconjugation of bile acids results in impaired digestion and absorption of lipids and fat-soluble vitamins—A, D, and E. However, vitamin K status is optimal due to bacterial synthesis of vitamin K [16].
- Vitamin B12 deficiency is noted due to defective absorption and bacterial consumption of the vitamin. However, folate levels may be elevated secondary to bacterial synthesis of folate [16].
- Iron, thiamine, and nicotinamide deficiency are also reported rarely, but the mechanism by which this happens is unknown [16].

Management

- Avoidance of antimotility agents such as opioids.
- Promotility agents such as erythromycin and amoxicillin-clavulanic acid can be tried.
- Broad-spectrum antibiotics are used to treat SIBO as both aerobic and anaerobic bacteria are involved. Rifaximin, an antibiotic with poor intestinal absorption is well studied in SIBO and

is also found to be effective in the management of methane producers. Antibiotic stewardship is recommended while using this mode of management [16].

- Identification and management of nutritional deficiencies are imperative [15].
- Since carbohydrates serve as a substrate for the bacteria, restricting carbohydrates may theoretically benefit the condition. However, there are no studies to support this hypothesis [16].
- Although low FODMAP diets may help improve symptoms in patients with IBS which is commonly associated with SIBO, their role in management of SIBO is unclear [16].
- Fat restriction is beneficial only in patients with fat malabsorption [16].
- Elemental diets can be considered in the management of SIBO since the macronutrients in elemental diet are predominantly absorbed in the proximal small bowel. A small study using elemental diet for 2 weeks showed improvement in symptoms and normalization of the breath test [17]. The practicality of using elemental diets is limited by their high cost and palatability.
- Although probiotic use has been shown to improve intestinal barrier function and modulate immune response, some studies show increased symptoms (bloating) and adverse events such as lactic acidosis and cognitive impairment which improve upon stopping the probiotic. Hence, the use of probiotics in the management of SIBO should be individualized [15].

Gastroparesis

- Gastroparesis is defined as delay in gastric emptying in the absence of mechanical obstruction. Children present with various symptoms including nausea, vomiting, epigastric pain, and early satiety which accounts for a significant reduction in the quality of life [18].

- The common causes of gastroparesis in children are idiopathic, postinfection, postsurgical, and diabetes among others [18]. Medications such as anticholinergics and opiates can also delay gastric emptying.
- The pathophysiology of gastroparesis is poorly understood and includes factors such as impaired fundic accommodation, diminished antral contractions, altered myoelectric activity of the stomach, and reduced pyloric compliance [19]. Although the number of interstitial cells is reduced in gastroparesis, the extent of reduction doesn't correlate with symptom severity [19].
- Gastroparesis is diagnosed by establishing delay in gastric emptying and ruling out mechanical obstruction [19].
- Although various modalities such as stable isotope breath test and wireless motility capsule are available to study the gastric emptying, gastric emptying scintigraphy is well-accepted modality despite its shortcomings such as absence of a standard protocol and normative values in children.
- Gastroparesis is managed by dietary modifications, optimizing glycemic control, and medical and surgical therapies.

Nutritional Impact

- In the case of malnutrition or poor weight status, catch-up growth may be needed.
- Focus on fluid intake and rehydration is important. Some individuals have intolerance to fluids as well.
- Due to symptom severity and the consequences of impaired motility (e.g., SIBO), the nutritional intake in children declines. Additionally, low stomach acidity secondary to medications also contributes to malnutrition including nutritional deficiencies of iron, vitamin B12, calcium, and vitamin D. Other micronutrient deficiencies include vitamins E, K and folate, magnesium, and potassium [18].

Management

- Normal gastric emptying relies on factors such as food consistency, composition, and volume. Diet modification is the first step in the management of gastroparesis [18].
- In general, foods that cause symptoms in patients with gastroparesis include foods that are fatty, acidic, spicy, and rich in roughage [20].
- Nutritional recommendations for kids with gastroparesis include diets low in fat, fiber, and refined carbohydrates based on the theoretical influence of these factors on gastric emptying. It is also shown that medium-chain triglycerides (MCT) empty faster than long-chain fatty acids (LCT) in preterm infants [21].
- In addition to slowing gastric emptying, fiber (especially insoluble fiber) can also cause phytobezoar in the setting of impaired gastric emptying. Low-fiber diets are hence recommended for patients with gastroparesis. The degree of tolerance to fiber varies from person to person, and hence the fiber recommendation must be individualized [22].
- Consuming small particle size foods such as those that can be easily mashed with a fork, chewing food well before swallowing, and reducing the food particle size using a blender can all be helpful in these children [18].
- Liquid or pureed foods can be used in patients unable to tolerate solid foods, as these empty faster than solids. Blenderizing foods into smoothies or using nutritional supplements can also be tried [19].
- Taking small frequent meals can help meet calorie requirements and improve tolerance. Additionally, sitting or standing for about 2 hours after meals can also improve gastric emptying [22].
- If oral intake cannot meet calorie and fluid requirements, enteral feeding should be considered. Post pyloric feeding (naso or gastro-duodenal and jejunal tube feeds) that bypasses

the stomach is preferred in these patients [18]. Continuous feeds over 24 hours can be initiated and slowly advanced to reach goal calorie and fluid requirements. A cyclic regimen can be introduced later, depending on patient tolerance [22].

- Polymeric formulas with no fiber can be tried first in these patients. Blenderized formula is another option, and it is preferred by many patients due to its natural constituents and better tolerance [19].
- Parenteral nutrition is considered when oral and enteral feeds are not tolerated, leading to significant malnutrition. Patients and parents should be educated on the indications and possible risks associated with parenteral nutrition before initiation as well as the need to stop parenteral nutrition as early as possible. Oral and enteral nutrition should be continued and gradually increased as tolerated, while continuing parenteral nutrition and the parenteral nutrition should be weaned and stopped as soon as nutritional needs are met via oral or enteral means [19].
- Prokinetics to accelerate gastric emptying and antiemetics are often used to treat gastroparesis. When symptoms are not well controlled, neuromodulators can also be tried [23].
- Pyloric botulinum toxin injection and gastric neurostimulator are other management options for the patients who fail nutrition and pharmacological management [23].

Pediatric Intestinal Pseudo Obstruction (PIPO)

- PIPO (previously known as chronic intestinal pseudo-obstruction of childhood or CIPO) is a disabling motility disorder that affects the neuromuscular apparatus of the gastrointestinal tract (GIT). It is diagnosed when patients fulfill at least 2 of the following criteria [24].

  - Objective measure of small intestinal neuromuscular involvement (manometry/histopathology, transit studies).
  - Recurrent and/or persistently dilated loops of small intestine with air fluid levels.
  - Genetic/metabolic abnormalities associated with PIPO.
  - Dependence on enteral feeding/parenteral nutrition for maintenance of adequate nutrition and/or growth.
- Its prevalence is about 3.7 per one million in children under 15 years of age [25]. Depending on the age of onset, location of dysmotility, the extent and severity of GIT involved, the clinical manifestation varies [24].
- PIPO in children varies from their adult counterparts with respect to age of onset, type of dysmotility (myopathic vs neuropathic), and association with urological involvement and malrotation. Additionally, the pediatric pseudo-obstruction is predominantly primary and can be congenital, while it is predominantly secondary to other underlying conditions in adults. Patients with PIPO also require more specialized nutrition support (enteral and parenteral) than their adult counterparts [24].
- Investigations should be geared toward excluding mechanical obstruction, identifying potential secondary causes, and finding pathophysiologic features that may help direct management [26].
- Antroduodenal manometry can be a helpful adjunct in those unresponsive to medical therapy with the presence of phase III of the migrating motor complex excluding PIPO. Full-thickness biopsies may be useful in detecting neuropathy, myopathy, or abnormalities in the interstitial cells of Cajal, though our understanding of the histopathology remains limited [26].
- The primary focus of management of PIPO involves maintaining adequate nutrition, protecting and improving the gut motility, improving symptoms, and treating complications. Improving nutritional status plays a vital role in management of PIPO, as improved nutrition promotes better GI motor function in the unaffected GI tract and boosts outcomes [25].

Nutritional Assessment

- In addition to the disabling symptoms which lead to poor feeding and malnutrition, the dysmotility associated with SIBO can also contribute to malnutrition in kids with PIPO.
- Serial growth parameters such as weight, height, mid-upper arm circumference, and triceps skin fold should be measured. Due to waterlogging in intestinal segments with dysmotility, fluid and electrolyte losses from decompressive enterostomies, relying only on the weight parameter may not be accurate [25].
- Nutritional evaluation should focus on electrolyte imbalances, anemia, renal function, calcium, and bone mineral density [25].

Management

- Whenever possible, oral nutrition should be encouraged if it is tolerated and there is no contraindication for swallowing.
- Feeding should be tailored to suit the patient's skills and the extent and severity of dysmotility involved.
- Low-fat diets are preferred. MCTs accelerate small bowel motility compared to LCTs in healthy individuals [27, 28]. MCTs are also found to have shorter gastric emptying times than LCTs in preterm babies [21].
- Water-soluble fibers are found to delay gastric emptying, and they also hamper glucose and lipid absorption in the small intestine. In addition to delaying gastric emptying, insoluble fibers also have the potential to form phytobezoars in the stomach if the stomach motility is affected. It is thus advisable to not give fibers to patients with PIPO [24].
- ESPGHAN recommends starting with polymeric formula and switch to hydrolyzed or elemental formula if polymeric formula is not tolerated.

- Blenderized diets are found to improve tolerance and abdominal symptoms in adult studies. It also improves the richness and diversity of fecal microbiota in medically complex patients, which may contribute to the improved symptoms in patients with PIPO [29].
- Due to the faster emptying of whey predominant breast milk compared to polymeric formula, breast milk is the best choice for patients diagnosed during the prenatal and neonatal period. If breast milk is not an option, commercial whey-based formula can be used to lessen the risk of lacto-bezoar with casein-based formula.
- In patients with gastroparesis, liquid meals should be offered as liquid emptying is often preserved. Bite size and dissolvable foods such as sugar puffs and wafers can be used in patients who tolerate oral feeds.
- When oral feeding is not tolerated, enteral feeds should be considered. Gastric feeding is preferred if gastric dysmotility is ruled out. A gastrostomy is recommended for decompression in patients with PIPO, and this can also be used to administer feeds.
- In patients with gastroparesis and those who do not tolerate gastric feeding, jejunal feeds should be initiated. Tolerance to jejunal feeds is better if MMCs are present on antroduodenal manometry [30].
- About a third of patients with PIPO require parenteral nutrition. This should be started only in genuine cases of intolerance to oral and enteral nutrition.
- Weaning to enteral and oral nutrition can be achieved with time in 38–62% of patients [31]. Predictors for long-term parenteral nutrition include onset before 1 year of age, presence of midgut volvulus, urinary tract involvement, and myopathic features on antroduodenal manometry or histopathology.
- Poor prognostic factors include neonatal onset, acute onset, urinary tract involvement, and requirement for surgery [32]. A myopathic pattern on antroduodenal manometry and patients presenting in infancy are poor prognostic indicators [33].

Gastroesophageal Reflux Disease

- NASPGHAN and ESPAGHAN guidelines define gastroesophageal reflux disease (GERD) as the passage of gastric contents into esophagus with or without regurgitation/vomiting resulting in troublesome symptoms and complications that affects daily functioning [34].
- The prevalence of GERD gradually decreases from about 26% at 3 months of age to about 3% at 6 months of age [35].
- Risk factors for developing GERD in children include obesity, asthma, prematurity, and congenital abdominal malformations such as diaphragmatic hernia, esophageal atresia, and gastroschisis [36].
- The symptoms of GERD vary with age and include feeding refusal, failure to thrive, regurgitation with or without vomiting, heartburn, epigastric pain, dysphagia, and hematemesis. Non-GI symptoms such as wheezing, cough, hoarseness, apnea spells, brief resolved unexplained events, recurrent otitis media, and pneumonia are also reported [34].
- The utility of upper GI radiography, ultrasound, and endoscopy in the evaluation of GERD is to identify predisposing factors (e.g., hiatal hernia), rule out mimickers of GERD (e.g., malrotation, pyloric stenosis, eosinophilic esophagitis) and to evaluate the consequences of GERD (e.g., erosive esophagitis) [34].
- Combined pH and multichannel intraluminal impedance studies (pH-MII) are the most sensitive modality for diagnosing GERD [36]. pH-MII is superior to pH alone studies due to its ability to evaluate both acid and nonacid refluxes, associate symptoms with reflux, and to differentiate between swallow and reflux-related drops in pH [34]. The pH-MII is also useful in determining the effect of acid suppression therapy, correlating persistent symptoms and esophagitis with acid/ non-acid reflux and differentiating GERD and nonerosive reflex disease from hypersensitive esophagus and functional heartburn [34].

Nutritional Management

- No increased nutritional needs.
- Most infants improve with non-pharmacological management and pharmacological management is indicated in children who do not respond to conservative management [36].
- Elevation of the head to 40 degrees and left lateral position have shown improvement in GERD [37]. However, to prevent sudden infant death, the best positioning for infants is supine.
- Small volume and frequent feeds are recommended to provide adequate daily total volume and calories. Care should be taken to avoid overfeeding, which can worsen GERD.
- Thickening of feeds is often attempted and is found to reduce the visible regurgitation. However, the pH-MII parameters don't seem to show improvement for both acid and nonacid reflux.
- Cereal-based or commercial thickeners can be used to thicken formula. Due to good solubility, affordability, and low incidence of clogging nipples, rice cereal is preferred over other food cereals. The FDA put forward a warning on rice cereal due to high arsenic content and proposed to keep the levels of arsenic below 100 parts per billion. Cereals cannot be used to thicken breast milk due to the possibility of mammary amylase digesting the cereal.
- Commercial thickeners may be carob bean, xanthan gum, or corn starch based [38]. Carob beans thickeners can be used for infants over 42 weeks of gestational age and xanthan gum and other thickeners are approved only for children over 1 year due to concerns of necrotizing enterocolitis. Both carob bean and xanthan gum can be used to thicken breast milk [38].
- The thickening of formula/ breast milk should be guided by a physician or dietician.
- Cow's milk protein elimination should be tried if modifying the feed consistency and volume don't help as it is difficult to distinguish cow's milk protein allergy (CMPA) from GERD. In formula-fed babies, extensively hydrolyzed for-

mula should be trialed for at least 2 weeks and symptom improvement evaluated. Amino acid-based formula should be reserved for patients with refractory and or severe symptoms. Breastfeeding mothers should avoid all forms of dairy including casein and whey for 2 weeks to eliminate cow's milk protein in breast milk [34].

- The probiotic Lactobacillus *reuteri* DSM17938 has shown improvement in crying times and regurgitation in infants but has not shown improvement in the classic symptoms of GERD [39].
- Earlier introduction of pureed foods to infants closer to 4–6 months if developmentally appropriate, may provide some relief.
- Additional considerations for infants include formula mixing methods/recipe, feeding schedules, and positioning post feeds (holding the infant upright for 30 minutes after feeds).
- Children/adolescents should: avoid reflux triggers including acidic foods, greasy foods, citrus, caffeine, chocolate, and spicy foods.
  - Achieving a healthy weight status may also help improve GERD symptoms.
- Despite no clear evidence of benefit with acid suppression, proton pump inhibitors (PPIs) for 4–8 weeks are often used as first line in the management of GERD, and H2 blockers are used when a PPI is contraindicated or not available. When these pharmacological interventions fail and before considering anti-reflux surgery, baclofen can be tried [34].
- Transpyloric feeds (naso or gastro jejunal) have been shown to reduce apnea/bradycardia in premature neonates [40] and reduce aspiration pneumonia in children with neurological comorbidities comparable to fundoplication [41].
- Anti-reflux surgery is reserved for those with severe life-threatening complications of GERD, refractory symptoms despite pharmacological therapy, conditions that are high risk for GERD-related complications and those dependent on chronic pharmacotherapy for relief of symptoms [34].

Functional Diarrhea

- The Rome foundation defines functional diarrhea as painless passage of four large unformed stools daily with symptoms lasting over 4 weeks. The onset is between 6 months and 60 months of age, and there is no failure to thrive if the calorie intake is adequate [2]
- -These children do not have weight loss or hematochezia, and they are able to maintain normal activity and appetite.
- -The treatment includes reassurance, dietary modification, and avoidance of restrictive diets [42].

Nutrition Management

- Diarrhea does not necessarily result in increased energy or protein needs. In cases of malnutrition or poor weight status, catch-up growth may be needed.
- Consider evaluating sodium, potassium magnesium, phosphorus, chloride, and zinc.
- Focus on fluid intake and rehydration is important.
- Restore fluid and electrolyte balance.
- To decrease GI motility, avoid simple carbohydrates such as lactose sucrose, and fructose found in dairy products, refined white grains, fruit juice, and foods with added sugars. Also avoid sugar alcohols such as sorbitol, xylitol, mannitol, and sucralose found in sugar-free alternatives and caffeine.
- Avoid high fiber and gas-producing foods such as nuts, beans, corn, broccoli, cauliflower, brussels sprouts, and cabbage.
- Incorporate stool-thickening foods such as oatmeal, rice cereal, or pectin.

References

1. Shava U, Srivastava A, Mathias A, Kumar N, Yachha SK, Gambhir S, et al. Functional dyspepsia in children: A study of pathophysiological factors. J Gastroenterol Hepatol. 2021;36(3):680–6.
2. Hyams JS, Di Lorenzo C, Saps M, Shulman RJ, Staiano A, Van Tilburg M. Childhood functional gastrointestinal disorders: child/adolescent. Gastroenterology. 2016;150(6):1456–68. e2
3. Koppen IJ, Vriesman MH, Saps M, Rajindrajith S, Shi X, van Etten-Jamaludin FS, et al. Prevalence of functional defecation disorders in children: a systematic review and meta-analysis. J Pediatr. 2018;198(121–30):e6.
4. Drossman DA, Tack J. Rome foundation clinical diagnostic criteria for disorders of gut-brain interaction. Gastroenterology. 2022;162(3):675–9.
5. Nurko S, Benninga MA, Solari T, Chumpitazi BP. Pediatric aspects of nutrition interventions for disorders of gut-brain interaction. Official J Am College Gastroenteroll ACG. 2022;117(6):995–1009.
6. Waseem S, Rubin L. A comprehensive review of functional dyspepsia in pediatrics. Clin J Gastroenterol. 2022;15(1):30–40.
7. Morariu I-D, Avasilcai L, Vieriu M, Lupu VV, Morariu B-A, Lupu A, et al. Effects of a Low-FODMAP Diet on Irritable Bowel Syndrome in Both Children and Adults—A Narrative Review. Nutrients. 2023;15(10):2295.
8. Thapar N, Benninga MA, Crowell MD, Di Lorenzo C, Mack I, Nurko S, et al. Paediatric functional abdominal pain disorders. Nat Rev Dis Primers. 2020;6(1):89.
9. Jo'rayev S. Functional dyspepsia and its treatment in children. Академические исследования в современной науке. 2022;1(17):41–8.
10. Medow MS, Thek KD, Newman LJ, Berezin S, Glassman MS, Schwarz SM. β-galactosidase tablets in the treatment of lactose intolerance in pediatrics. Am J Dis Child. 1990;144(11):1261–4.
11. Shulman RJ, Hollister EB, Cain K, Czyzewski DI, Self MM, Weidler EM, et al. Psyllium fiber reduces abdominal pain in children with irritable bowel syndrome in a randomized, double-blind trial. Clin Gastroenterol Hepatol. 2017;15(5):712–9. e4.
12. Romano C, Comito D, Famiani A, Calamarà S, Loddo I. Partially hydrolyzed guar gum in pediatric functional abdominal pain. World J Gastroenterol: WJG. 2013;19(2):235.
13. Tabbers M, DiLorenzo C, Berger M, Faure C, Langendam M, Nurko S, et al. Evaluation and treatment of functional constipation in infants and children: evidence-based recommendations from ESPGHAN and NASPGHAN. J Pediatr Gastroenterol Nutr. 2014;58(2):258–74.

14. Bae SH, Son JS, Lee R. Effect of fluid intake on the outcome of constipation in children: PEG 4000 versus lactulose. Pediatr Int. 2010;52(4):594–7.
15. Opatowska M, Gmitrzuk J, Malinka Z, Wiśniewska K, Jachymek A, Jakubiec J, et al. SIBO in pediatric population: literature review on pathogenesis, symptoms, diagnosis and treatment. Quality Sport. 2024;15:52152.
16. Adike A, DiBaise JK. Small intestinal bacterial overgrowth: nutritional implications, diagnosis, and management. Gastroenterol Clin. 2018;47(1):193–208.
17. Pimentel M, Constantino T, Kong Y, Bajwa M, Rezaei A, Park S. A 14-day elemental diet is highly effective in normalizing the lactulose breath test. Dig Dis Sci. 2004;49:73–7.
18. Jackman L, Arpe L, Thapar N, Rybak A, Borrelli O. Nutritional Management of Pediatric Gastrointestinal Motility Disorders. Nutrients. 2024;16(17):2955.
19. Limketkai BN, LeBrett W, Lin L, Shah ND. Nutritional approaches for gastroparesis. Lancet Gastroenterol Hepatol. 2020;5(11):1017–26.
20. Wytiaz V, Homko C, Duffy F, Schey R, Parkman HP. Foods provoking and alleviating symptoms in gastroparesis: patient experiences. Dig Dis Sci. 2015;60:1052–8.
21. Siegel M, Krantz B, Lebenthal E. Effect of fat and carbohydrate composition on the gastric emptying of isocaloric feedings in premature infants. Gastroenterology. 1985;89(4):785–90.
22. Krasaelap A, Kovacic K, Goday PS. Nutrition management in pediatric gastrointestinal motility disorders. Nutr Clin Pract. 2020;35(2):265–72.
23. Lu PL, Di Lorenzo C. Gastroparesis in the pediatric patient: children are not little adults. Gastrointest Disorder. 2020;2(2):8.
24. Thapar N, Saliakellis E, Benninga MA, Borrelli O, Curry J, Faure C, et al. Paediatric intestinal pseudo-obstruction: evidence and consensus-based recommendations from an ESPGHAN-led expert group. J Pediatr Gastroenterol Nutr. 2018;66(6):991–1019.
25. Pescarin M, Day H, Thapar N, Jackman L, Saliakellis E, Lindley KJ, et al. Optimizing nutrition in pediatric intestinal pseudo-obstruction syndrome. Neurogastroenterol Motility. 2023;35(5):e14562.
26. Arbizu R, Freiberg B, Rodriguez L. Lower gastrointestinal functional and motility disorders in children. Pediatr Clin. 2021;68(6):1255–71.
27. Verkijk M, Vecht J, Gielkens H, Lamers C, Masclee A. Effects of medium-chain and long-chain triglycerides on antroduodenal motility and small bowel transit time in man. Dig Dis Sci. 1997;42:1933–9.
28. Ledeboer M, Masclee A, Jansen J, Lamers C. Effect of equimolar amounts of long-chain triglycerides and medium-chain triglycerides on small-bowel transit time in humans. J Parenter Enter Nutr. 1995;19(1):5–8.

29. Gallagher K, Flint A, Mouzaki M, Carpenter A, Haliburton B, Bannister L, et al. Blenderized enteral nutrition diet study: feasibility, clinical, and microbiome outcomes of providing blenderized feeds through a gastric tube in a medically complex pediatric population. J Parenter Enter Nutr. 2018;42(6):1046–60.
30. Di Lorenzo C, Flores AF, Buie T, Hyman PE. Intestinal motility and jejunal feeding in children with chronic intestinal pseudo-obstruction. Gastroenterology. 1995;108(5):1379–85.
31. Papadatou B, Ferretti F, Gambarara M, Diamanti A, De Peppo F, Bagolan P, et al., editors. Clinical heterogeneity of chronic intestinal pseudo-obstruction. Transplantation proceedings. Elsevier; 1997.
32. Faure C, Goulet O, Ategbo S, Breton A, Tounian P, Ginies J-L, et al. Chronic intestinal pseudoobstruction syndrome clinical analysis, outcome, and prognosis in 105 children. Dig Dis Sci. 1999;44:953–9.
33. Fell J, Smith V, Milla P. Infantile chronic idiopathic intestinal pseudo-obstruction: the role of small intestinal manometry as a diagnostic tool and prognostic indicator. Gut. 1996;39(2):306–11.
34. Rosen R, Vandenplas Y, Singendonk M, Cabana M, DiLorenzo C, Gottrand F, et al. Pediatric gastroesophageal reflux clinical practice guidelines: joint recommendations of the North American Society for Pediatric Gastroenterology, Hepatology, and Nutrition and the European Society for Pediatric Gastroenterology, Hepatology, and Nutrition. J Pediatr Gastroenterol Nutr. 2018;66(3):516–54.
35. Sintusek P, Mutalib M, Thapar N. Gastroesophageal reflux disease in children: What's new right now? World J Gastrointestinal Endos. 2023;15(3):84.
36. Friedman C, Sarantos G, Katz S, Geisler S. Understanding gastroesophageal reflux disease in children. Jaapa. 2021;34(2):12–8.
37. Vandenplas Y, De Schepper J, Verheyden S, Devreker T, Franckx J, Peelman M, et al. A preliminary report on the efficacy of the Multicare AR-Bed in 3-week–3-month-old infants on regurgitation, associated symptoms and acid reflux. Arch Dis Child. 2010;95(1):26–30.
38. Duncan DR, Larson K, Rosen RL. Clinical aspects of thickeners for pediatric gastroesophageal reflux and oropharyngeal dysphagia. Curr Gastroenterol Rep. 2019;21:1–9.
39. Indrio F, Di Mauro A, Riezzo G, Civardi E, Intini C, Corvaglia L, et al. Prophylactic use of a probiotic in the prevention of colic, regurgitation, and functional constipation: a randomized clinical trial. JAMA Pediatr. 2014;168(3):228–33.
40. Misra S, Macwan K, Albert V. Transpyloric feeding in gastroesophageal-reflux–associated apnea in premature infants. Acta Paediatr. 2007;96(10):1426–9.

41. Srivastava R, Downey EC, O'Gorman M, Feola P, Samore M, Holubkov R, et al. Impact of fundoplication versus gastrojejunal feeding tubes on mortality and in preventing aspiration pneumonia in young children with neurologic impairment who have gastroesophageal reflux disease. Pediatrics. 2009;123(1):338–45.
42. Keating JP. Chronic diarrhea. Pediatr Rev. 2005;26(1):5–14.
43. Scarlata K. Accessed 23 Jan 2025. Available from: https://www.todaysdietitian.com/newarchives/072710p30.shtml.
44. University M. Accessed 23 Jan 2025. Available from: https://www.monashfodmap.com/about-fodmap-and-ibs/.
45. NIDDK. Accessed 23 Jan 2025. Available from: https://www.niddk.nih.gov/health-information/digestive-diseases/irritable-bowel-syndrome/eating-diet-nutrition.

Index

A
Abetalipoproteinemia, 94, 362
Absorption, 91–93
  iron, 134–135
Aceruloplasminemia, 144, 202
Acid suppression, 472
Acute kidney injury (AKI)
  definition, 601
  nutrition considerations and recommendations, 602–603
    macronutrients, 604
    micronutrients, 605–606
  stages of, 602
Acute recurrent pancreatitis (ARP)
  clinical investigations, 502
  clinical presentation, 502
  diagnostic criteria, 502
  etiology, 502
  management, 503, 504
Acute respiratory distress syndrome (ARDS)
  asthma, 597, 598
  growth assessment, 595
  invasive ventilation, 595
  mechanical ventilation, 594
  noninvasive ventilation, 595
  protein requirements, 596
Acyanotic lesions, 380–382
Adolescents, 10–11, 14
Adolescents (aged 13-18 years), 10–11
Adult beriberi, 255, 256
Adult thiamine deficiency, 261
Albumin infusion, 552
Albuminemia, 607
Almond milk, 53
Alpha lipoic acid (ALA)
  cellular transport, 338
  definition, 335–336
  dose recommendations and potential use, 337
  future research, 338
  physiology, 336
  sources, 337
Americans with Disabilities Act (ADA), 415
Aminoacids
  conditionally essential, 100
  essential, 98–99
  non-essential, 99
Amino acid transport disorders, 104–106
  Blue diaper syndrome, 107–108
  cystinuria, 108
  Hartnup disorder, 107
  lysinuric protein intolerance, 108–109
Amoxicillin-clavulanic acid, 649
Anorexia nervosa, 626

K. Radhakrishnan (ed.), *Handbook of Clinical and Practical Pediatric Nutrition*, https://doi.org/10.1007/978-3-031-97759-6

Anticoagulants, CoQ10, 332
Antidiarrheal therapy, 472
Anti-emetics, 444
Antigen-presenting cells (APCs), 516
Anti-reflux formula, 52
Anti-sterility factor, 359
Asthma, 597, 598
Ataxia with vitamin E deficiency (AVED), 362
Atransferrinemia, 144
Autoimmune enteropathy, 123
Autoimmune protocol diet (AIP), 436
Avoidant/restrictive food intake disorder (ARFID), 307, 627
  definition, 446
  treatment, 447, 448
  vs. PFD, 447

B

Basal metabolic rate (BMR), 17–19
Bile-acid-binding resin, 472
Binge eating disorder (BED), 627
Biotinidase deficiency, 289, 292
Biotin (vitamin B7/H)
  bacterial sources, 291
  cofactor, 289
  cycle, 290
  deficiency, 291
  definition, 289
  dietary sources, 290
  functions, 290
  future aspects, 293
  recommendations for dosage intake, 292, 293
  secondary biotin deficiency, 292
Blenderized diets, 656
Blenderized foods, 560
Blood glucose
  manganese, 220–221
  monitoring, 404
Blue diaper syndrome, 107–108
Bone matrix homeostasis, 183
Bowel obstruction, 473
Breastfed assessment and treatment, 42–43
Bronchopulmonary dysplasia (BPD), 593, 594
Brown-Vialetto-Van Laere Syndrome Type 1 (hRFT-1), 266, 269
Bulimia nervosa, 626
B vitamins, 40

C

Calcium
  dietary calcium absorption and storage, 155–156
  dietary calcium intake, 153–155
  hypercalcemia, 162
  hypocalcemia
    infancy and childhood, 160–162
    neonatal hypocalcemia, 159
  physiology and homeostasis, 156–159
  supplementation, 534
Carbohydrates, 582
  absorption of simple sugars, 114–116
  classification, 112
  digestion, 114–115
  disaccharides, 112
  disorders of carbohydrate digestion, 117
    fructose malabsorption, 120, 121
    glucose-galactose malabsorption, 121
    lactose malabsorption and intolerance, 118–119
    mucosal disorders, 122–123
    primary disorders, 117
    secondary disorders, 117
    sucrase-isomaltase enzyme deficiency, 119

Trehalose deficiency, 121
DRI, 113
monosaccharides, 112
oligosaccharides, 112
polysaccharides, 112
requirements across all ages, 113
simple sugars, 111
starches, 113
Carnitine, 76, 78
deficiency
in cardiovascular disease, 323
CPT1, defects in, 321
CPT2 deficiency, 321
future directions research potential, 323–324
inborn errors of metabolism, 322
OCTN2 carnitine transporter, 320
primary carnitine deficiency, 320
secondary carnitine deficiency, 321–322
supplementation, 322–323
role of, 318
synthesis, 318–320
Carotenoids, 344, 345
Celiac disease, 122
clinical aspects of, 515, 516
follow up, 539
GF diet, 515
gluten-free diet
allergen labeling, 526, 527
antibodies, 538, 539
cross contamination, 527–530
education, 522
financial cost, 536
food labeling, 524–526
goal of, 522
grains and derivatives, 523
natural alternatives, 524
nutritional cost, 531–535
social cost, 536–538
high-risk groups, 521, 522
screening and diagnosis
gluten challenge, 520
gluten consumption, 518
HLA testing, 519
indications, 517
Marsh scoring system, 519
non-biopsy, 519, 520
specificity and sensitivity, 518
TTG IgA, 518
symptoms of, 516, 517
Centers of Disease Control (CDC) growth charts, 7, 10–13
Cerebral palsy, 561, 562
Ceruloplasmin, 221, 225
Charcot-Marie tooth disease, 567
Childhood, hypocalcemia, 160–162
Cholecalciferol (vitamin D3), 351
Cholesterol, manganese, 221
Chromium (Cr), 235, 243, 244
Chronic kidney disease (CKD)
definition, 606
nephrotic syndrome, 610
nutrition considerations and recommendations, 608–609
renal tubulopathies, 611–612
stages of, 606, 607
Chronic liver disease
dietary recommendations, 455–457
energy and protein needs, 457–459
history and physical exam, 452–454
maldigestion and malabsorption, 452
metabolic risks and evaluation, 454, 455
nutrient metabolism, 452
poor intake, 451
Chylomicron retention disorder, 94

Chylothorax, 389
Coagulation abnormalities, 549
Cobalt, 235, 240–241
Coconut milk, 53
Coenzyme A (CoA), 277–279
Coenzyme Q10 (CoQ10)
absorption and metabolism, 330
drug interactions, 332
future aspects, 332
history, 327
physiology, 327–328
primary deficiency, 328, 329
safety, 331
secondary deficiency, 329
side effects, 331
sources and available dosage forms, 330–331
Complete proteins, 98
Complex carbohydrates, 112
Conditionally essential amino acids, 100
Congenital disorder of glycosylation type IIn (CDG2N), 225
Congenital heart disease (CHD)
acyanotic lesions, 380–382
complications, 389–391
cyanotic lesions, 380
definition, 377
feeding practices, protocols and nutritional needs, 384–388
heart failure and transplantation, 391, 392
incidence, 377, 379
nutrition assessment and malnutrition, 382–384
nutrition monitoring and evaluation, 388, 389
stratification, 378–379
Congenital lactase deficiency, 117, 118
Congenital myopathies, 566, 567
Congenital sucrase-isomaltase deficiency (CSID), 119
Continuous glucose monitors (CGM), 404
Copper (Cu)
ATP7A and ATP7B, 199, 200
catalytic cofactor, 196
deficiency, 201–202
dietary sources, 196–198
functions/uses, 200
genetic disorders, 202
Huppke Brendal syndrome, 208
MEDNIK syndrome, 207
Menkes disease, 204, 205
metabolism, 198–200
deficiency, 202
duodenum, 198
excess, 202
liver, 199
portal circulation, 198
target tissues/organs, 199–200
occipital horn syndrome, 206
Wilson disease, 203–205
Cows milk based formula, 50
CPT1, defects in, 321
CPT2 deficiency, 321
Crohn's disease (CD), 428
Crohn's disease exclusion diet (CDED), 434
Cyanocobalamin (vitamin B12)
acute and chronic, 302–303
assessment, 300–301
clinical presentation, 298
dietary sources, 296
digestion and metabolism, 297–298
etiology, 299–300
future research applications, 303
management, 301–302
RDA, 296
role of, 298, 300
Cyanotic lesions, 380
Cyproheptadine, 444
Cysteine, 76, 79
Cystic fibrosis (CF), 505, 590–593
Cystinuria, 108

D

Dapagliflozin, 405
Dermal synthesis, vitamin D, 352
Diabetes
advocacy, 414
cause of, 397
college, 412
diagnostic criteria, 398
DKA, 407
etiology of, 398
HHS, 407
hyperglycemia, 406
hypoglycemia, 406
pediatric diabetes, nutrition assessment
carbohydrate counting, 410, 411
energy needs, 408
principles of, 408–410
protein needs, 408
type 1 diabetes, 412
school/daycare, 412
sports, 413
surveillance, 414
T1D
clinical presentation of, 401
definition, 399–400
insulin therapy, 403, 404
laboratory evaluation, 401, 402
management, 402, 403
medications, 400
stages of, 400
technology, 404, 405
T2D, 405, 406
definition, 399
telehealth, 413
Diabetic ketoacidosis (DKA), 407
Diacylglycerol (DAG) deficiency, 94
Diet elimination, 489
Dietary reference intakes (DRI), 3, 8, 9, 14, 17, 18, 22, 31–33
protein, 100
Dietary sources
folic acid, 306
vitamin B_6, 285–286
vitamin B12, 296
vitamin C, 314
Digestible Indispensable Amino Acid Score (DIAAS), 101
Digestion, 91, 92
carbohydrates, 114–115
protein
disorders of, 106
gastric, 102
jejunal and ileal digestion, 103
oral, 102
pancreatic and duodenal, 102–103
1,25-dihydroxyvitamin-D (1,25 OHD), 351
Disaccharides, 112
Disorders of carbohydrate digestion, 117
fructose malabsorption, 120, 121
glucose-galactose malabsorption, 121
lactose malabsorption and intolerance, 118–119
mucosal disorders, 122–123
primary disorders, 117
secondary disorders, 117
sucrase-isomaltase enzyme deficiency, 119
Trehalose deficiency, 121
Disorders of gut brain interaction (DGBI)
definition, 643, 644
functional diarrhea, 646–647, 660
gastroparesis, 650–653
GERD, 657–659
management, 645, 647, 648
nutritional impact, 644, 645
PIPO, 653–656
SIBO, 648–650

Distal hereditary motor neuropathy, 202
Distal ileum, 464
Divalent metal transporter 1 (DMT1), 222
Donor milk, 578, 579
Duchenne muscular dystrophy (DMD), 555, 563, 564
Ductal dependent pulmonary blood flow, 385
Dynamic contrast-enhanced magnetic resonance lymphangiography (DCMRL), 550
Dyslipidaemia, 275

E

Eating disorders
- DSM-5, 625–628
- grazing, compulsive subtype, 629
- grazing, non-compulsive subtype, 629
- history, 629, 630
- inpatient nutritional insufficiency protocol, 634
  - medical criteria, 635
  - refeeding syndrome, 635, 636
  - supplement requirements, 635
- laboratory evaluation, 632–633
- monitoring and growth expectations, 640
- nutrition assessment, 633, 634
- outpatient nutrition counseling, 638
  - meal plan, 638, 639
- physical examination, 631
- prognosis, 640, 641
- RED-S, 629
- SCOFF, 631
- vitamin/mineral deficiencies, 636, 637

Ebb phase, 21
Electrolytes, 74, 78, 583, 584
Elemental formula, 51, 54
Empagliflozin, 405
Endomysial antibody, 518
Energy needs for infants, 3
Enteral feeding tubes, 559
Enteral formulas, 552
Enteral nutrition (EN), 468, 478, 576, 577
Enteral nutrition support
- bolus feeds, 65
- continuous feeds, 65
- enteral tubes, 59
  - gastro-Jejunal tube, 63
  - G tube, 62
  - ND/NJ tube, 61
  - NG tube, 60
- formula delivery techniques, 64–65
- formula selection considerations, 63–64
- long term complications, 65, 66
  - considerations/monitoring, 66
  - transitioning to oral feeds, 67
- placement feeding tube, 58–61

Enteral nutrition therapy (EEN), 434
Enteral option, 301
Enterocyte intracellular iron, 135
Enterocyte monosaccharide transporters, 116
Enterokinase deficiency, 106
Enzymatic deficiency, 268
Eosinophilic esophagitis (EoE), 488, 489
Eosinophilic gastrointestinal disorders (EGIDs), 488
Ergocalciferol (vitamin D2), 351
Erythromycin, 649
Essential fatty acid deficiency (EFAD), 90–91, 551
Essential fatty acids, 88–89
- deficiency (EFAD), 90–91, 551
- synthesis, 89–90

Everolimus, 552

Exocrine pancreatic insufficiency (EPI), 122
causes, 506
clinical manifestations, 505
definition, 504
diagnosis, 508, 509
etiology, 505–508
treatment, 508, 510
Extensively hydrolyzed formula, 51
Extra skeletal effects, of vitamin D, 356–357

F

Failure to thrive (FTT)
definition, 441
diagnosis, 441
etiology, 442, 443
treatment, 443, 444
Fat
absorption, 92–93
classification, 86
digestion, 91–93
essential fatty acids, 88–89
deficiency, 90–91
synthesis, 89–90
malabsorption, 93–94
requirements across ages, 88
transport, 92
types, 85–88
Fat restriction, 650
Fat-soluble vitamins, 552
Fazio-Londe syndrome, 269
Feeding approaches, 469
Feeding disorder
ARFID
definition, 446
treatment, 447, 448
vs. PFD, 447
PFD, 444, 445
Feeding problems, 474
Feeding protocols, 577, 578
Feeding/solids, infants, 4
Fermentable oligosaccharides, disaccharides, monosaccharides and polyols (FODMAP), 645
Ferritin, 134, 136–138, 140
Ferroportin, 135
Ferrous iron, 135, 136
Fiber, 113
Flavin adenine dinucleotide (FAD), 266–269
Flavin mononucleotide (FMN), 266, 267, 269
Flow phase, 21
Fluid calculations, 23
Folate deficiency
diagnosis, 309
genetic causes, 307–308
inadequate intake or malabsorption, 307
management of, 309
medication, 308
other causes of, 308
signs and symptoms, 309
Folic acid
absorption and metabolism, 306
dietary sources, 306
folate deficiency
diagnosis, 309
genetic causes, 307–308
inadequate intake or malabsorption, 307
management of, 309
medication, 308
other causes of, 308
signs and symptoms, 309
future research, 310
physiology, 305–306
Fontan-associated protein-losing enteropathy, 547, 548
Food allergies
IgE-mediated allergies, 486, 487
resolution, 487
vs. non-IgE mediated allergies, 488–492
non-IgE mediated allergies
dietary management, 492
food protein, 491

Food allergies (*cont.*)
FPIAP, 493
FPIES, 494
vs. IgE mediated allergies, 488–492
pollen food allergy syndrome, 487
Food protein induced allergic proctocolitis syndrome (FPIAP), 493
Food protein induced enterocolitis syndrome (FPIES), 494
Foremilk, 39
Fortification, 43–44
Fortified foods, vitamin D, 352
Fructose malabsorption, 120, 121
Functional constipation (FC), 644
Functional diarrhea, 646–647, 660
Functional dyspepsia (FD), 644
Functional iron deficiency, 138

G
Gastric digestion, 102
Gastric Tube (GT), 59, 64
Gastroesophageal reflux disease (GERD)
definition, 657
nutritional management, 658, 659
pH-MII, 657
prevalence, 657
risk factors, 657
symptoms, 657
Gastro-Jejunal tube (GJT), 59, 64
Gastroparesis
causes, 651
definition, 650
management, 652, 653
modality, 651
nutritional impact, 651
pathophysiology, 651
Gliadin, 516
Glucagon-like Peptide-2 (GLP-2), 473
Glucagon-like-peptide-1 (GLP-1), 405
Glucose-galactose malabsorption, 121
Gluten-free (GF) diet, 515, 520
allergen labeling, 526, 527
antibodies, 538, 539
cross contamination, 527–530
education, 522
financial cost, 536
food labeling, 524–526
goal of, 522
grains and derivatives, 523
natural alternatives, 524
nutritional cost, 531–535
social cost, 536–538
Goat's milk, 53
Graft versus host disease (GVHD), 548, 619, 620

H
Hartnup disorder, 107
Hematopoietic stem cell transplant (HSCT), 618
Heme iron, 129
Hemp milk, 53
Henoch-Schönlein purpura, 549
Hepcidin, 135, 137
High calorie formula, 52
High MCT oil formula, 52, 54
High protein diet, 552
Hindmilk, 39
HLA testing, 519
Holliday-Segar method, 23
Holocarboxylase synthetase (HCLS), 292
Human milk, 578–581
components, 39–40
composition, 39–40
contraindications, 45
donor breastmilk safety considerations and recommendations, 46
early cessation, 44

enrichment recipes, 44
fed baby with poor weight gain, 42–43
feeding and benefits, 38
feeding initiation and continuation, 41
fortification and enrichment, 43–44
healthcare providers· resources for, 46
medication safety, resources for, 46
production, 38–39
reason for, 45
recommend intakes and volumes, 41
safe storage, sharing, and handling, 42
Human milk fortifiers (HMF), 50, 580
Human riboflavin transporter 2 (hRFt-2), 266
Hypercalcemia, 162
Hyperglycemia, 406
Hyperglycemic hyperosmolar state (HHS), 407
Hypermagnesemia
causes, 189–190
clinical manifestations, 190–191
definition, 189–192
evaluation, 191–192
management, 192
Hypermanganesemia with dystonia 1 (HMNDYT1), 224, 225
Hypermetabolism, 66
Hyperphosphatemia, 172, 173
Hypertrophic gastropathy, 549
Hypoalbuminemia, 549
Hypoallergenic formulas, 51, 54
Hypobetalipoproteinemia, 94
Hypocalcemia
infancy and childhood, 160–162
neonatal hypocalcemia, 159
Hypoglycemia, 406
Hypomagnesemia
causes, 184–186
clinical manifestations, 186
definition, 184
evaluation, 186–187
management, 188–189
Hypometabolism, 66
Hypoparathyroidism, 160, 161
Hypophosphatemia, 171–174
Hypoxia inducible factor-1 (HIF-1a), 312

I

IBD anti-inflammatory diet (IBD-AID), 436
IgE-mediated allergies, 486, 487
Ileocecal valve (ICV), 465
Immune deficiencies, 549
Inborn errors of metabolism, 322
Incomplete proteins, 98
Indirect calorimetry (IC), 21–23, 32
Infancy, hypocalcemia, 160–162
Infant formula, 50–55
Infantile beriberi, 254–255
Infants, 3–6
Inflammatory bowel disease (IBD), 123, 548
classifications, 427
Crohn's disease, 428
IBD-U, 429
nutrition, 430–432
energy/protein needs, 437
healthy eating/mediterranean diet, 432, 433
induction/maintenance therapy, 433, 435–437
social/environmental, 438
supplementation, 437
research in, 438
ulcerative colitis, 429
Insoluble fiber, 113
Insulin pumps, 405
Intestinal absorption, 180–181
Intestinal disorders, 442

Intestinal failure associated liver disease (IFALD), 473
Intrauterine growth restriction (IUGR), 586
Intravenous fat emulsions (IVFE), 583
Intravenous lipid (ILE) emulsions, 72
Iodine
  metabolism, 236–238
  RDA, 239, 240
Iodine deficiency (ID), 238, 239
Iodine deficiency disorder (IDD), 235, 238, 239
Iron, 40
  heme and non-heme, 131, 146–147
  implication in health and disease
    aceruloplasminemia, 144
    atransferrinemia, 144
    deficiency and anemia, 138–142
    iron overload, 142–143
    lead poisoning, 144
  infants, 6
  matabolism
    absorption, 134–135
    regulation, 137
    transport, distribution, and storage, 136–137
  metabolism, overview, 133–138
  overload, 142–144
  in pediatrics, 130
  pregnant and lactating patients, 131
  recommended dietary allowance and tolerable upper intake levels, 145
  recycling, 137–138
  regulation, 137
  role and function, 132–133
  sources and bioavailability, 129–131
Iron transport, distribution, and storage, 136–137
Irritable bowel syndrome (IBS), 643

J

Jejunal and ileal digestion, 103
Jejunal tube (JT), 59

K

Keshan disease, 229
Kwashiorkor, 30

L

Lactase, 535
Lactose malabsorption and intolerance, 118–119
Lipase, 498, 508
Lipase and colipase deficiency, 93
Long-acting insulin, 403
Long chain triglyceride (LCT), 551
Long term anticonvulsant therapy, 291
Loperamide, 472
Low-fat diet, 551
Low lactose formula, 51
Lysinuric protein intolerance (LPI), 108–109

M

Magnesium
  evaluation of, 183
  future aspects, 192–193
  hypermagnesemia
    causes, 189–190
    clinical manifestations, 190–191
    definition, 189–192
    evaluation, 191–192
    management, 192
  hypomagnesemia, 184–189
    causes, 184–186
    clinical manifestations, 186
    definition, 184

evaluation, 186–187
management, 188–189
measurement, 183
nutritional Sources of, 181–182
physiology
body distribution, 178–179
functions, 179–180
hemostasis, 180
recommended dietary allowance, 177, 178
Malnutrition, 24–26, 30
biochemical data, 28–31
illness and non-illness related, 26
laboratory tests, 29
macro and micro-nutrient deficiencies, 27–28
pediatric malnutrition criteria, 25
types of, 30
waterlow criteria, 24
Manganese (Mn), 74, 77, 78
absorption, metabolism and excretion, 222–224
blood glucose, 220–221
CDG2N, 225
cholesterol, 221
exposure, storage, and excretion, 221–223
growth, bones and collagen, 220
HMNDYT1, 224
HMNDYT2, 224–225
MnSOD, 220
RDA table, 222
symptoms, 224
Marasmus, 30
Marsh scoring system, 519
Medium chain fat (MCT), 390, 391
Medium chain triglyceride (MCT), 551
MEDNIK syndrome, 202
Ménétrier's disease, 549
Menkes disease (MD), 204, 205
Metabolic bone disease (MBD), 174, 474
Metformin, 405
Micronutrient deficiencies, 474
Micronutrients, 74–78
Mid-upper arm circumference (MUAC), 24
Miliaria crystallina, 223
Milk and milk alternatives, 53
Minerals, 584, 585
Molybdate transporter1 (MOT1), 241
Molybdate transporter 2 (MOT2), 241
Molybdenum, 235, 241–243
Molybdenum cofactor deficiency (MoCD), 242
Monosaccharides, 112
Monounsaturated fatty acids, 86
Mucosal disorders, 122–123, 442
Mucosal injury, 548, 549
Multiple carboxylase deficiency, 292
Multiple daily injection (MDI), 403
Multivitamins (MVI), 74, 76

N
NADPH epoxidase (NAXE), 275
NADPH oxidoreductase-like protein (NAXD), 275
Nasoduodenal (ND) tube, 59, 61
Nasojejunal (NJ) tube, 59
Neonatal gastrointestinal (GI) tract
colon, rectum, and anus, 572, 573
development, 569
esophagus, 570
small intestine, pancreas, and biliary system, 571, 572
stomach, 570, 571
Neonatal hypocalcemia, 159
Nephrotic syndrome, 610
Neuromuscular disorders (NMD)
cerebral palsy, 561, 562
Charcot-Marie tooth disease, 567

Neuromuscular disorders (NMD) (*cont.*)
complications, 555
congenital myopathies, 566, 567
DEXA scan, 557
DMD, 555, 563, 564
energy requirements, 558
enteral tube feeds, 559
feeding ability and nutritional status, 558
formula selection, 559–561
multidisciplinary approach, 556
nutritional assessment, 557
SFT, 557
spinal muscular atrophy, 564, 565
Niacin (vitamin B3)
deficiency, 273
digestion and metabolism, 272
medince, role in, 275
newer role/developmental research, 275
RDA, 272–273
toxicity, 274
Nicotinamide adenine dinucleotide (NAD), 272, 274, 275
Nicotinamide adenine dinucleotide phosphate (NADP), 272, 274, 275
Non-essential amino acids, 99
Non-heme iron, 129, 130
Nutrition assessment
clinical cases, 31–33
energy calculations, 20–23
illness and non-illness related, 26
malnutrition, 24–26
biochemical data, 28–31
laboratory tests, 29
macro and micro-nutrient deficiencies, 27–28
types of, 30
waterlow criteria, 24
pediatric malnutrition criteria, 25
protein calculations, 23–24
Nutritional vitamin D deficiency Rickets, 354

O

Oat milk, 53
Occipital horn syndrome, 206
OCTN2 carnitine transporter, 320
Octreotide, 552
Oligosaccharides, 112, 115
Oral aversion, 474
Oral digestion, 102
Organic formula, 52
Osteocalcin, 369
Osteopenia, 174
Other specified feeding and eating disorders (OSFED), 628

P

Pancreatic and duodenal digestion, 102–103
Pancreatic disorders
acute pancreatitis
classification, 498
clinical investigations, 500
clinical presentation, 499
diagnosis, 498
etiology, 498, 499
management, 500, 501
ARP and chronic pancreatitis
clinical investigations, 502
clinical presentation, 502
diagnostic criteria, 502
etiology, 502
management, 503, 504
EPI
causes, 506
clinical manifestations, 505
definition, 504
diagnosis, 508, 509
etiology, 505–508
treatment, 508, 510
incidence, 497

Pancreatic enzyme replacement therapy (PERT), 508
Pantothenate kinase-associated neurodegeneration (PKAN), 279
Pantothenic acid (vitamin B5)
  assessment, 279
  deficiency, 278–279
  dietary sources, 277–278
  digestion and metabolism, 278
  future studies, 279
  PKAN, 279
  RDA, 277–278
  toxicity, 279
Parental formulations, 301
Parenteral nutrition (PN), 386, 468, 477, 621
  associated complications, 77
  calculations, 78–79
  carnitine, 76
  cysteine, 76
  lock therapy, 79–80
  micronutrients, 74–78
  monitoring, evaluation, and clinical considerations, 78
  nutrient composition, 72–74
  pediatric indications, 70–71
  prematurity
    advancement, 581
    macronutrients, 582, 583
    micronutrients, 583–586
  route of administration, 70
Pediatric feeding disorder (PFD)
  definition, 444, 445
  vs. ARFID, 447
Pediatric formula, 54
Pediatric intestinal failure (PIF), 461
  absorption, complications, and adaptation, 462–463, 465
  anthropometrics, 466, 476
  clinical management, 466
  colon loss, 465
  complications, 473–475
  diet/nutrition support, 477, 478
  distal intestinal loss, 464, 465
  etiology, 462
  fluid and energy needs, 477
  laboratory assessment, 479–481
  laboratory monitoring, 470, 471
  nutrition intervention
    macronutrients, micronutrients, 466, 467, 470
    route of, 468, 469
    solid food introduction, 469
  outcomes, 482
  pharmacological therapy, 472, 473
  post-transplantation, 476
  proximal intestinal loss, 464
  research, 482
  small bowel transplantation, 476
  small intestine length, 464
  surgical interventions, 475
  vitamin/mineral supplements, 479
Pediatric intestinal pseudo obstruction (PIPO), 653
  antroduodenal manometry, 654
  investigations, 654
  management, 654–656
  nutritional assessment, 655
  prevalence, 654
  pseudo-obstruction, 654
Pediatric malnutrition criteria, 25
Pediatric obesity
  classification, 417, 418
  clinical assessment, 420
  comorbidities and medical complications, 418
  medical and surgical management, 423, 424
  risk factors, 419
  treatment, 420–422
  weight loss goals, 423
Pellagra, 271, 273–275
Peterson's failure to thrive (FTT), 18, 19, 31

pH and multichannel intraluminal impedance studies (pH-MII), 657
Phosphorus
body distribution, 165–166
dietary sources, 167
hormonal control of serum phosphorus levels, 169–170
hyperphosphatemia, 172, 173
hypophosphatemia, 171–173
intestinal absorption, 168–169
lab evaluation, 173
osteopenia/MBD of maturity, 174
primary hyperphosphatemia, 170–171
receptors, 168
recommended dietary allowance, 168
renal excretion, 169
sensing, 170
serum concentration, 166
Physical activity co-efficient, 21
Phytobezoar, 652
Pollen food allergy syndrome, 487
Polysaccharides, 112
Polyunsaturated fatty acids (PUFAs), 86, 88
Premature formulas, 50
Prematurity
anthropometric assessment, 575, 576
donor milk, 578, 579
enteral nutrition, 576, 577
feeding protocols, 577, 578
human milk, 578–581
parenteral nutrition
advancement, 581
macronutrients, 582, 583
micronutrients, 583–586
Pre-term infant formula, 50
Primary carnitine deficiency, 320
Primary intestinal lymphangiectasia (PIL), 547
Probiotics, 650
Progressive encephalopathy with brain edema or leukoencephalopathy-1 (PEBEL1), 275
Progressive encephalopathy with brain edema and leukoencephalopathy-2 (PEBEL2), 275
Protein
absorption, 103, 104
assessing optimal protein intake, 101
critically ill patients, 101
definition, 97–101
digestion, 101
disorders of, 106
gastric, 102
jejunal and ileal digestion, 103
oral, 102
pancreatic and duodenal, 102–103
DRI, 100
specific enzyme deficiencies, 106–107
Protein-losing enteropathy (PLE), 390
causes and pathophysiology, 545, 546
definition, 545
diagnosis, 550, 551
lymphatic abnormalities, 547, 548
mucosal injury, 548, 549
pathophysiological consequences, 549
symptoms, 545
treatment
dietary modifications, 551, 552
pharmacological interventions, 552
surgical and interventional approaches, 553
Prothrombin time (PT), 371
Pulmonary disorders

acute and chronic respiratory distress
asthma, 597, 598
growth assessment, 595
invasive ventilation, 595
mechanical ventilation, 594
noninvasive ventilation, 595
protein requirements, 596
BPD, 593, 594
cystic fibrosis, 590–593
Pyridoxal 5'-phosphate (PLP), 281, 282, 284
Pyridoxal (PL), 281, 282
Pyridoxamine 5'-phosphate (PMP), 281, 282
Pyridoxamine (PM), 281, 282
Pyridoxine-dependent epilepsy (PDE), 284
Pyridoxine 5'-phosphate (PNP), 281, 282
Pyridoxine (PN), 281–283

R
Recombinant human PTH (rh-PTH), 161
Recommended dietary allowances (RDAs), 534
cyanocobalamin (vitamin B12), 296
iodine, 239, 240
magnesium, 177, 178
manganese, 222
niacin (vitamin B3), 272–273
pantothenic acid (vitamin B5), 277–278
phosphorus, 168
selenium, 229
thiamine, 261
vitamin A, 346
vitamin B_6, 286
Refeeding syndrome, 66, 585, 586, 635, 636
Reference protein, 98
Registered dietitian (RD), 615
Relative energy deficiency in sport (RED-S), 629
Renal excretion, 169, 182–183
Renal formula, 52
Renal tubulopathies, 611–612
Resting energy expenditure (REE), 20
Retinyl esters, 344, 345
Riboflavin (vitamin B2)
assessment, 267–268
deficiency, 268, 269
dietary sources, 265
digestion and metabolism, 266–267
function of, 267
future aspects, 269
toxicity, 269
Rifaximin, 649
Rogers syndrome, 257

S
Sarcopenia, 455
Saturated fatty acids, 86
Schofield, 19
Schofield equation, 18
Secondary biotin deficiency, 292
Secondary carnitine deficiency, 321–322
Secondary lactose intolerance, 118
Secondary lymphangiectasia, 547
Selective IgA deficiency, 522
Selenium
absorption and metabolism, 229
deficiency, 229–230
diagnosis and treatment, 230, 231
dietary sources, 228–229
future aspects, 231
physiologic functions, 227, 228
RDA, 229
toxicity, 231
Semi-vegetarian diet, 436
Short acting insulin, 404
Short bowel syndrome (SBS), *see* Pediatric intestinal failure (PIF)
Sinusoidal obstruction syndrome (SOS), 618

Sirolimus, 552
Skin fold thickness (SFT), 557
Small bowel transplantation, 476
Small intestinal bacterial overgrowth (SIBO), 472
  definition, 648, 649
  management, 649, 650
  nutritional impact, 649
Sodium-glucose cotransporter 2 (SGLT2) inhibitors, 405
Soluble fiber, 113
Soy formula, 51
Soy milk, 53
Specialty formula, 55–56
Specific carbohydrate diet (SCD), 433, 436
Spinal muscular atrophy, 564, 565
Standard pediatric electrolyte doses, 75
Starches, 113
Stem cell transplantation
  cancer diagnosis, 617, 618
  GVHD, 619, 620
  HSCT, 618
  impacts of chemotherapy, 616
  long term impacts of cancer treatment, 621, 622
  micronutrient deficiencies, 616
  parenteral nutrition, 621
  symptoms, 615
  types of cancer, 615
  VOD/SOS, 618
Steroids, 552
Stool alpha-1-antitrypsin (A1AT), 550
Sucrase-isomaltase enzyme deficiency, 119
Systemic lupus erythematosus (SLE), 549

T

Teduglutide, 473
Telehealth, 413
Thermic effect of food (TEF), 20
Thiamine (vitamin B1)
  absorption and transport, 251
  biologic activity, 252–253
  chemical structure, 250
  clinical manifestations, 254, 255
    adult beriberi, 255, 256
    infantile beriberi, 254–255
    Wernicke-Korsakoff syndrome, 256, 257
  dietary sources, 250, 251
  future aspects, 261, 262
  history, 249, 250
  laboratory diagnosis, 258–262
  metabolism dysfunction syndromes, 257–258
  risk factors, 253–257
  treatment, 261–262
Thiamine diphosphate (ThDP), 252, 257, 260, 262
Thiamine metabolism dysfunction syndrome 1 (thiamine-responsive megaloblastic anemia syndrome), 257
Thiamine metabolism dysfunction syndrome 2 (biotin/thiamine-responsive encephalopathy type), 257
Thiamine metabolism dysfunction syndrome 3 (microcephaly Amish type), 258
Thiamine metabolism dysfunction syndrome 4 (bilateral striatal degeneration and progressive polyneuropathy), 258
Thiamine metabolism dysfunction syndrome 5 (episodic encephalopathy type), 258
Thiamine monophosphate (ThMP), 251
Tissue transglutaminase (TTG), 516
Toddlers (aged 1-4 years)
  feeding skills, 7
  growth charts, 7–9
  macronutrient, 8
  nutrients, 8

Total body water (TBW), 30
Total energy expenditure (TEE), 19, 20
Total parenteral nutrition (TPN), 223
Trace elements, 74
Transcobalamin II deficiency, 299
Transport, 92
Trehalose deficiency, 121–122
Triglycerides, 85
Trypsin deficiency, 102, 106, 107
Tubular disorders, 611–612
Type 1 diabetes (T1D), 412
 clinical presentation of, 401
 definition, 399–400
 insulin therapy, 403, 404
 laboratory evaluation, 401, 402
 management, 402, 403
 stages of, 400
 technology, 404, 405
Type 2 diabetes (T2D), 399, 405, 406

U
Ubiquinol, 328–331
Ubiquinone, 327, 328, 330, 331
Ulcerative colitis (UC), 429

V
Veno-occlusive disease (VOD), 618
Ventricular assist device (VAD), 392
Vitamin A
 deficiency, 345–347
 derivatives, 344
 digestion, absorption, transport and stores, 345
 dosing in deficiency states, 346
 future research, 349
 recommended daily allowance, 346
 roles, 343
 sources, 344–345
 status assessment, 347
 toxicity, 348
  acute toxicity, 348
  chronic toxicity, 348–349
 uses of, 349
Vitamin B_6 (pyridoxine)
 absorption, metabolism, and physiological role, 282–283
 deficiency, 283
 dietary sources, 285–286
 enzymes and role, 282, 283
 future aspects, 286
 metabolic and cellular functions, 281
 PDE, 284
 RDA, 286
 supplementation, 285
 toxicity, 285
 treatment, 283–284
Vitamin B12, 235, 240, 241
Vitamin C
 areas of research, 315
 body stores and absorption, 313
 clinical manifestations, 313–315
 dietary sources, 314
 dosage, 314
 monitoring in children, 315
 physiologic functions, 311–313
 recommended dietary intake, 314
Vitamin D, 40, 535
 causes of, 355
 deficiency states, 160, 354
 extra skeletal effects, 356–357
 future aspects, 357
 infants, 6
 nutritional deficiency Rickets, 354
 physiology, 351–353
 recommended intake, 352
 treatment, 353
 VDDR, type-1 and type-2, 355–356
Vitamin D-dependent Rickets (VDDR), type-1 and type-2, 355–356

Vitamin E
 deficiency, 361–363
 etiologies, 362
 future aspects, 364
 measurements and dosing, 363
 metabolism and transport, 360–361
 natural sources, 360
 physiology, 361
 supplementation, 360
 toxicity, 364
 treatment, 363–364
Vitamin K, 40
 deficiency, 370–372
 forms, 368
 gut microbiome, 372
 history of, 367
 metabolic cycle, 369
 in newborns, 370
 physiology, 368, 369
 toxicity of, 372
Vocal cord injury, 389

W
Waterlow criteria, 24
Weight loss, 615
Wernicke encephalopathy (WE), 256
Whole Cow's milk, 53
Williams syndrome, 162
Wilson disease (WD), 203–205
World Health Organization (WHO), 3, 20, 33

Y
Young children, 9–10

Z
Zinc
 physiological roles and function of, 211–213
 roles and function of, 212
Zofran, 444